Working with Emotion in Cognitive-Behavioral Therapy

Working with Emotion in Cognitive-Behavioral Therapy

Techniques for Clinical Practice

edited by
Nathan C. Thoma
Dean McKay

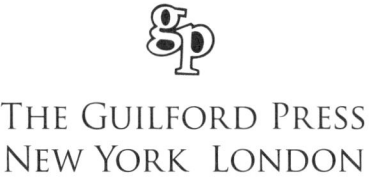

The Guilford Press
New York London

© 2015 The Guilford Press
A Division of Guilford Publications, Inc.
72 Spring Street, New York, NY 10012
www.guilford.com

All rights reserved

No part of this book may be reproduced, translated, stored in
a retrieval system, or transmitted, in any form or by any means,
electronic, mechanical, photocopying, microfilming, recording,
or otherwise, without written permission from the publisher.

Printed in the United States of America

This book is printed on acid-free paper.

Last digit is print number: 9 8 7 6 5 4 3 2 1

The authors have checked with sources believed to be reliable in their
efforts to provide information that is complete and generally in accord
with the standards of practice that are accepted at the time of publication.
However, in view of the possibility of human error or changes in
behavioral, mental health, or medical sciences, neither the authors, nor
the editors and publisher, nor any other party who has been involved in
the preparation or publication of this work warrants that the information
contained herein is in every respect accurate or complete, and they are
not responsible for any errors or omissions or the results obtained from
the use of such information. Readers are encouraged to confirm the
information contained in this book with other sources.

Library of Congress Cataloging-in-Publication Data

Working with emotion in cognitive-behavioral therapy : techniques for clinical
practice / edited by Nathan C. Thoma and Dean McKay.
      p. ; cm.
   Includes bibliographical references and index.
   ISBN 978-1-4625-1774-9 (alk. paper)
   I. Thoma, Nathan C., editor. II. McKay, Dean, 1966– editor.
   [DNLM: 1. Cognitive Therapy—methods. 2. Emotions. 3. Professional–
Patient Relations. WM 425.5.C6]
   RC489.C63
   616.89'142—dc23
                                                                    2014022749

About the Editors

Nathan C. Thoma, PhD, is Clinical Instructor of Psychology at Weill Cornell Medical College. His clinical interests center on integrating experiential, interpersonal, and relational approaches into cognitive-behavioral therapy, and he has undergone advanced training in emotion-focused therapy and schema therapy. Dr. Thoma has written on a variety of topics related to psychotherapy research, including an article in the *American Journal of Psychiatry* that the journal's editors named as one of the seven most important articles in 2012. He is a Diplomate of the Academy of Cognitive Therapy and serves as Member-at-Large and Membership Chair for the New York City Cognitive Behavioral Therapy Association.

Dean McKay, PhD, ABPP, is Professor of Psychology at Fordham University, where he is a faculty member in the Doctoral Training Program in Clinical Psychology. His research focuses primarily on obsessive–compulsive disorder and related conditions for all age groups. Dr. McKay is board certified in cognitive-behavioral psychology and clinical psychology by the American Board of Professional Psychology and serves on the board of directors of its cognitive-behavioral therapy specialty. He also serves on the Scientific Advisory Board of the International Obsessive–Compulsive Disorder Foundation and the Scientific Council of the Anxiety and Depression Association of America. Dr. McKay is President of the Association for Behavioral and Cognitive Therapies (2013–2014 term). He is the author of more than 195 articles, book chapters, and books, and is founder and codirector of a group private practice in White Plains, New York.

Acknowledgments

This book was developed from a wide range of ideas the editors have entertained over the past several years. We have both taken the position that clients are best served when our interventions are based on a scientific foundation. If we are to be truly objective, we should set aside our preconceived theoretical biases and understand the data on hand. Numerous therapeutic traditions lay claim to being efficacious, but none have "cornered the market" on efficacy. However, all therapeutic approaches involve emotional processing as part of behavior change.

This book is clearly intended as a cognitive-behaviorally oriented book. However, many of the contributors have drawn from theories other than cognitive-behavioral in making recommendations that meet the challenge of helping clients change both behavior and emotion. This has resulted in a text that is more eclectic than the typical cognitive-behavioral book for clinicians. We hope that this cross-theoretical approach will be useful as you apply the principles herein with your clients.

We are grateful for the efforts of our contributors, a distinguished group of researchers and practitioners. We would like to give special mention to one contributor, Leigh McCullough, who agreed to coauthor a chapter (Chapter 7), despite her grave illness at the time. We were extremely honored by her contribution and were saddened that she passed away before the book was published. We are thankful that this book contains a chapter that bears her name.

We would like to thank Senior Editor Jim Nageotte at The Guilford Press for his hard work and sage guidance as we developed this book from a proposal to the finished volume you hold in your hands. The production team at Guilford collectively deserves great praise for their professionalism in making this book possible.

Nathan C. Thoma would like to thank his wife, Raya, for her steadfast support throughout the process of putting this book together. He also thanks Aaron Heller, Stephen Kosloff, and Brian Pilecki for their helpful comments on the Introduction, as well as Christian S. Chan for discussions that helped crystallize the unifying themes of the book.

Dean McKay would like to thank his wife, Dawn, for her incredible support and patience through the years, dating back to college. What a great ride it's been!

Contributors

Arnold Arntz, PhD, Department of Clinical Psychology, University of Amsterdam, Amsterdam, The Netherlands

Christian S. Chan, PhD, Department of Psychology, The University of Hong Kong, Pokfulam, Hong Kong

David M. Clark, PhD, Department of Experimental Psychology, University of Oxford, Oxford, United Kingdom

Rick A. Cruz, MA, Department of Psychology, Utah State University, Logan, Utah

Susan Daflos, PhD, Vancouver CBT Centre, Vancouver, British Columbia, Canada

Thane M. Erickson, PhD, Department of Psychology, Seattle Pacific University, Seattle, Washington

Andrew P. Fleming, PhD, Department of Psychiatry and Behavioral Sciences, University of Washington, Seattle, Washington

David M. Fresco, PhD, Department of Psychology, Kent State University, Kent, Ohio

Christopher K. Germer, PhD, Division of Psychology, Harvard Medical School, Boston, Massachusetts

Paul Gilbert, PhD, Mental Health Research Unit, University of Derby, Derby, United Kingdom

Leslie S. Greenberg, PhD, Department of Psychology, York University, Toronto, Ontario, Canada

Adele M. Hayes, PhD, Department of Psychology, University of Delaware, Newark, Delaware

Steven C. Hayes, PhD, Department of Psychology, University of Nevada, Reno, Reno, Nevada

Julia E. Hitch, PhD, private practice, Seattle, Washington

Robert J. Kohlenberg, PhD, ABPP, Department of Psychology, University of Washington, Seattle, Washington

Jessica Kraus, MA, Clinical Psychology Program, New School for Social Research, New York, New York

Robert L. Leahy, PhD, American Institute for Cognitive Therapy, New York, New York

Rachel Lunt, PhD, Vancouver CBT Centre, Vancouver, British Columbia, Canada

Offer Maurer, PhD, The Center for Academic Studies, Or-Yehuda, Israel; Israeli Institute of Schema Therapy, Tel-Aviv, Israel

Leigh McCullough, PhD (deceased), Harvard Medical School, Boston, Massachusetts

Adam McGuire, MS, Department of Psychology, Seattle Pacific University, Seattle, Washington

Dean McKay, PhD, ABPP, Department of Psychology, Fordham University, Bronx, New York

Douglas S. Mennin, PhD, Department of Psychology, Hunter College, New York, New York

Michelle G. Newman, PhD, Department of Psychology, The Pennsylvania State University, University Park, Pennsylvania

Rachel Ojserkis, MA, Department of Psychology, Fordham University, Bronx, New York

Kristin A. R. Osborn, MA, Department of Psychiatry, Harvard Medical School, Boston, Massachusetts

Mia Skytte O'Toole, MSc, PhD fellow, Department of Psychology and Behavioral Sciences, Aarhus University, Aarhus, Denmark

Eshkol Rafaeli, PhD, Department of Psychology, Gonda Multidisciplinary Brain Research Center, Bar-Ilan University, Ramat Gan, Israel; Israeli Institute of Schema Therapy, Tel-Aviv, Israel

C. Beth Ready, PhD, Department of Psychology, University of Delaware, Newark, Delaware

Jeremy D. Safran, PhD, Clinical Psychology Program, New School for Social Research, New York, New York

Dennis Tirch, PhD, American Institute for Cognitive Therapy, New York, New York

Nathan C. Thoma, PhD, Department of Psychiatry, Weill Cornell Medical College, New York, New York

Mavis Tsai, PhD, Department of Psychology, University of Washington, Seattle, Washington

Pål G. Ulvenes, PhD, Research Institute, Modum Bad Psychiatric Center, Vikersund, Norway

Jennifer C. Plumb Vilardaga, PhD, VA Puget Sound HealthCare System, Seattle, Washington

Mattthieu Villatte, PhD, Evidence-Based Practice Institute, Seattle, Washington

Bruce E. Wampold, PhD, ABPP, Department of Counseling Psychology, University of Wisconsin–Madison, Madison, Wisconsin; Research Institute, Modum Bad Psychiatric Center, Vikersund, Norway

Maureen Whittal, PhD, Vancouver CBT Centre, Vancouver, British Columbia, Canada

Jennifer Wild, DClinPsy, Department of Experimental Psychology, University of Oxford, Oxford, United Kingdom

Carly Yasinski, MA, Department of Psychology, University of Delaware, Newark, Delaware

Contents

Introduction   1
Nathan C. Thoma and Dean McKay

PART I. ACCEPTANCE AS ENGAGEMENT: NOTICING, ALLOWING, AND BEING WITH EMOTION

1. Mindfulness: It's Not What You Think   11
   Christopher K. Germer and Christian S. Chan

2. Understanding and Taking Advantage of Experiential Work in Acceptance and Commitment Therapy   32
   Jennifer C. Plumb Vilardaga, Matthieu Villatte, and Steven C. Hayes

3. Compassion-Focused Therapy: An Introduction to Experiential Interventions for Cultivating Compassion   59
   Dennis Tirch and Paul Gilbert

PART II. EXPOSURE: EVOKING AND STAYING WITH DIFFICULT EMOTIONS

4. Exposure in Experiential Context: Imaginal and *In Vivo* Approaches   83
   Dean McKay and Rachel Ojserkis

5. Behavioral Experiments: Using Experiences to Test Beliefs 105
 Susan Daflos, Rachel Lunt, and Maureen Whittal

 6. Application of Exposure and Emotional Processing Theory 121
 to Depression: Exposure-Based Cognitive Therapy
 Adele M. Hayes, C. Beth Ready, and Carly Yasinski

 7. Creating Change through Focusing on Affect: 146
 Affect Phobia Therapy
 Kristin A. R. Osborn, Pål G. Ulvenes, Bruce E. Wampold, and Leigh McCullough

 ### PART III. USING IMAGERY TO CONNECT WITH EMOTIONS AND TRANSFORM MALADAPTIVE SCHEMAS AND BELIEFS

 8. Imagery Rescripting for Personality Disorders: 175
 Healing Early Maladaptive Schemas
 Arnoud Arntz

 9. Imagery Rescripting for Posttraumatic Stress Disorder 203
 Arnoud Arntz

 10. Experiential Exercises and Imagery Rescripting in Social 216
 Anxiety Disorder: New Perspectives on Changing Beliefs
 Jennifer Wild and David M. Clark

 ### PART IV. EMOTION-FOCUSED APPROACHES: CAPTURING AND ENHANCING IN-SESSION EMOTION AS A STEP TOWARD CHANGE

 11. Integrating Emotion-Focused Therapy 239
 into Cognitive-Behavioral Therapy
 Nathan C. Thoma and Leslie S. Greenberg

 12. Working with Modes in Schema Therapy 263
 Eshkol Rafaeli, Offer Maurer, and Nathan C. Thoma

 13. Emotional Schema Therapy 288
 Robert L. Leahy

14. Emotion Regulation Therapy: An Experiential Approach 310
to Chronic Anxiety and Recurring Depression
*Mia Skytte O'Toole, Douglas S. Mennin,
and David M. Fresco*

PART V. WORKING WITH INTERPERSONAL PROCESS: USING CLIENTS' AND THERAPISTS' EMOTIONAL REACTIONS TO EACH OTHER AS VEHICLES FOR CHANGE

15. Relational Techniques in a Cognitive-Behavioral 333
Therapy Context: "It's Bigger Than the Both of Us"
Jeremy D. Safran and Jessica Kraus

16. Adding an Interpersonal–Experiential Focus 356
to Cognitive-Behavioral Therapy for Generalized
Anxiety Disorder
*Thane M. Erickson, Michelle G. Newman,
and Adam McGuire*

17. Functional Analytic Psychotherapy: Using Awareness, 381
Courage, Love, and Behaviorism to Promote Change
*Mavis Tsai, Andrew P. Fleming, Rick A. Cruz,
Julia E. Hitch, and Robert J. Kohlenberg*

Conclusion: Experiential Methods, Cognitive-Behavioral 399
Therapy, and Next Steps in Emotional Engagement
in Treatment
Dean McKay and Nathan C. Thoma

Index 405

Introduction

Nathan C. Thoma
Dean McKay

Since the introduction of the cognitive model for psychotherapy over 50 years ago (Beck, 1963), countless studies have documented the efficacy of cognitive-behavioral therapy (CBT). There is now a wide range of empirically supported protocols designed to target specific diagnoses (Barlow, 2014). However, these protocols are not a panacea. For many patients they do not completely ameliorate symptoms, and additionally relapse in some disorders is not uncommon. One hypothesized avenue by which CBT treatments may succeed more universally is by facilitating clients' deepening of their affective experience. Notably, this is an approach that has traditionally been associated more strongly with therapies other than CBT, such as psychodynamic therapy or existential/humanistic therapies (Blagys & Hilsenroth, 2002; Goldfried, 2013). Yet, in recent years, interest in finding effective means of engaging with emotion in CBT has surged.

Advances in the scientific understanding of the interrelatedness of emotion, thought, and behavior along with the continued evolution of clinical knowledge have led researchers and clinicians alike to strive for therapeutic approaches that provide what has been called *corrective emotional experience* (Alexander & French, 1946; Pachankis & Goldfried, 2007). In particular, a variety of evidence has come to suggest that actively working to intensify contact with emotions within therapy sessions can be effective in reducing clients' suffering outside of session. Such approaches see emotion as a vehicle for change rather than solely as a target for change. Thus, *experiential* techniques—those aimed at actively engaging with emotion rather than focusing exclusively on reducing it—have seen extensive development, refinement, and empirical testing within the past decade. The aim of this book is to present to practicing clinicians a sampling of the state of the art in experiential approaches to working with emotion that can be applied within a CBT framework. We hope to provide immediate clinical utility as well as whet readers' appetites for further exploration of these promising approaches.

Since the time of Ancient Greece, Western culture has held rationality in high regard, showing a fascination with the potential for reason to guide or even overpower the primitive, brutish forces of the emotions. Plato, one of the founders of Western philosophy, depicted reason as a charioteer steering two horses, which were meant to represent the noble and ignoble passions (Griswold, 2010). Later, the Stoics took such a perspective even further, holding that a person who had achieved moral and intellectual perfection would not even experience emotions such as fear, envy, lust, or even passionate love (Baltzly, 2012). Modern Western cultural epochs since that time, from the Scientific Revolution through the Enlightenment and the Industrial Revolution, have all cherished the value of reason in explaining, predicting, and manipulating the world around us. Clearly rationality has shown itself to be a powerful faculty. It would be tempting to think that rationality could and should be applied to solve all possible problems, including that of taming our unruly emotional experiences within. However, a variety of findings suggest that reason and emotion may not be as readily separable as Western cultural conceptions have traditionally assumed.

To illustrate, take the case example cited in Damasio (1994) of a man with a brain lesion that disrupted his emotion system, while leaving his rational faculties intact. This man, who seemed charming, intelligent, and articulate, was nonetheless incapable of making a simple decision about which date to choose for his next appointment. Without being fully connected to his emotions, the man lost an important compass for navigating even the simplest of tasks.

Emotions provide what Damasio calls "somatic markers," which signify to us what is important or of value (Damasio, 1994). Along these lines, a new paradigm gaining a strong foothold in the cognitive sciences, known as the embodied mind perspective, holds that all abstract reasoning is built out of embodied experience, arising from the senses and grounded in the emotions, rather than existing as a separable faculty that is privy to a disembodied and objective view of the world (see Lakoff & Johnson, 1999).

Emotions are inextricably woven into cognition. They provide a rapid, preverbal system of danger assessment (LeDoux, 1996); mark salience in laying down memories (Panksepp, 1998); influence interpersonal signaling and communication (Sroufe, 1996); aid in social competence (Mayer & Salovey, 1997); and interact with conscious thought to create narratives that situate the self in the world over time (Angus & Greenberg, 2011). From an evolutionary perspective, emotions are seen as fundamentally necessary and adaptive (Izard, 1991). Emotions provide information that orients the human organism to important needs along with the motivation to interact with the environment to satisfy those needs (Frijda, 1986).

While emotions can be seen as fundamentally adaptive, emotional problems arise when emotions are underregulated, overregulated, or misplaced owing to relating more to past experiences than to the present. Beck (1976) developed an approach to address these difficulties, known as cognitive therapy, based on recruiting rationality to reflect upon reality, gain a more accurate perspective, and thus bring emotion more in tune with the actual situation. Yet, in that a variety of scientific theories have come to view emotion and reason as integral aspects of higher-order cognitive-affective mental structures, some CBT theorists have argued that relying on rational reflection alone is bound to remain incomplete (Samoilov & Goldfried, 2000). Indeed, a common client stuck point in CBT is the oft-heard complaint, "Rationally, I get that it's not true [that I'm a fraud, or failure, etc.], but it still feels true."

Cognitive therapy has clearly moved the enterprise of psychotherapy forward, through codifying a specific method of alleviating suffering, empirically testing that method, and building a substantial evidence base. And clinically speaking, working with clients to build coping skills through increasing metacognitive awareness can be a powerful platform for strengthening emotional resilience. However, a variety of evidence now supports the notion of not only using rationality to tame and attenuate negative emotion but using emotion itself as an entry point into dysfunctional cognitive-affective networks.

Drawing upon Lang's (1977) bioinformational model, Foa and Kozak's (1986) emotional-processing theory proposed that in order to modify excessive fear responses, it is necessary first to activate the underlying fear circuitry in order to make it available for modification. Next, additional information with elements that are incompatible with the existing fear-related information must be added so that new, updated circuitry can be formed. The basic tenets of this theory have been validated at the neurobiological level in animal models in a process known as *reconsolidation update*. In this process, existing, learned fear circuitry is rendered labile and modifiable when it is first reactivated through invoking elements of the originating fear stimulus (see Tronson & Taylor, 2007). This principle has been applied at the clinical level most explicitly in exposure therapy for the anxiety disorders. We propose that the same principle—that of activating emotion in order to enhance the modification of the underlying cognitive-affective mental structures—can be a powerful basis for a variety of interventions across a plurality of emotional difficulties.

Evidence suggests that emotional arousal and expression are related to a positive outcome in a variety of psychotherapies. High emotional arousal at the start of treatment along with between-session habituation has been linked to positive outcomes in exposure therapy for anxiety disorders (e.g., Borkovec & Sides, 1979; Jaycox, Foa, & Morral, 1998). A meta-analysis of process–outcome studies of short-term psychodynamic therapy (PDT) in mixed clinical samples showed a significant effect for the relationship between expression of affect and outcome at posttreatment (Diener, Hilsenroth, & Weinberger, 2007). In the treatment of depression, midtreatment emotional arousal predicted positive outcome in emotion-focused therapy (EFT) and client-centered therapy (CCT; Missirlian, Toukmanian, Warwar, & Greenberg, 2005). Techniques that evoke and explore emotion have been found to be related to outcomes across both PDT and CBT (Jones & Pulos, 1993).

It appears likely that something more than simply arousing and venting emotions in general is important to maximize therapeutic change. For example, until recently, it was believed that exposure therapy produced change through extinction and habituation within exposure sessions. However, more recent evidence implies that habituation may be less important than building distress tolerance and the acceptance of emotion (Arch, Wolitzky-Taylor, Eifert, & Craske, 2012; Bluet, Zoellner, & Feeney, 2014; Craske et al., 2008). Additionally, accommodation of new meanings derived through the experience of emotion also appears to be important in exposure therapy (Sobel, Resick, & Rabalais, 2009). In experiential therapy for depression, Missirlian et al. (2005) found that clients' ability to make meaning of their aroused emotion added to outcome over and above midtreatment emotional arousal. Further, Auszra, Greenberg, and Herrmann (2013) demonstrated that it is the quality of the awareness of emotion that is experienced, along with the clients' attitude toward it, that relates most strongly to outcome and helps determine whether the aroused emotion will be productive. Measures of in-session emotional processing that center on attending to, accepting, and differentiating cognitive-affective experience are related to outcome in EFT, CCT, and CBT (Castonguay, Goldfried, Wiser, Raue, & Hayes, 1996; Goldman, Greenberg, & Pos, 2005; Pos, Greenberg, & Warwar, 2009; Watson & Bedard, 2006).

Thus it appears that in order to create a *corrective* emotional experience for clients, it is necessary to help clients attend to their emotion, accept it, and draw new meaning from it. While the Rogerian, client-centered conditions of empathy, positive regard, and genuineness on the part of the therapist can help clients feel and express their emotions, evidence suggests that adding active techniques that guide clients through specific emotional-processing tasks can significantly improve outcome both at posttreatment and long-term follow-up (Ellison, Greenberg, Goldman, & Angus, 2009). Yet it also remains important that therapists implement emotionally evocative techniques in a manner that maintains a strong alliance between them and their clients, even in highly structured procedures such as prolonged exposure (McLaughlin, Keller, Feeney, Youngstrom, & Zoellner, 2014). In this book, we present a variety of approaches aimed at helping clients engage with their emotions, using active techniques that are grounded in empirical evidence and that can be implemented in ways that promote a strong sense of connectedness between therapists and clients.

This book has been divided into five parts. Part I centers on the acceptance of emotion and of all aspects of experience. This part includes chapters on acceptance and commitment therapy (ACT), the integration of mindfulness practice into CBT, and a focus on self-acceptance and self-compassion through compassion-focused therapy. Approaches centering on mindfulness and acceptance have been met with a veritable flood of interest on the part of clinicians in recent years. The chapters herein provide concise, vivid clinical illustrations that exemplify this important work.

Part II elaborates on applications of exposure to emotion. Notably, the chapter on imaginal and *in vivo* exposure therapy provides guidance not only on nuanced ways to enhance client emotional engagement in exposure work but also addresses common emotional challenges that may arise for therapists in the context of administering exposures. Additionally, a chapter is included on the use of exposure within depression, which can be considered a relatively new application, arising from programmatic research. We have reached outside of CBT to include a chapter on affect phobia therapy (APT), an evidence-based model of psychodynamic therapy that incorporates learning theory and deliberate exposure to adaptive affect as a source of healing. Last, this part includes a chapter on behavioral experiments—another mainstay of traditional CBT. We have included it here since behavioral experiments rely on experiences (rather than Socratic questioning) to change beliefs, and thus can be considered an experiential approach to change that holistically engages both cognition and affect.

Part III includes three chapters that all demonstrate applications of a procedure known as *imagery rescripting*, in which clients are first exposed imaginally to traumatic memories and then are asked to behave in new ways within the imagined scene. This procedure adds a new twist to the implementation of exposure therapy and is proposed to work via different mechanisms. The chapters cover the application of imagery rescripting to personality disorders, posttraumatic stress disorder (PTSD), and social anxiety. The latter chapter also fits the imagery procedures into a larger package of experiential and cognitive work for social anxiety.

Part IV features approaches that seek to work with emotions that arise organically in session and then further enhance emotional processing as well as self-regulation strategies. We include EFT, a research-driven, time-limited humanistic therapy that engages clients in exercises aimed at expressing underlying needs and resolving emotional blocks to getting those needs met. Another chapter that incorporates emotion-focused work discusses working with schema modes, an approach arising from schema therapy. Schema mode work can be considered an update to Jeffrey Young's (Young, Klosko, & Weishar, 2003) original schema model, providing a model of conceptualization that is geared toward a particular emphasis on experiential work within session, such as use of imagery and Gestalt-style "chair work." The chapter on emotional schema therapy elaborates an extension of cognitive restructuring that focuses on patient attitudes toward emotion. Last, the chapter on emotion regulation therapy demonstrates ways of working with generalized anxiety disorder (GAD) and anxious depression. This approach is meant to extend traditional CBT methods of working with chronic anxiety to address the maladaptive emotion regulation strategies that entrenched symptoms such as pervasive worry and rumination can entail.

Finally, Part V brings together methods of working with therapist and client emotional reactions to each other. A chapter on relational techniques discusses an approach from psychodynamic therapy that makes the process of alliance rupture and repair the central focus of the therapy. The authors have conducted promising research on adding such work as a supplementary module when traditional CBT falters because of difficulties in the alliance. A chapter on interpersonal and experiential focus for GAD details an integrative approach that combines psychodynamic relational work and exercises from EFT with CBT. The final chapter covers functional analytic psychotherapy (FAP), an approach that views interpersonal transactions between the client and therapist through a behavioristic lens. Unafraid to advocate for explicit expressions of love, compassion, and caring for clients, FAP exemplifies a warm, lively manner that injects an unmistakable sense of vitality into the act of delivering psychotherapy.

For each chapter, authors elaborate on the theory behind their approach, provide a brief review of the evidence for the approach, and describe its clinical application in a way that paints a picture of what therapists actually do and say, relying on clinical examples when possible. In that the book is meant to be of practical clinical value, we asked authors to emphasize the latter in particular. Authors also included a limitations and future directions section, demarcating emerging frontiers of further clinical and research development. Each chapter ends with a list of additional resources, including instructional books, websites, and DVDs, so that clinicians may use the present volume as a jumping-off point as they seek to expand their clinical repertoire and to further grow as therapists.

We hope that you enjoy reading this book as much as we have enjoyed the privilege of putting it together. We ourselves are thoroughly grateful to the authors for the learning experiences they afforded us as editors of their valuable work.

References

Alexander, F. F., & French, T. M. (1946). *Psychoanalytic therapy: Principles and application*. Oxford, UK: Ronald Press.
Angus, L., & Greenberg, L. (2011). *Working with narrative in emotion focused therapy: Changing stories, healing lives*. Washington, DC: American Psychological Association Press.

Arch, J. J., Wolitzky-Taylor, K. B., Eifert, G. H., & Craske, M. G. (2012). Longitudinal treatment mediation of traditional cognitive behavioral therapy and acceptance and commitment therapy for anxiety disorders. *Behaviour Research and Therapy, 50*(7–8), 469–478.

Auszra, L., Greenberg, L. S., & Herrmann, I. (2013). Client emotional productivity—Optimal client in-session emotional processing in experiential therapy. *Psychotherapy Research, 23*(6), 732–746.

Barlow, D. H. (2014). *Clinical handbook of psychological disorders* (5th ed.). New York: Guilford Press.

Baltzly, D. (2012). Stoicism. In *The Stanford encyclopedia of philosophy* (winter ed.). Retrieved from *http://plato.stanford.edu/archives/win2012/entries/stoicism*.

Beck, A. T. (1963). Thinking and depression: I. Idiosyncratic content and cognitive distortions. *Archives of General Psychiatry, 9*(4), 324–333.

Beck, A. T. (1976). *Cognitive therapy and the emotional disorders*. Oxford, UK: International Universities Press.

Blagys, M. D., & Hilsenroth, M. J. (2002). Distinctive features of cognitive-behavioral therapy: A review of the comparative psychotherapy process literature. *Clinical Psychology Review, 22*(5), 671–706.

Bluett, E. J., Zoellner, L. A., & Feeny, N. C. (2014). Does change in distress matter?: Mechanisms of change in prolonged exposure for PTSD. *Journal of Behavior Therapy and Experimental Psychiatry, 45*(1), 97–104.

Borkovec, T. D., & Sides, J. (1979). The contribution of relaxation and expectance to fear reduction via graded imaginal exposure to feared stimuli. *Behaviour Research and Therapy, 17*, 529–540.

Castonguay, L. G., Goldfried, M. R., Wiser, S., Raue, P. J., & Hayes, A. M. (1996). Predicting the effect of cognitive therapy for depression: A study of unique and common factors. *Journal of Consulting and Clinical Psychology, 64*(3), 497–504.

Craske, M. G., Kircanski, K., Zelikowsky, M., Mystkowski, J., Chowdhury, N., & Baker, A. (2008). Optimizing inhibitory learning during exposure therapy. *Behaviour Research and Therapy, 46*(1), 5–27.

Damasio, A. R. (1994). *Descartes' error: Emotion, rationality and the human brain*. New York: Putnam.

Diener, M. J., Hilsenroth, M. J., & Weinberger, J. (2007). Therapist affect focus and patient outcomes in psychodynamic psychotherapy: A metaanalysis. *American Journal of Psychiatry, 164*, 936–941.

Ellison, J. A., Greenberg, L. S., Goldman, R. N., & Angus, L. (2009). Maintenance of gains following experiential therapies for depression. *Journal of Consulting and Clinical Psychology, 77*(1), 103–112.

Foa, E. B., & Kozak, M. J. (1986). Emotional processing of fear: Exposure to corrective information. *Psychological Bulletin, 99*(1), 20–35.

Frijda, N. H. (1986). *The emotions*. Cambridge, UK: Cambridge University Press.

Goldfried, M. R. (2013). Evidence-based treatment and cognitive-affective-relational-behavior therapy. *Psychotherapy, 50*, 376–380.

Goldman, R. N., Greenberg, L. S., & Pos, A. E. (2005). Depth of emotional experience and outcome. *Psychotherapy Research, 15*, 248–260.

Griswold, C. L. (Ed.). (2010). *Self-knowledge in Plato's Phaedrus*. State College: Pennsylvania State Press.

Izard, C. E. (1991). *The psychology of emotions*. New York: Plenum Press.

Jaycox, L. H., Foa, E. B., & Morral, A. R. (1998). Influence of emotional engagement and habituation on exposure therapy for PTSD. *Journal of Consulting and Clinical Psychology, 66*, 185–192.

Jones, E. E., & Pulos, S. M. (1993). Comparing the process in psychodynamic and cognitive-behavioral therapies. *Journal of Consulting and Clinical Psychology, 61*, 306–316.

Lakoff, G., & Johnson, M. (1999). *Philosophy in the flesh: The embodied mind and its challenge to Western thought*. New York: Basic Books.

Lang, P. J. (1977). Imagery in therapy: An information processing analysis of fear. *Behavior Therapy, 8*(5), 862–886.

LeDoux, J. E. (1996). *The emotional brain: The mysterious underpinnings of emotional life*. New York: Simon & Schuster.

Mayer, J. D., & Salovey, P. (1997). What is emotional intelligence? In P. Salovey & D. Sluyter (Eds.), *Emotional development and emotional intelligence: Implications for educators* (pp. 3–31). New York: Basic Books.

McLaughlin, A., Keller, S. M., Feeny, N. C., Youngstrom, E. A., & Zoellner, L. A. (2014). Patterns of therapeutic alliance: Rupture–repair episodes in prolonged exposure for posttraumatic stress disorder. *Journal of Consulting and Clinical Psychology, 82*(1), 112–121.

Missirlian, T. M., Toukmanian, S. G., Warwar, S. H., & Greenberg, L. S. (2005). Emotional arousal, client perceptual processing, and the working alliance in experiential psychotherapy for depression. *Journal of Consulting and Clinical Psychology, 73*, 861–871.

Pachankis, J. E., & Goldfried, M. R. (2007). An integrative, principle-based approach to psychotherapy. In S. G. Hofmann & J. Weinberger (Eds.), *The art and science of psychotherapy* (pp. 49–68). New York: Routledge/Taylor & Francis.

Panksepp, J. (1998). *Affective neuroscience: The foundations of human and animal emotions*. New York: Oxford University Press.

Pos, A. E., Greenberg, L. S., & Warwar, S. H. (2009). Testing a model of change in the experiential treatment of depression. *Journal of Consulting and Clinical Psychology, 77*(6), 1055–1066.

Samoilov, A., & Goldfried, M. R. (2000). Role of emotion in cognitive-behavior therapy. *Clinical Psychology: Science and Practice, 7*(4), 373–385.

Sobel, A. A., Resick, P. A., & Rabalais, A. E. (2009). The effect of cognitive processing therapy on cognitions: Impact statement coding. *Journal of Traumatic Stress, 22*(3), 205–211.

Sroufe, L. A. (1996). *Emotional development: The organization of emotional life in the early years*. New York: Cambridge University Press.

Tronson, N. C., & Taylor, J. R. (2007). Molecular mechanisms of memory reconsolidation. *Nature Reviews Neuroscience, 8*(4), 262–275.

Watson, J., & Bedard, D. (2006). Clients' emotional processing in psychotherapy: A comparison between cognitive behavioral and process experiential therapies. *Journal of Consulting and Clinical Psychology, 74*, 152–159.

Young, J. E., Klosko, J. S., & Weishar, M. E. (2003). *Schema therapy: A practitioner's guide*. New York: Guilford Press.

PART I

ACCEPTANCE AS ENGAGEMENT

Noticing, Allowing,
and Being with Emotion

CHAPTER 1

Mindfulness

It's Not What You Think

Christopher K. Germer
Christian S. Chan

> When we make pain the enemy, we solidify it. This resistance is where our suffering begins.
> —Ezra Bayda

Lauren had suffered from panic attacks for most of her adult life. She explained in the intake interview that she had tried just about everything to get rid of her anxiety, including relaxation, cognitive restructuring, exposure therapy, insight-oriented psychotherapy, and medication. With the help of therapy she managed to go from being housebound to keeping a job, but she dreaded getting up in the morning to white-knuckle her drive to work. "Why am I still so anxious despite doing all the right things?" Lauren wondered aloud. She had recently read about the benefits of mindfulness and hoped that mindfulness might provide an answer.

From a mindfulness point of view, Lauren would remain a fugitive from her anxiety as long as she tried to get rid of it. The dictum is "What you resist, persists." We create problems in our lives to the extent that we fight against difficult sensations and emotions. For example, struggling with sleeplessness may lead to chronic insomnia and trying not to grieve can result in depression. Conversely, "What you can feel, you can heal." Our difficulties subside when we allow them into our lives, gradually and safely. What would it take for Lauren to allow the sensations of anxiety to come and go in her body, and to let her fears of having a heart attack simply be "thoughts" without catastrophizing them?

Two key questions in the case conceptualization of a mindfulness-based therapist are (1) What pain is the client resisting? and (2) How can I help the client develop a more accepting *relationship* to his or her pain? In Lauren's case, she was resisting the experience of anxiety, and the therapist's task was to help her gradually open to it. That is a tall order, especially with panic disorder where clients feel they're fighting for their lives. Therefore, mindfulness-based therapy moves in stages toward acceptance. We start with *exploring* (turning toward discomfort with curiosity), and then move to *tolerating* (safely enduring discomfort), then to *allowing* (letting discomfort come and go), and finally to *welcoming* (embracing difficult experiences as part of life). The stages of acceptance correspond to a gradual loosening of resistance.

Lauren was invited by her therapist to *explore* the nonthreatening tensions that resided in her body but didn't presage a panic attack. Then she learned to *tolerate* anxiety by focusing on her breathing rather than her catastrophic thinking. Thereafter, Lauren discovered that she could disentangle from her panic when she learned to name her emotions and *allow* them to be there ("That's loneliness." "That's fear."). Finally, she began to *welcome* the opportunity to surf the waves of anxiety rather than being tumbled over by them, savoring her newfound freedom. This entire process corresponded to a radically new relationship to anxiety.

Background and Theory

There are many definitions of "mindfulness," all of which are inadequate to the task because mindfulness is a preconceptual, preverbal experience of direct awareness. Mindfulness can't be put into words. There is a subtle difference, for example, between knowing that a car backfired outside your office and consciously *feeling* the sound in your body. Similarly, you may see a flash of green at your door before you notice it is the green dress of the woman you are expecting for your next appointment. Mindfulness is the first moment of sensory experience, the earliest stage of information processing, before we have a chance to think further about it or to formulate our ideas into words. In this regard, mindfulness is profoundly experiential.

A basic definition of *mindfulness* is "moment-by-moment awareness." Other definitions include "keeping one's consciousness alive to the present reality" (Hanh, 1976, p. 11); "the clear and single-minded awareness of what actually happens to us and in us at the successive moments of perception" (Nyanaponika, 1972, p. 5); and "the awareness that emerges through paying attention, on purpose, in the present moment, and non-judgmentally to the unfolding of experience moment by moment" (Kabat-Zinn, 2003, p. 145).

Although the word *mindfulness* is an English translation of the Buddhist Pali word *sati*, even different traditions within Buddhist psychology do not agree on the meaning of mindfulness (Williams & Kabat-Zinn, 2011). In modern scientific psychology, we have arrived at our definitions by looking for commonalities found in various training programs (Carmody, 2009) or by investigating what seems to be useful to patients in mindfulness-oriented treatment. In a consensus opinion among experts, Bishop et al. (2004) proposed a two-component model of mindfulness. "The first component involves the self-regulation of attention so that it is maintained on immediate experience, thereby allowing for increased recognition of mental events in the present moment. The second component involves adopting a particular orientation towards one's experience that is characterized by curiosity, openness, and acceptance" (p. 232). A shorthand definition of mindfulness in the therapeutic context is "awareness of present experience with acceptance" (Germer, 2013).

Mindfulness can be understood as a *process* (defined above) and a *practice*, such as meditation. Three types of meditation practices are typically taught under the umbrella of "mindfulness meditation" in the West (Salzberg, 2011): (1) focused attention, (2) open monitoring, and (3) loving-kindness and compassion. Focused attention calms the mind by returning again and again to a single object, such as the breath; open monitoring cultivates equanimity in the face of challenges, using methods such as labeling emotions or scanning the body for sensations; and loving-kindness and compassion meditation adds an element of care, comfort, and soothing to our awareness. Meditation can occur formally (e.g., sitting meditation) or informally throughout the day.

The first two types of meditation are attention-regulation strategies that are currently the primary focus of clinical research (Carmody et al., 2009). Over the past few years, however, there has been growing interest in loving-kindness and compassion (Hofmann, Grossman, & Hinton, 2011). Neurological evidence suggests that the mental skills cultivated by all three meditation types represent overlapping, yet distinct, brain processes (Brewer et al., 2011; Desbordes et al., 2012; Lee et al., 2012; Lutz, Slagter, Dunne, & Davidson, 2008). Preexisting brain function may even predict which kind of meditation an individual prefers (Mascaro, Rilling, Negi, & Raison, 2013).

Mindfulness in Cognitive-Behavioral Therapy

We are currently in the third generation of cognitive-behavioral therapy (CBT) (Hayes, 2011). The first generation was behavior therapy, focusing on classical Pavlovian conditioning and contingencies of reinforcement.

The second was cognitive therapy aimed at altering dysfunctional thought patterns. The third generation is mindfulness, acceptance, and compassion-based psychotherapy, in which our *relationship* to experience, often intense and disturbing emotions, shifts during the course of therapy.

In this new approach, we are interested in more than cognitions. In a critical review of the evidence, Longmore and Worrell (2007) challenged a key tenet of cognitive therapy that "all therapies alter dysfunctional cognitions," and they found that (1) cognitive *interventions* like behavioral activation, cognitive therapy, exposure, and response prevention did not add significant value to one therapy over another; and (2) cognitive *change* was not causal in improving symptoms, that is, changes in the content of thinking occured as readily in noncognitive therapies. From a mindfulness perspective, the possibility exists that we were unknowingly helping our clients cultivate mindfulness whenever we asked them to monitor their thoughts and behaviors and explore the antecedents and consequences of their beliefs.

Mindfulness-based therapy is designed to establish a new relationship to *all* experience, including emotions, cognitions, sensations, behaviors, and intentions. Learning to hold any difficult experience in mindful awareness, without resistance, dismantles the scaffolding that maintains psychological problems. Progress in mindfulness-based treatment is a process of gradually opening to and feeling unpleasant experience.

Mindfulness training also *refines* our awareness. The power of mindful awareness to dismantle symptoms becomes most evident when we have the capacity to witness how our symptoms subtly arise upstream as we process information. In Lauren's case, for example, she was invited to drop her attention into her body and see how her heart naturally sped up and slowed down before it mushroomed into a panic attack, which dissipated her reactivity. Similarly, if we can witness the arising of difficult emotions as a change in physical sensations or compulsive urges as a shift in intention—if we can get *underneath* our symptoms—then we have more choice in how we behave in the world.

Mindfulness, Acceptance, and Compassion

When mindfulness is in full bloom—when we feel calm and vibrant amid the full range of our thoughts, feelings, and sensations—our experience is permeated with acceptance and compassion. Particularly in the clinical arena, however, mindfulness is usually tinged by distressing emotions, such as in "worried attention" or "sad attention." That is when we need to intentionally activate acceptance and compassion to become more mindful. Acceptance is "active nonjudgmental embracing of experience in the here and now" (Hayes, Follette, & Linehan, 2004, p. 21) and compassion is "basic kindness, with deep awareness of the suffering of oneself and other living beings, coupled with the wish and effort to alleviate it" (Gilbert, 2009, p. xiii). Acceptance and compassion contribute a tone of warmth and affection to our awareness.

Since the advent of mindfulness-based treatments in the 1990s, acceptance has typically focused on *moment-to-moment experience* (nonresistance and nonavoidance of sensations, emotions, and thoughts) (Kabat-Zinn, 1990; Hayes, Strosahl, & Wilson, 1999; Linehan, 1993a; Segal, Williams, & Teasdale, 2013). However, earlier giants in the field of psychotherapy such as William James, Sigmund Freud, B. F. Skinner, and Carl Rogers all considered *self*-acceptance to be psychologically beneficial (Williams & Lynn, 2010). Modern compassion-based treatments are staunchly reclaiming the *experiencer* as an important object of acceptance (Germer & Neff, 2013; Gilbert, 2010a) in addition to moment-to-moment *experience*.

Self-compassion is central to mindfulness and compassion-based treatment. Self-compassion may be considered the heart of mindfulness when we meet suffering. Mindfulness says, "*Open* to your suffering with spacious awareness and it will change." Self-compassion adds, "*Be kind to yourself* in the midst of suffering and it will change." Mindfulness asks, "What do I *know*?" and self-compassion asks, "What do I *need*?" Together, mindfulness and self-compassion comprise a state of warm-hearted, connected presence during difficult moments in our lives.

Although the definitions of mindfulness, acceptance, and compassion differ, the capacity to "be with" our experience in a mindful manner engages not only higher cortical processes of awareness, but also our emotions. If we turn away from our experience with disgust, or hide from ourselves in shame, we cannot be mindful. Alternatively, learning to hold our emotions and ourselves in affectionate awareness opens the mind to new possibilities and positive changes (Fredrickson, Cohn, Coffey, Pek, & Finkel, 2008.)

Evidence

The research literature on mindfulness has been growing exponentially over the past 10 years. As seen in Figure 1.1, there were 421 peer-reviewed articles on mindfulness indexed in PsychINFO through 2005, whereas there are now over 2,400 articles as of 2012. Additionally, there are now over 60 mindfulness treatment and research centers in the United States alone.

The effectiveness of mindfulness-based treatments is well established. We have structured interventions for treating a broad range of mental and physical disorders, randomized controlled trials supporting these interventions, and numerous reviews and meta-analyses of those studies (Chen et

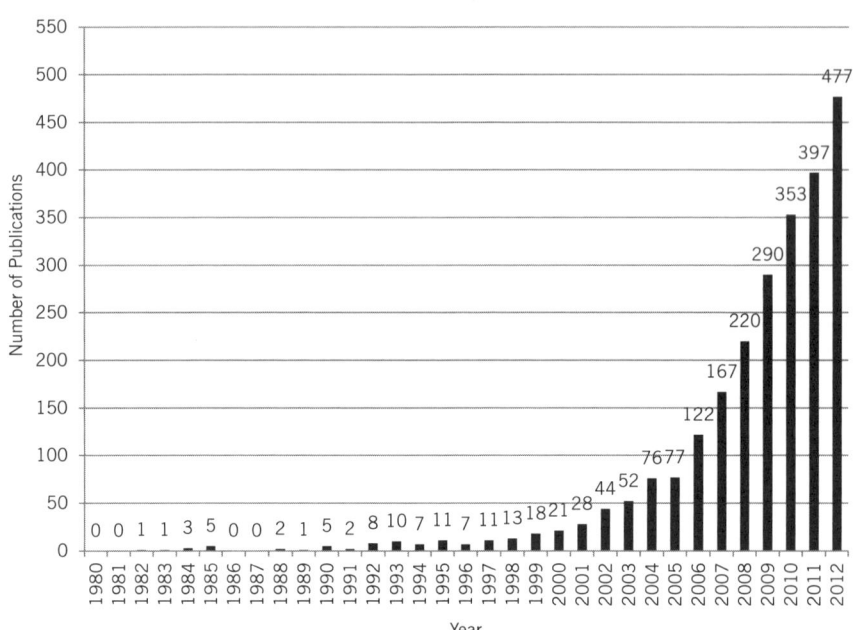

FIGURE 1.1. Research publications on mindfulness, 1980–2012. Figure provided by David S. Black, PhD, Institute for Prevention Research, Keck School of Medicine, University of Southern California, and reprinted by permission of the author (*www.mindfulexperience.org*).

al., 2012; Chiesa, Calati, & Serretti, 2010; Davis & Hayes, 2011; Fjorback, Arendt, Ornbol, Fink, & Walach, 2011; Greeson, 2009; Grossman, Niemann, Schmidt, & Walach, 2004; Hoffmann et al., 2011; Hoffman, Sawyer, Witt, & Oh, 2010; Keng, Smoski, & Robins, 2011; Khoury et al., 2013; Piet & Hougaard, 2011; Rubia, 2009; Vollestad, Nielsen, & Nielsen, 2012). See *www.mindfulexperience.org* for a comprehensive, mindfulness research database with monthly updates.

The four, most frequently cited, empirically supported, mindfulness-based treatment programs are mindfulness-based stress reduction (MBSR; Kabat-Zinn, 1990), mindfulness-based cognitive therapy (MBCT; Segal, Williams, & Teasdale, 2013), dialectical behavior therapy (DBT; Linehan, 1993a), and acceptance and commitment therapy (ACT; Hayes et al., 1999). The latter two programs do not emphasize mindfulness meditation per se, but are based on the principles of mindfulness and acceptance. There are many other mindfulness programs that have grown out of these templates, or were developed for specific populations, conditions, or skills training, such as mindfulness-based relapse prevention (Witkiewitz & Bowen, 2010); mindfulness-based eating awareness training (Kristeller & Wolever, 2011); mindfulness-based cognitive therapy for children (Semple, Lee, Rosa, & Miller, 2010); mindfulness-based stress reduction for teens (Biegel, Brown, Shapiro, & Schubert, 2009); mindfulness and acceptance-based behavioral treatment of anxiety (Roemer, Orsillo, & Salters-Pedneault, 2008); mindfulness-based relationship enhancement (Carson, Carson, Gil, & Baucom, 2004); mindful self-compassion training (Neff & Germer, 2013); and compassion-focused therapy (Gilbert, 2010a, 2010b, 2010c).

Mechanisms of Action

There is good evidence that mindfulness interventions can be helpful for a variety of problems, such as anxiety, depression, emotion dysregulation, low self-esteem, attentional difficulties, and chronic pain. A key question in the mindfulness literature is "How does mindfulness actually work?" What are the internal mechanisms that enable clients to live their lives more fully and meaningfully? Mindfulness may be considered a mechanism of action in its own right, but a variety of subprocesses correlated with identifiable brain regions seem to be active when we're being mindful. Hölzel and colleagues (2011) identified six mechanisms for which we find corresponding brain activity during mindfulness meditation:

1. *Attention regulation*—stability of awareness in spite of competing input.
2. *Body awareness*—noticing subtle sensations, being conscious of one's emotions.
3. *Emotion regulation*—decreased reactivity, not letting emotional reactions interfere with performance.
4. *Reappraisal*—seeing difficulties as meaningful or benign, rather than as all bad.
5. *Exposure*—global desensitization to "whatever is present in the field of awareness."
6. *Flexible sense of self*—disidentification with emotions, increasing adaptivity.

Additional mechanisms with empirical support include *self-compassion* (Hölzel et al., 2011; Neff, 2011; Neff & Germer, 2013); *values clarification* (sense of purpose) and *flexibility* (cognitive, emotional, and behavioral adaptiveness) (Hayes et al., 1999; Shapiro, Carlson, Astin, & Freedman, 2006); *emotion differentiation* (awareness of emotional experiences) (Hill & Updegraff, 2012); and *metacognitive awareness* (Corcoran, Farb, Anderson, & Segal, 2010). These mechanisms of action seem to map nicely to a variety of psychological disorders. For example, mindful attention regulation for attention deficit disorder (van der Oord, Bögels, & Peijnenburg, 2012), body awareness for eating disorders (Kristeller & Wolever, 2011), and self-compassion for shame-based disorders (Gilbert & Proctor, 2006).

Currently, the field of CBT has largely adopted the core processes of mindfulness even in treatments where the word *mindfulness* is not used. One example is the unified protocol for the transdiagnotic treatment of emotional disorders by David Barlow and colleagues (Farchione et al., 2012). It consists of four modules familiar to mindfulness-oriented therapists: (1) increasing emotional awareness, (2) facilitating flexibility in appraisals, (3) identifying and preventing behavioral avoidance, and (4) identifying situational and interoceptive exposure to emotion cues.

Overall, mindfulness appears to be an underlying, *transdiagnostic*, psychological process that alleviates a broad spectrum of disorders. We now explore ways that mindfulness practices and processses can be applied to the clinical context.

Application

As we noted, a variety of structured treatment protocols have been developed for mindfulness-based treatment of psychological disorders. We will now describe a heuristic for applying mindfulness into individual treatment—the "three P's"—matching *person*, *process*, and *practice*. Mindfulness-based clinicians are encouraged to understand each of these elements and keep them in mind during treatment.

Mindfulness-based treatment is decidedly idiographic—it depends on moment-to-moment fluctuations within the *person* in his or her context. A common instruction of mindfulness meditation is "pay attention to what is most salient and alive in your field of awareness." This instruction pertains to mindfulness-based treatment as well, and translates into the therapeutic question: "What emotional pain is the client resisting?" Furthermore, a client's painful emotions are nestled in values. For example, unemployment might be welcomed by a person who values free time, but it could be devastating for someone who wants to provide for his or her family. By understanding what emotional pain a client is resisting and what he or she values, we can begin to understand the client and tailor treatment appropriately.

And as mentioned earlier, mindfulness seems to work through a variety of change *processes*, or mechanisms of change. Understanding these change processes is a lens through which the clinician can begin to design an intervention. For example, cultivating body awareness may help a client disentangle from obsessive thinking, regulating attention away from a panic attack can reduce anxiety to a manageable level, exposure (nonavoidance) to traumatic memories through the cultivation of spacious awareness may facilitate desensitization, and self-compassion training could ameliorate the destructive impact of shame.

Finally, there are *practices*—practical exercises and instructions—that clinicians can teach their clients to help them cultivate a more mindful, accepting relationship to their emotional pain (see also Germer, Siegel, & Fulton, 2013; Pollak, Pedulla, & Siegel, 2014; Siegel, 2010). The three general types of mindfulness practices mentioned earlier are focused attention, open monitoring, and compassion. Clincians might ask: Could focusing on the movement of the breath in the body help to defuse a volatile domestic situation? Might monitoring self-judgments reduce a depressed person's self-critical thinking? Would a client stricken with grief over the suicide of a friend find relief by repeating the compassionate phrase "May I learn to forgive myself?"

By matching the three P's—person, process, and practice—the mindfulness-based clinician can customize mindfulness for individual therapy. A clinical example follows.

Clinical Example

Ed was a 29-year-old, single, gay male who referred himself to treatment for depression. His chief complaints included 2 years of low moods, hypersomnia, lack of energy despite sufficient sleep, impaired concentration, and low self-esteem. He described general discontent that stemmed, in part, from his inability to find his "true calling." Ed lamented being single and worried that he would never find true love ("the one"). At the time of intake, Ed was self-employed as a freelance commercial music composer. His father was a Chilean American and his mother was a white European American. Due to his father's work, Ed moved from one continent to another throughout his childhood. He described himself as a "third-culture kid," an identity he saw as core to his personality.

My (C. S. C.) original CBT treatment plan focused on identifying Ed's automatic thoughts, using the Dysfunctional Thought Record, and then systematically adjusting his lifestyle with an emphasis on sleep regulation and reintroducing pleasurable activities, especially those that would provide additional social support. At intake, Ed requested that the course of treatment be brief because he was intending to leave fairly soon for a year or two in Chile, although he had not set a specific date for his departure.

Ed's depressed mood apparently worsened after his father's death a few years prior. Ed had difficulty with his traditionally minded father ever since Ed came out as a gay man at age 16. Around the same time, Ed rebelled against his parents, experimented with drugs, and lived lavishly with his parents' money. He managed to complete college with a degree in music but soon thereafter he tried to earn a living by making music and it became a chore for him. After the death of his father, Ed found sporadic jobs and had difficulty maintaining them. More recently, he worked for an NGO and did what he considered meaningful work, but resigned within a year, saying that his employer, whom he initially admired, disappointed him. Thereafter, Ed survived with freelance work and money inherited from his father, which he felt guilty spending. His relationship with his mother, who lived in a different geographic area, was reasonably good. Although Ed and his mother did not see each other on a regular basis, they tried to stay in touch with one another.

My initial efforts at treating Ed's depression were fraught with difficulty. Ed claimed to enjoy the structured, interactive, and collaborative approach of CBT, which he contrasted with his previous "talk" therapy, but he was reluctant to adhere to the homework assignments. He did not put much effort into the behavioral activation exercises either. He dismissed the weekly assignments as rigid and described them as routines that could not teach him anything he did not already know.

Person

In the three-P model, we first try to identify what sensations, thoughts, or emotions a person is struggling with (i.e., resisting/not accepting) and what he or she values in life (see also Hayes et al., 1999; Orsillo & Roemer, 2011). Ed found it difficult to accept that he had not found the "right" career path and the "right" person for a long-term romantic relationship. Upon further probing, it also became clear that he resented his father for not accepting him for who he was ("What kind of father would reject his own son because he is gay?!"), and behind his anger was a lingering sense of sadness for their estranged relationship and shame for living off his father's money.

When asked what he valued, Ed said he liked "being useful" and "engaging in work that is meaningful and exciting." What he could not accept was to live a routinized life. When asked about pleasurable activities, Ed reported that he enjoyed cooking and traveling. We discovered that his love for cooking stemmed from the social interaction that the activity provides, especially when he prepared food for his friends. Scheduled dinner parties lifted his mood. As for traveling, he despised tourists and described himself as a traveler who, unlike a typical tourist, immersed himself in the host culture. He was looking forward to leaving everything behind and going on his next voyage.

Process

What change process might help Ed to begin to lead a more meaningful, productive life? As mentioned above, treatment began in a traditional CBT manner by inviting Ed to monitor the thoughts that made him depressed and what triggered them. For example, Ed said he felt most depressed when he stayed in bed too long in the morning. This led to an "unproductive day," in which he "wasted time doing nothing." He would then stay up all night to make up for lost time, but low energy and motivation would prevent him using the extra time productively. This cycle frequently resulted in the recurring thought "I'm wasting my life." I suggested to Ed that we collaborate on a daily schedule that would include work, leisure, and rest. Ed rejected the idea of living by a schedule because he believed schedules were for "businessman and boring people" and not free-wheeling individuals like himself.

It gradually became clear that Ed's rigid way of viewing himself as an unstructured, countercultural person was interfering with achieving his goals in life. Therefore, developing a more *flexible sense of self* began to emerge as a possible therapeutic change process.

Ed refused to get an office job, even though he needed the money, because office jobs were "mundane" and "boring," a contradiction to his identity. Another example of a rigid sense of self was his identity as "third-culture kid" ("We are constantly restless") and the need to get away from wherever he was. I suggested that perhaps his trips were in a way a form of avoidance or escape from certain responsibilities and aspects of life that are not "exciting." This was met with hostile defensiveness and caused a breach, albeit brief, in our alliance.

Furthermore, Ed's rigid sense of self seemed to be a reaction to the anger, sadness, and shame he felt in relationship to his father. Since his father had passed away, there was no chance for healing that relationship, but perhaps Ed could find a new relationship to the emotions themselves? Could he become more aware of his emotions, and gradually desensitize to the distress they elicit, through awareness of how they manifest in his body, rather than engaging in endless arguments in his mind with his father? Therefore, *body awareness of emotion* appeared to be another change process that might help Ed release the exhausting and destructive power of anger, and perhaps *self-compassion* for sadness and shame (Gilbert & Proctor, 2006).

Practice

After using the Dysfunctional Thought Record, Ed reported that he was glad to discover how his thoughts made him more depressed, but he found it difficult to separate his thoughts from his feelings ("This is just how I feel, no matter what!") or to change his thoughts. Similarly, initial efforts to engage him in pleasurable activities were not entirely successful ("They don't excite me the way I expected"). Given the difficulties we met in the effort to help altering Ed's thoughts, feelings, and behaviors, mindfulness meditation appeared to be a potentially beneficial alternative route to bring about changes. Perhaps, through the more intimate self-monitoring practice of mindfulness meditation, Ed could begin to distinguish between his thoughts and emotions, and see his emotions as simply emotions, not facts bearing directly on his self-identity or self-worth.

Ed had some prior exposure to meditation practice. He was therefore receptive to mindfulness meditation in the therapeutic context. We began with 3 minutes of mindful breathing during the therapy session, which gradually was increased to 10 minutes, and eventually to 20 minutes per sitting. Ed was encouraged to practice in the same manner at home by setting aside a fixed time of the day for his practice. It was a time when he was not easily disturbed or tired. Like all behavioral exercises, this one was not without its challenges, so weekly monitoring was implemented and obstacles discussed and tackled in session.

Over time, Ed learned to "sit with" difficult emotions, especially anger, sadness, and shame, both in and between sessions. When those emotions became too intense in meditation, Ed shifted his attention to his breathing (focused attention) to calm down. Then he explored where in his body the emotions of anger, sadness, and shame expressed themselves most readily (anger was tension in his belly; sadness was heartache, and shame was hollowness in the head region), and he learned to "allow and soften" those emotions—allowing them to come and go as sensations in the body, and softening or relaxing the muscles where the emotions were felt. Through this practice of finding and transforming emotion in the body, Ed's anger, sadness, and shame were slowly brought down to manageable levels.

Mindfulness appears also to help increase flexibility in sense of self. Ed's self-concept (free-spirited, third-culture, gay man) gradually began to soften through mindfulness practice. By keeping his attention more often with moment-to-moment experience (experiential processing) rather than obsessively promoting and protecting his rigid sense of self (narrative processing; Farb et al., 2007), Ed found he had more creative energy at his disposal to think in adaptive ways about his life. After 2 months, Ed agreed to search for a day job and found one. This led to further improvement because he was able to recognize some of his inaccurate assumptions about "cubical jobs." Ed remarked, "Just having a place to go to each morning does wonders!"

Ed returned again and again to the topic of his father in therapy. His anger, sadness, and shame seemed to be driven by the conviction that his father did not love him, especially as a gay man. Self-compassion is considered an antidote to sadness and shame, so we folded loving-kindness meditation with self-compassion phrases into his meditation practice. Ed used the phrases "May I be free from sadness," "May I be free from shame," "May I be kind to myself," and "May I be kind to others." These phrases helped Ed to shift his attention from his father and how angry he was with him to his own emotional pain and his natural longing to be loved by his father. The phrases validated, over and over, how painful it was to feel rejected, and how important it was to Ed to be seen, heard, and appreciated for who he was. Since his father had passed away, Ed was finally giving to himself what he desperately wanted to receive from his father.

Over time, through intentional softening of the pain and anger associated with his father, Ed's frame of reference began to expand and he was able to entertain the possibility that perhaps his father, with his traditional upbringing, did not know how to handle that fact that his son was gay. Ed reported an incident that he had not previously shared with anyone. Ed had apparently visited his father in the hospital a few days before his father died. Knowing his father's condition, Ed overcame his anger and told his father that he loved him. His father wept and replied, "Hearing this is the best medicine I can ever take!" Although his father never explicitly reciprocated Ed's verbal expression of love, Ed felt it was implied in his father's words. Ed's growth in therapy since starting meditation exercises, particularly this important shift in how he viewed his father, enabled him to look beyond his anger toward his father and to contact healing feelings such as forgiveness and even love. From that point onward, we focused on cultivating those feelings by expanding Ed's loving-kindness meditation to include his father, imagining him in the afterlife: "May you and I both be happy and free from suffering."

Our treatment ended when Ed finally left for Chile. Prior to his departure, his attitude toward the trip had also shifted as a result of a more flexible understanding of his identity. In session, we explored explicitly the goals he hoped to accomplish through this trip. The cultivation of acceptance allowed Ed to entertain the possibility that he had been using traveling as avoidance. Through the practice of nonjudgmental observation of his thoughts and feelings, Ed was able to be honest with himself and, in turn, to explore his deep desires and yearning. Traveling was no longer simply an expression of his restless nature, but an opportunity to enjoy the freedom of a foreign culture to practice new forms of self-care, self-identity, and self-expression.

Strategies for Helping Clients Build and Maintain a Meditation Practice

Mindfulness meditation may be practiced *informally* during the day, such as by taking a mindful breath, or *formally* in sitting meditation (Germer, 2013). Ultimately, however, mindfulness-based therapists are trying to help their clients be more aware and accepting of moment-to-moment experience, not to transform them into good meditators. The mindfulness-based CBT therapist needs to be flexible and collaborative to determine which practices fit each individual client, including how to use the therapy relationship to enhance a client's mindfulness. For a more detailed consideration of how to integrate formal and informal meditation into therapy, see Pollak et al. (2014).

Habits, especially good ones, are hard to develop. It is especially difficult to develop a formal mindfulness practice. Formal meditation is like going to the mental gym, and progress in mindfulness appears to be "dose-dependent" (Lazar et al., 2005; Pace et al., 2009; Rubia, 2008). Therefore, if a client has a taste for it, meditation should be encouraged. In Ed's case, his earlier meditation habit had fallen by the wayside. It was easy to engage him in meditation with the support of therapy, but as the weeks progressed his practice waned again. We needed to carefully monitor, in a nonjudgmental, nonshaming way, the conditions under which he practiced and didn't practice. Most important, we needed to manage Ed's expectations. The assumptions that clients have about meditation largely determines if they will practice formal meditation. Below are some tips that many clients (and clinicians!) find helpful in maintaining a regular meditation practice.

Start Small

Our ideas about the length of time we should be meditating can make the practice unnecessarily burdensome. It helps to apply the "3-minute rule"—to simply *begin*. This is how Ed reengaged in meditation, and over time he developed a taste for it and extended his periods of practice.

Make It Pleasant

When we practice correctly, meditation feels like a vacation rather than yet another task to squeeze into a busy day. It helps to ask oneself, "What can I let go of to make meditation less like work and more like play?" "Can I shed the need to be relaxed or to concentrate better, and just *be*?" "Am I trying to achieve a particular state, or can I simply open myself more fully to the state I'm in?" The point is to make meditation more pleasant and self-reinforcing.

Connect to Core Values

Does meditation have a place in what you consider a meaningful and valuable life? For example, do you want to be awake and aware of the beauty of each passing moment so you don't feel you've wasted your life preoccupied with problems? Do you want to be happy? Is it important to you to be as compassionate as possible? Reminding ourselves of our core values may be an incentive to meditate rather than answering e-mails or reading the newspaper every morning.

Good Will, Not Good Feelings

When we meditate, we are likely to feel good, bad, or even nothing at all. Meditation cultivates a new relationship to all these feelings. One way that meditation works is by desensitizing difficult emotions that inevitably arise during states of calmness. When we meet difficult emotions with loving awareness rather than with fear or anger, we usually feel better as an inevitable by-product. The point of meditation is long-term emotional well-being, but we need to let go of the need to feel good during meditation itself in order to achieve that salubrious state.

Social Support

Meditation can feel quite lonely for some people, so they lose interest. Some suggestions to make meditation less solitary are to meditate with your cat or dog, listen to guided meditations, connect to other meditators in real time with a mobile phone application like the *Insight Timer*, join an online meditaton support group, read a passage from a book, listen to a talk by an inspiring teacher before practicing, meet weekly with a practice group, or go on retreat.

Physical Support

Make a cozy, attractive space in your home dedicated to meditation. Include objects that have very special meaning to you. It helps to practice roughly the same time each day so that you get entrained to move toward your meditation space rather than beginning other activities. It is also important that you are comfortable while meditating. You will not meditate very long if it is physically painful. Try to find a chair that you like, or if you want to sit on a cushion or bench, make sure your posture is properly adjusted to support your body without effort.

Future Directions

Considering the broad range of mindfulness practices available to clinicians, there do not seem to be any specific counterindications for mindfulness-based treatment, only limitations due to insufficient understanding of a client, the change processes, or the practices. For example, it is unwise to recommend open-monitoring sitting meditation to a recently traumatized client who wants to relax because it will probably activate traumatic memories. Instead, establishing safety through grounding techniques such as feeling the soles of the feet would be a more useful first step.

Some clients feel that mindfulness is not for them because they cannot meditate. However, taking a breath and asking a few simple questions is often all that is required: "What am I sensing?" "What am I feeling?" "What am I thinking?" "What am I doing?" Clients should also be encouraged to become their own best teacher, perhaps by asking "What do I need now?" As Mary Oliver (1986) eloquently expressed it, "You only have to let the soft animal of your body love what it loves" (p. 14).

Meditation, and mindfulness in particular, is now one of the most thoroughly researched psychotherapeutic methods available to clinicians (Black, 2013; Smith, 2004; Walsh & Shapiro, 2006). Research on the influence of mindfulness meditation on brain structure and function, combined with findings from cognitive, affective, and social research, are uncovering key mechanisms of action for mindfulness, which, in turn, are being targeted for particular psychological disorders (Jha, 2013). Their effectiveness might vary across contexts and disorders, but the sheer volume of randomized, controlled clinical trials and meta-analyses of those trials demonstrates that mindfulness-based treatment is now a well-established treatment modality (Germer, 2013). Limitations to the research remain, however. For example, the effect sizes of the randomized controlled trials are generally not large, many of the sample sizes are relatively small, and there is some likelihood of publication bias (Bohlmeijer, Prenger, Taal, & Cuijpers, 2010; Eberth & Sedlmeier, 2012; see also funnel plots in Hofmann et al., 2010).

Although research demonstrates positive effects of engaging in mindfulness practice, there will always be ambiguity and room for clinical wisdom in mindfulness-based treatment. Mindfulness-based treatment is a uniquely complex undertaking insofar as it is about transforming a particular client's relationship to his or her moment-to-moment experience, all of which is constantly changing. Furthermore, clinical practice occurs in a social context and "the therapy relationship accounts for why clients improve (or fail to improve) as much as the particular treatment method" (Norcross & Lambert, 2011, p. 2). There is even preliminary evidence that a clinician's personal meditation practice has a positive impact on treatment outcome (Grepmair et al., 2007).

How can we best prepare ourselves to become mindfulness-based psychotherapists? Most fundamentally, we should continue to hone our clinical skills—to understand psychopathology, explore the latest theories and research, develop interpersonal skills, cultivate cultural sensitivity—*and practice mindfulness meditation*. During the early evolution of MBCT, the program developers did not practice meditation themselves, and the results were disappointing (Segal et al., 2013). Soon thereafter, they visited a MBSR class (on which the MBCT program is based) and were surprised to notice that the MBSR teachers were not trying to "fix" their clients, they behaved like fellow travelers on the path to emotional well-being, they seemed unintimidated by strong emotions in their clients, and mostly they inquired into the precise nature of each student's experience without suggesting it should be otherwise. In their tone and style of conversation, MBSR teachers modeled for their students how to practice mindfulness. This approach to teaching—embodying the practice and modeling for others—is now an intrinsic part of both MBCT and MBSR, two of the most widely practiced mindfulness training programs available today.

Whither mindfulness-based treatment? Mindfulness is an ancient Buddhist practice to know the mind, shape the mind, and free the mind (Nyanaponika, 1965) and the convergence of that ancient Eastern psychology and Western psychology has just begun. In light of the burgeoning research, we can expect to further refine the change processes and practices relevant to clinical practice. We will surely develop creative new techniques to address the needs of specific populations and diagnostic groups, perhaps targeting interventions to alter specific dysfunctional brain patterns. More generally, since mindfulness appears to be an underlying change process in psychological treatment as well as a set of practices designed to promote emotional well-being, it has the potential to draw clinical practitioners and scientists closer together, as well as integrate the professional and private lives of clinicians.

Further Resources

Books for Clinicians

- See Germer, Siegel, and Fulton (2013) for the best-selling professional text on mindfulness and psychotherapy.
- For a companion to the clinical text mentioned above, see Pollak, Pedulla, and Siegel (2014).
- See Hayes, Follette, and Linehan (2004) for an overview of mindfulness and acceptance in the cognitive-behavioral tradition.

Books for Clients

- For a jargon-free, empirically based, primer on the psychology and practice of mindfulness, see Baer (2013).
- For a step-by-step guide to applying mindfulness and self-compassion to manage difficult emotions, see Germer (2009).
- See Williams, Teasdale, Segal, and Kabat-Zinn (2007) for the essential reader on mindfulness-based cognitive therapy for depression.

Mindfulness Meditations

- To address everyday problems with mindfulness, go to *www.Mindfulness-Solution.com*.
- To cultivate mindful presence, go to *www.TaraBrach.com*.
- To develop mindful self-compassion, go to *www.MindfulSelfCompassion.org*.

References

Baer, R. (2013). *Practicing happiness: How mindfulness can free you from psychological traps and help you build the life you want.* London: Constable.

Biegel, G. M., Brown, K. W., Shapiro, S. L., & Schubert, C. M. (2009). Mindfulness-based stress reduction for the treatment of adolescent psychiatric outpatients: A randomized clinical trial. *Journal of Consulting and Clinical Psychology, 77*(5), 855–866.

Bishop, S. R., Lau, M., Shapiro, S., Carlson, L., Anderson, N. D., Carmody, J., et al. (2004). Mindfulness: A proposed operational definition. *Clinical Psychology: Science and Practice, 11*(3), 230–241.

Black, D. (2013). Research publications on mindfulness, 1980–2012. Retrieved May 20, 2013, from *www.mindfulexperience.org/mindfo.php*.

Bohlmeijer, E., Prenger, R., Taal, E., & Cuijpers, P. (2010). The effects of mindfulness-based stress reduction therapy on mental health of adults with a chronic medical disease: A meta-analysis. *Journal of Psychosomatic Research, 68*(6), 539–544.

Brewer, J. A., Worhunsky, P. D., Gray, J. R., Tang, Y. Y., Weber, J., & Kober, H. (2011). Meditation experience is associated with differences in default mode network activity and connectivity. *Proceedings of the National Academy of Sciences of the United States of America, 108*(50), 20254–20259.

Carmody, J. (2009). Evolving conceptions of mindfulness in clinical settings. *Journal of Cognitive Psychotherapy: International Quarterly, 23*(3), 270–280.

Carmody, J., Baer, R., Lykins, E., & Olendzki, N. (2009). An empirical study of the mechanisms of mindfulness in a mindfulness-based stress reduction program. *Journal of Clinical Psychology, 65,* 613–626.

Carson, J. W., Carson, K. M., Gil, K. M., & Baucom, D. H. (2004). Mindfulness-based relationship enhancement. *Behavior Therapy, 35*(3), 471–494.

Chen, K., Berger, C., Manheimer, E., Forde, D., Magidson, J., Dachman, L., et al. (2012). Meditative therapies for reducing anxiety: A systematic review and meta-analysis of randomized controlled trials. *Depression and Anxiety, 29,* 545–562.

Chiesa, A., Calati, R., & Serretti, A. (2011). Does mindfulness training improve cognitive abilities?: A systematic review of neuropsychological findings. *Clinical Psychology Review, 31,* 449–464.

Corcoran, K. M., Farb, N., Anderson, A., & Segal, Z. V. (2010). Mindfulness and emotion regulation: Outcomes and possible mediating mechanisms. In A. M. Kring & D. M. Sloan (Eds.), *Emotion regulation and psychopathology: A transdiagnostic approach to etiology and treatment* (pp. 339–355). New York: Guilford Press.

Davis, D. M., & Hayes, J. A. (2011). What are the benefits of mindfulness?: A practice review of psychotherapy-related research. *Psychotherapy, 48*(2), 198–208.

Desbordes, G., Negi, L., Pace, T., Wallace, A., Raison, C., & Schwartz, E. (2012). Effects of mindful-attention and compassion meditation training on amygdala response to emotional stimuli in an ordinary, non-meditative state. *Frontiers in Human Neuroscience, 6,* 292.

Eberth, J., & Sedlmeier, P. (2012). The effects of mindfulness meditation: A meta-analysis. *Mindfulness, 3,* 174–189.

Farb, N. A., Segal, Z. V., Mayberg, H., Bean, J., McKeon, D., Fatima, Z., et al. (2007). Attending to the present: Mindfulness meditation reveals distinct neural modes of self-reference. *Social Cognitive and Affective Neuroscience, 2*(4), 313–322.

Farchione, T., Fairholme, C., Ellard, K., Boisseau, C., Thompson-Hollands, J., Carl, J., et al. (2012). Unified protocol for transdiagnostic treatment of emotional disorders: A randomized controlled trial. *Behavior Therapy, 43*(3), 666–678.

Fjorback, L., Arendt, M., Ornbol, E., Fink, P., & Walach, H. (2011). Mindfulness-based stress reduction and mindfulness-based cognitive therapy—a systematic review of randomized controlled trials. *Acta Psychiatrica Scandinavica, 123*(2), 102–119.

Fredrickson, B. L., Cohn, M. A., Coffey, K. A., Pek, J., & Finkel, S. M. (2008). Open hearts build lives: Positive emotions, induced through loving-kindness meditation, build consequential personal resources. *Journal of Personality and Social Psychology, 95*, 1045–1062.

Germer, C. K. (2009). *The mindful path to self-compassion: Freeing yourself from destructive thoughts and emotions.* New York: Guilford Press.

Germer, C. K. (2013). Mindfulness: What is it? What does it matter? In C. K. Germer, R. D. Siegel, & P. R. Fulton (Eds.), *Mindfulness and psychotherapy* (2nd ed., pp. 3–35). New York: Guilford Press.

Germer, C. K., & Neff, K. (2013). Self-compassion in clinical practice. *Journal of Clinical Psychology, 69*(8), 856–867.

Germer, C. K., Siegel, R. [D.], & Fulton, P. (Eds.). (2013). *Mindfulness and psychotherapy* (2nd ed.). New York: Guilford Press.

Gilbert, P. (2009). *The compassionate mind: A new approach to life's challenges.* Oakland, CA: New Harbinger.

Gilbert, P. (2010a). Compassion focused therapy. *International Journal of Cognitive Therapy, 3*, 95–210.

Gilbert, P. (2010b). *Compassion focused therapy: The CBT distinctive features series.* London: Routledge.

Gilbert, P. (2010c). An introduction to compassion focused therapy in cognitive behavior therapy. *International Journal of Cognitive Therapy, 3*(2), 97–112.

Gilbert, P., & Proctor, S. (2006). Compassionate mind training for people with high shame and self-criticism: Overview and pilot study of a group therapy approach. *Clinical Psychology and Psychotherapy, 13*, 353–379.

Greeson, J. (2009). Mindfulness research update: 2008. *Complementary Health Practice Review, 14*(1), 10–18.

Grepmair, L., Mietterlehner, F., Loew, T., Bachler, E., Rother, W., & Nickel, N. (2007). Promoting mindfulness in psychotherapists in training influences the treatment results of their patients: A randomized, double-blind, controlled study. *Psychotherapy and Psychosomatics, 76*, 332–338.

Grossman, P., Niemann, L., Schmidt, S., & Walach, H. (2004). Mindfulness-based stress reduction and health benefits: A meta-analysis. *Journal of Psychosomatic Research, 57*, 35–43.

Hahn, T. W. (1976). *The miracle of mindfulness.* Boston: Beacon Press.

Hayes, S. C. (2011). Open, aware, and active: Contextual approaches as an emerging trend in the behavioral and cognitive therapies. *Annual Review of Clinical Psychology, 7*(1), 141–168.

Hayes, S. C., Follette, V. M., & Linehan, M. M. (Eds.). (2004). *Mindfulness and acceptance: Expanding the cognitive-behavioral tradition.* New York: Guilford Press.

Hayes, S. C., Strosahl, K. D., & Wilson, K. G. (1999). *Acceptance and commitment therapy: An experiential approach to behavior change.* New York: Guilford Press.

Hill, C., & Updegraff, J. (2012). Mindfulness and its relationship to emotion regulation. *Emotion, 12*(1), 81–90.

Hofman, S., Grossman, P., & Hinton, D. (2011). Loving-kindness and compassion meditation: Potential for psychological interventions. *Clinical Psychology Review, 31*, 1126–1132.

Hofman, S., Sawyer, A., Witt, A., & Oh, D. (2010). The effect of mindfulness-based therapy on anxiety and depression: A meta-analytic review. *Journal of Clinical and Consulting Psychology, 78*(2), 169–183.

Hölzel, B. K., Lazar, S. W., Gard, T., Schuman-Olivier, Z., Vago, D. R., & Ott, U. (2011). How does mindfulness meditation work?: Proposing mechanisms of action from a conceptual and neural perspective. *Perspectives on Psychological Science, 6*(6), 537–559.

Jha, A. (2013, April 13). *Neural mechanisms of mindfulness: Emerging models.* Paper presented at the 11th annual International Scientific Conference, Center for Mindfulness in Medicine, Health Care, and Society, University of Massachusetts, Norwood, MA.

Kabat-Zinn, J. (2003). Mindfulness-based interventions in context: Past, present, and future. *Clinical Psychology: Science and Practice, 10*(2), 144–156.

Keng, S., Smoski, M., & Robins, C. (2011). Effects of mindfulness on psychological health: A review of empirical studies. *Clinical Psychology Review, 31*, 1041–1056.

Khoury, B., Lecomte, T., Fortin, G., Masse, M., Therien, P., Bouchard, V., et al. (2013). Mindfulness-base therapy: A comprehensive meta-analysis. *Clinical Psychology Review, 33*, 763–771.

Kristeller, J., & Wolever, R. (2011). Mindfulness-based eating awareness training for treating binge eating disorder: The conceptual foundation. *Eating Disorders, 19*(1), 49–61.

Lazar, S. W., Kerr, C. E., Wasserman, R. H., Gray, J. R., Greve, D. N., Treadway, M. T., et al. (2005). Meditation experience is associated with increased cortical thickness. *NeuroReport, 16*(17), 1893–1897.

Lee, T., Leung, M., Hou, W., Tang, J., Yin, J., So, K., et al. (2012). Distinct neural activity associated with focused-attention meditation and loving-kindness meditation. *PLOS ONE, 7*(8), e40054.

Linehan, M. M. (1993a). *Cognitive-behavioral treatment of borderline personality disorder.* New York: Guilford Press.

Linehan, M. M. (1993b). *Skills training manual for treating borderline personality disorder.* New York: Guilford Press.

Longmore, R., & Worrell, M. (2007). Do we need to challenge thoughts in cognitive behavior therapy? *Clinical Psychology Review, 27*(2), 173–187.

Lutz, A., Slagter, H. A., Dunne, J. D., & Davidson, R. J. (2008). Attention regulation and monitoring in meditation. *Trends in Cognitive Sciences, 12*(4), 163–169.

Mascaro, J. S., Rilling, J. K., Negi, L. T., & Raison, C. L. (2013). Pre-existing brain function predicts subsequent practice of mindfulness and compassion meditation. *NeuroImage, 69*, 35–42.

Neff, K. D. (2011). *Self-compassion: Stop beating yourself up and leave insecurity behind.* New York: Morrow.

Neff, K.D., & Germer, C. (2013). A pilot study and randomized controlled trial of the Mindful Self-Compassion program. *Journal of Clinical Psychology, 69*(1), 28–44.

Norcross, J. C., & Lambert, M. J. (2011). Evidence-based therapy relationships. In J. C. Norcross (Ed.), *Psychotherapy relationships that work* (2nd ed., pp. 3–21). New York: Oxford University Press.

Nyanaponika, T. (1965). *The heart of Buddhist meditation.* York Beach, ME: Red Wheel/Weiser.

Nyanaponika, T. (1972). *The power of mindfulness.* San Francisco: Unity Press.

Oliver, M. (1986). *Dream work.* Boston: Atlantic Monthly Press.

Orsillo, S. M., & Roemer, L. (2011). *The mindful way through anxiety: Break free from worry and reclaim your life.* New York: Guilford Press.

Pace, T., Negi, L., Adams, D., Cole, S., Sivilli, T., Brown, T., et al. (2009). Effect of compassion meditation on neuroendocrine, innate immune and behavioral responses to psychosocial stress. *Psychoneuroendocrinology, 34*(1), 87–98.

Piet, J., & Hougaard, E. (2011). The effect of mindfulness-based cognitive therapy for prevention of relapse in recurrent major depressive disorder: A systematic review and meta-analysis. *Clinical Psychology Review, 31*(6), 1032–1040.

Pollak, S. M., Pedulla, T., & Siegel, R. D. (2014). *Sitting together: Essential skills for mindfulness-based psychotherapy.* New York: Guilford Press.

Roemer, L., Orsillo, S. M., & Salters-Pedneault, K. (2008). Efficacy of an acceptance-based behavior therapy for generalized anxiety disorder: Evaluation in a randomized controlled trial. *Journal of Consulting and Clinical Psychology, 76*(6), 1083–1089.

Rubia, K. (2009). The neurobiology of meditation and its clinical effectiveness in psychiatric disorders. *Biological Psychiatry, 82,* 1–11.

Salzberg, S. (2011). *Real happiness: The power of meditation.* New York: Workman.

Segal, Z. V., Williams, J. M. G., & Teasdale, J. D. (2013). *Mindfulness-based cognitive therapy for depression* (2nd ed.). New York: Guilford Press.

Semple, R. J., Lee, J., Rosa, D., & Miller, L. F. (2010). A randomized trial of mindfulness-based cognitive therapy for children: Promoting mindful attention to enhance social–emotional resiliency in children. *Journal of Child and Family Studies, 19*(2), 218–229.

Shapiro, S., Carlson, L., Astin, J., & Freedman, B. (2006). Mechanisms of mindfulness. *Journal of Clinical Psychology, 62*(3), 373–386.

Siegel, R. D. (2010). *The mindfulness solution: Everyday practices for everyday problems.* New York: Guilford Press.

Smith, J. (2004). Alterations in brain and immune function produced by mindfulness meditation: Three caveats. *Psychosomatic Medicine, 66,* 148–152.

Van der Oord, S., Bögels, S., & Peijnenburg, D. (2012). The effectiveness of mindfulness training for children with ADHD and mindful parenting for their parents. *Journal of Child and Family Studies, 21,* 139–147.

Vøllestad, J., Nielsen, M., & Nielsen, G. (2012). Mindfulness- and acceptance-based interventions for anxiety disorders: A systematic review and meta-analysis. *British Journal of Clinical Psychology, 51*(3), 239–260.

Walsh, R., & Shapiro, S. (2006). The meeting of meditative disciplines and Western psychology: A mutually enriching dialogue. *American Psychologist, 61*(3), 227–239.

Williams, J. M., & Kabat-Zinn, J. (2011). Mindfulness: Diverse perspectives on its meaning, origins, and multiple applications at the intersection of science and dharma. *Contemporary Buddhism, 12*(1), 1–18.

Williams, J. M., & Lynn, S. (2010). Acceptance: An historical and conceptual review. *Imagination, Cognition and Personality, 30*(1), 5–56.

Williams, J. M. G., Teasdale, J. D., Segal, Z. V., & Kabat-Zinn, J. (2007). *The mindful way through depression: Freeing yourself from chronic unhappiness.* New York: Guilford Press.

Witkiewitz, K., & Bowen, S. (2010). Depression, craving, and substance use following a randomized trial of mindfulness-based relapse prevention. *Journal of Consulting and Clinical Psychology, 78*(3), 362–374.

CHAPTER 2

Understanding and Taking Advantage of Experiential Work in Acceptance and Commitment Therapy

Jennifer C. Plumb Vilardaga
Matthieu Villatte
Steven C. Hayes

Acceptance and commitment therapy (ACT) is an experiential approach to psychological treatment that is grounded in a systematic program of experimental science (Hayes, Strosahl, & Wilson, 1999, 2011) The applied theory that guides ACT, the psychological flexibility model, and the basic theory of language and cognition on which it is based, relational frame theory (RFT; Hayes, Barnes-Holmes, & Roche, 2001), can be used to see how to help clients develop an understanding about what they experience, how they respond to that experience, and how these different responses to experience relate to living a meaningful life. ACT uses a wide variety of exercises and therapist–client interactions that go beyond verbal discussion and literal explanation of experience, also known as experiential work, to do so. The purpose of this chapter is to explore the importance of experiential work from this theoretical perspective, and to provide some clinical tools for delivering and debriefing experiential exercises from an ACT perspective.

Theory

ACT is a modern contextual behavioral treatment model aimed at reducing human suffering through the cultivation of psychological flexibility. ACT therapists identify components of human suffering in terms of psychological rigidity (illustrated in Figure 2.1), and work to increase psychological flexibility through six interrelated core processes (illustrated in Figure 2.2). Clinicians help promote these psychological flexibility processes in ACT primarily through experiential exercises and metaphors as well as through listening, reflecting, questioning, and behavioral techniques (e.g., behavioral activation, behavioral monitoring, in-vivo exposure) found in any behavioral approach.

ACT is situated within a larger conceptual framework called contextual behavioral science (CBS) that guides scientific exploration and further refinement of the ACT work, but a full review of such work is beyond the scope of this chapter (see Hayes, Strosahl, & Wilson, 2011; Vilardaga, Hayes, Levin, & Muto, 2009, for more information). This larger framework situates all ACT work firmly within a behavioral framework with

Lack of Attention to the Present Moment: Inattention to current cues in environment, overattention to the past or feared future

Experiential Avoidance: Attempt to escape from or avoid difficult thoughts or feelings

Lack of Values Clarity: Lose contact with what we really want to be about in our lives

Psychological Rigidity

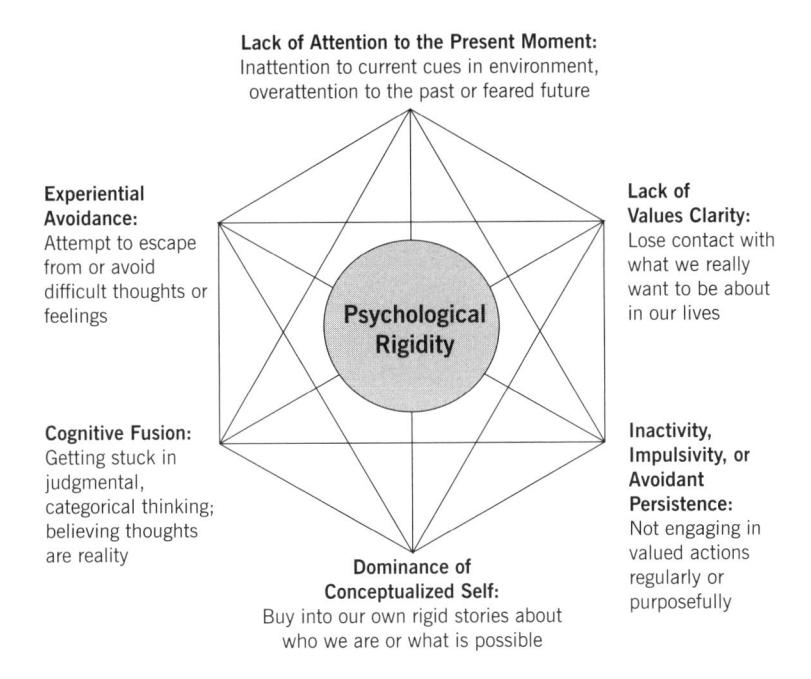

Cognitive Fusion: Getting stuck in judgmental, categorical thinking; believing thoughts are reality

Inactivity, Impulsivity, or Avoidant Persistence: Not engaging in valued actions regularly or purposefully

Dominance of Conceptualized Self: Buy into our own rigid stories about who we are or what is possible

FIGURE 2.1. Psychological rigidity as the ACT model of psychopathology. Copyright by Steven C. Hayes. Used by permission. The figure may be copied and reused freely.

Attention to the Present Moment:
Flexibly paying attention to what is happening here, now

Acceptance: Openness to experiences, even if they are uncomfortable

Values: Freely choosing what is most important in life

Psychological Flexibility

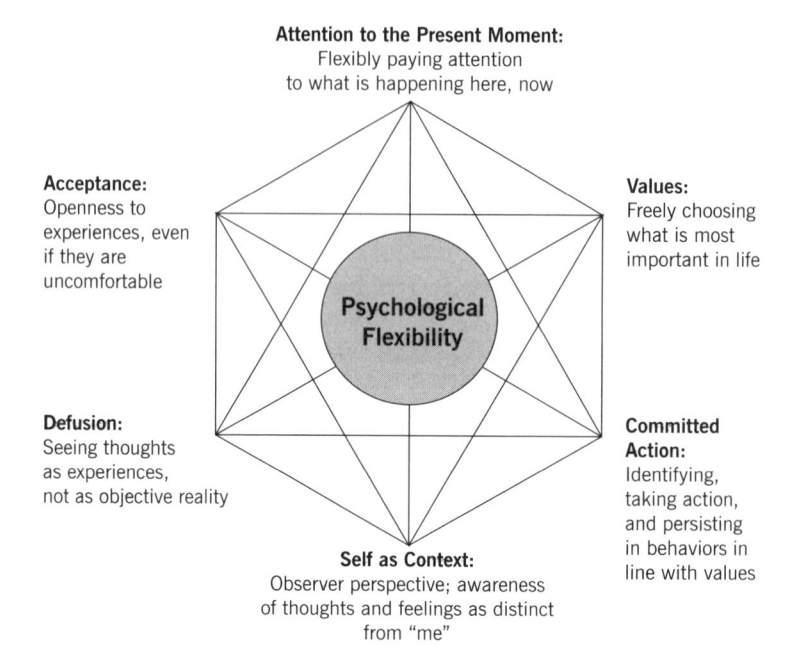

Defusion: Seeing thoughts as experiences, not as objective reality

Committed Action: Identifying, taking action, and persisting in behaviors in line with values

Self as Context: Observer perspective; awareness of thoughts and feelings as distinct from "me"

FIGURE 2.2. Psychological flexibility as the ACT model of intervention. Copyright by Steven C. Hayes. Used by permission. The figure may be copied and reused freely.

particular attention to the function (effect) and context (both a person's history of behaving and the current situation in which he or she behaves). From this perspective, ACT can be thought of as a way to create a healthy variation of behavior (through acceptance and defusion), deeply in touch with the current situational and historical context of one's life (through conscious perspective taking and flexible attention to the now), and to choose wise selection criteria for behavior (values) so as to develop behavioral patterns that are in service of such values (through committed action). In that sense the six processes of psychological flexibility can be thought of as contextually guided variation and selective retention at the psychological level. As such, ACT is not so much a technique as it is an inherently experiential approach based on a specific model of behaving (which includes thinking and feeling) in the world. That makes ACT extremely flexible as a technology and helps explain its broad applicability.

Experiential work, as opposed to verbally based discussions, is central to ACT in part because ACT originated from the experimental finding that verbal rules easily become overgeneralized, creating an insensitivity to direct experience (Zettle & Hayes, 1986). These experimental findings supported the development of a companion theory of language and cognition, RFT (Hayes et al., 2001). RFT, which is also situated within the CBS framework, helps researchers better address the importance of human language from within a behavioral perspective with behavioral goals. RFT research has increased understanding of the ways in which insensitivity, or the lack of awareness or response to changes in the environment, is a natural risk of human language. Essentially language allows for rapid judgments (that may not reflect the current environment as it is actually experienced), memories of things that happened in the past, and worries about a future that has not yet occurred—all of which can compete with awareness of and effective response to the current environment. The core idea of RFT is that symbolic relations (the basis of human cognition and language) are learned patterns of building, understanding, and responding to arbitrarily applicable relations among things (events, people, or psychological experiences). This has direct clinical implications.

For example, a client who thinks "I am weak" is applying a particular relational frame that has been derived from many previously learned examples of "is." As a result, a belief of this kind can construct a relation between the self and some unpleasant characteristic, which can then enter into networks of symbolic thought that may lead the client to avoid challenging activities (e.g., "If I am weak, then I can't accomplish challenging things"). Symbolic relations can also potentially transform the meaning and the impact of everything. In the previous example, perhaps the client heard once from a parent that he was weak, and it was enough to change the way he sees himself and influences whether or not he decides to engage in challenging activities. Symbolic relations change the way we interact with our inner and external worlds. As verbal rules increase in their dominance, such rules tend to become overextended. In other words, they become applied to more and more situations where these rules are not useful. As a result, the role of direct experience in influencing human behavior diminishes.

The ability of language and cognition to detach us from our direct experiences has both advantages and downsides, however. On the one hand, we can interact with things that are not immediately present, which allows us to plan future events or remember sweet memories and connect to meaningful areas of our lives in any kind of circumstances. On the other hand, we are never free from psychological pain because at any time we can contact aversive events from the past or anticipate future dangers even when the immediate context is not intrinsically threatening. This is typically what happens to clients who avoid situations triggering traumatic memories, for example.

There is a growing body of RFT research demonstrating that symbolic relations promote avoidance of previously unrelated experiences due to the transformation of their meaning (e.g., Hooper, Saunders, & McHugh, 2010). Such "symbolic generalization" spreads aversive histories and their resulting patterns of avoidance beyond our direct experience to quickly reach anything we can think of. We now know that people who have a specific phobia are much more likely to show such forms of symbolic generalization and resulting avoidance of stimuli that have not been directly learned as aversive (Dymond, Schlund, Roche, & Whelan, 2014).

The problematic impact of language and cognition goes beyond turning anything into potential targets of avoidance. Because symbolic relations can detach us from our direct experiences, we can persist in strategies that are not effective. For example, a client may think "I need to think of something else" when bothered by a traumatic memory and keep trying to distract herself even though the painful memory keeps coming back. Distraction itself may increase the frequency of the memory in the longer term but she has formulated a verbal rule that suggests it is the right thing to do. Symbolic rules create insensitivity to direct consequences of our actions, and research supports this idea. Hayes, Brownstein, Zettle, Rosenfarb, and Korn (1986) found that participants who had learned a task via verbal instruction showed effective responses more quickly at first, but participants who had to observe the consequence of their actions to master the task were better able to change their responses when the rules of the game changed without warning.

Many if not most psychological problems involve both response to events that are not physically present in the current context and persistence in unworkable behavioral strategies. For this reason, ACT contends that reconnecting clients with their direct experience can help them adjust their behavior in a more effective way and contact sources of meaning or satisfaction that might otherwise be overshadowed by symbolic events (Villatte, Villatte, & Monestes, 2014). The use of language is not abandoned—symbolic relations remain important in many ways such as in being able to follow the therapist in session, understanding the nature of experiential exercises, or generalizing therapy work to behavior in life outside the office. What is different is that language is used to guide and broaden the client's observation of his experience and to evaluate the effectiveness of his behavior with regard to his goals and values.

Empirical Evidence

Since being described in its modern form in 1999 (Hayes, Strosahl, & Wilson, 1999), ACT has been applied to many domains of human functioning (e.g., mental health, behavioral medicine, social topics such as prejudice and compassion, and work topics such as learning new methods or building effective work teams). A full review of ACT evidence is beyond the scope of this chapter; detailed scholarly reviews of the empirical literature can be found in Gaudiano (2011) and Hayes, Luoma, Bond, Masuda, and Lillis (2006).

Areas of particular strength include anxiety disorders (e.g., Arch et al.,

2012a), depression, (e.g., Bohlmeijer, Fledderus, Rokx, & Piertse, 2011) and both adolescent and adult chronic pain (e.g., Wetherell et al., 2011; Wicksell, Melin, Lekander, & Olsson, 2009). There is compelling evidence for ACT as a treatment for serious mental illness (Gaudiano, Nowlen, Brown, Epstein-Lubow, & Miller, 2013; White et al., 2011), substance abuse (Hayes et al., 2004; Smout et al., 2010), smoking cessation (Bricker, Mann, Marek, Liu, & Peterson, 2010; Gifford et al., 2011), diabetes management (Gregg, Callaghan, Hayes, & Glenn-Lawson, 2007), drug-resistant epilepsy (Lundgren, Dahl, Yardi, & Melin, 2008), cancer (Rost, Wilson, Buchanan, Hildebrandt, & Mutch, 2012), and improving or maintaining weight loss (Juarascio, Forman, & Herbert, 2010; Lillis, Hayes, Bunting, & Masuda, 2009).

As a result of these outcome studies, ACT has been listed as an evidence-based method by Division 12 of the American Psychological Association as having strong support for chronic pain and moderate support for several other areas, including mixed anxiety disorders, obsessive-compulsive disorder, depression, coping with psychosis and other areas (see *www.div12.org/PsychologicalTreatments/treatments.html*). It has been listed as an evidence-based practice on the Substance Abuse and Mental Health Services Administration (SAMHSA) National Registry of Evidence-Based Programs and Practices (see *http://nrepp.samhsa.gov/ViewIntervention.aspx?id=191*). Further, ACT has been applied nationally as a treatment for depression in the Department of Veterans Affairs, with initial positive results (Walser, Karlin, Trockel, Mazina, & Taylor, 2013).

Evidence for Components and Mediatiors of Change

Because of the centrality of these issues to the CBS strategy of treatment development, component studies and mediational studies have been frequently published on ACT. A recent meta-analysis of ACT component studies found 66 empirical studies on the treatment components suggested by the psychological flexibility model (Levin, Hildebrandt, Lillis, & Hayes, 2012). Significant positive effect sizes were observed for acceptance, defusion, present moment, values, mixed mindfulness components, and values plus mindfulness component interventions compared to inactive comparison conditions. Larger effect sizes were found for outcomes and comparisons that were theoretically specified. Interventions that included experiential methods (e.g., metaphors, exercises) were significantly more effective than rationales alone. Effect sizes did not differ between at-risk/distressed and convenience samples.

Mediation studies were summarized in Hayes and colleagues (2006), and several additional high-quality meditational studies have appeared since (e.g., Arch, Wolitzky-Taylor, Eifert, & Craske, 2012). Throughout the literature the evidence is consistent: ACT works in part by its impact on psychological flexibility, which in turn leads to positive clinical outcomes.

Clinical Application

The ACT model of psychopathology identifies key areas of human functioning that can become disrupted. It is a functional dimensional model, not a narrow "one-size-fits-all" conceptualization of psychopathology that is to be applied in its entirety to every client. ACT points to domains of functioning that individually or in combination contribute to reduce or enhance the ability of behavioral systems to evolve in a successful way. As a result, the model provides a helpful mapping of domains of functioning that can aid a clinician in developing an individualized case formulation, assessing both strengths and weaknesses with regard to each component of psychological flexibility. This assessment occurs throughout treatment in a dynamic and ongoing fashion. Individualized case formulation can then guide the selection of potential target behaviors in session based on the particular process the clinician seeks to either strengthen or reduce the negative impact of the process on client functioning.

ACT clinicians use the therapeutic environment to help clients explore their own behavior in terms of antecedents, experiences, responses, and consequences. Clinically this often takes the form of exploring difficult situations, the client's experiences, responses (both private and overt behavior), and the consequences of such responses. Consider the following questions: (1) "What was happening?"; (2) "What did you notice experiencing?"; (3) "What did you do in response to having that experience?"; and (4) "Did doing that get you closer to or further away from meaningful living?"

Let us examine each question separately. First, the question "What was happening?" helps a client begin to explore the contexts in which a given experience is likely to arise. Although many clients seeking help have a sense of when they tend to feel a particular way that is uncomfortable or behaviorally restricting, it can help the client to gain a greater sense of both the external events (such as intimate conversations in a relationship) and internal events (such as thoughts about failing an upcoming test) that are challenging.

Inviting clients to explore what they noticed about what they experienced can help the client to turn her attention to her private experiences more directly. By promoting a slow, deliberate exploration of body sensations, emotions, and thoughts, the client can strengthen her capacity for experiential awareness. For example, a client who says she felt a sense of danger might usefully notice that her hands formed a fist, her teeth clenched, and her stomach tightened as if she was about to be hit.

Asking clients to describe their response to their experiences provides opportunities to develop a conceptualization of potential clinical problems; from an ACT perspective, it is not the experience itself that is problematic, but the responses to it that limits meaningful living. Therefore, these questions are key to helping both client and clinician develop a conceptualization of the potential problem, but the problem cannot be fully explored until the consequence is also examined in terms of meaningful living.

Finally, then, asking about the short- and long-term consequences of a particular response ("Did doing that get you closer to or further away from meaningful living?") helps clients begin to orient from the problem being an uncomfortable or unwanted experience per se toward the idea that unhelpful responding to an experience is itself a problem. When the cost of doing so is cast in terms of the client's own values, he may become more aware of times that his behavior is not helping him to live a meaningful life. Such questions help clinicians explore a client's sense of values, which can sometimes be weak or lacking in clarity. If a client has difficulty determining if his behavior moves him closer to or further away from meaningful living or states that he does not know what meaningful living is, then this may indicate a weakness in values clarity as part of the case conceptualization. Rather than dive directly into values clarification, smaller, simpler ways to discuss meaning may be needed. For instance, clients may not have a strong sense of values early on in therapy, but may have a sense of "living as they would choose," "doing things they care about or enjoy," "living with purpose," or "living a fulfilling life."

Asking these four types of questions several times in several ways can thus help clients develop an understanding of how their behavior functions in their lives. However, it may be difficult for clients to recall and report on the antecedents, responses, and consequences for previous behaviors unless they have been paying particular attention in the moment. This is another way in which experiential exercises can be quite helpful. Rather than relying on distant memories in another context, in-session experiential exercises can allow the client to contact all of the parts of behavioral sequences in the immediate moment.

Engaging in eyes-closed experiential exercises in session can help the client focus on the antecedents, responses, and consequences without external distractions. Through the transformation of functions allowed by human symbolic ability, emotions experienced in the past ("there–then") can be experienced again in the present ("here–now"), and clients have an additional opportunity to attend to their responses to these experiences. Practicing experiential exercises provides opportunities for clients to be in better contact with their inner worlds, which can provide another opportunity to help the clients track which of their behaviors happen frequently, and how each functions in their lives in terms of meaningful living. Also, experiential exercises may help clients increase awareness of the experiences they have throughout the day, which without intentional examination may pass without being noticed. Finally, *how* clients engage in the in-session exercises in addition to the information gleaned from engaging in the exercises are important for helping to identify potential strengths and weaknesses in relation to the model. For instance, how easy is it for clients to attend to the present moment and engage in the exercise? Do they have difficulty identifying whether their response takes them closer or further away from meaningful living? Do they have a sense of what meaningful living is for them? Do clients tend to evaluate their experience, rather than simply notice or describe their experience? Do clients report rigid rules about how they should behave or what should be? Looking to answer these questions when engaging in experiential work can help both clients and clinicians develop individualized conceptualizations and hence a deeper understanding of the client's functioning.

Take for example a commonly used ACT metaphor, "Passengers on the Bus," which was originally printed in Hayes and colleagues (1999, pp. 157–158). Building on the printed version of the metaphor, clients can be encouraged to examine the particular uncomfortable experiences (thoughts, feelings, memories, etc.) as if they were "passengers" that arise while driving one's own "bus" and living one's life. Clients can be encouraged to name passengers with impactful names such as "Unrealistic Expectations" or "Scared-y Cat" and the ways in which the clients respond to each passenger is discussed in terms of where the client ends up "driving the bus": either toward meaningful living or away from it (by avoiding, engaging in self-criticism, or otherwise ignoring one's own valued behaviors). Clients are reminded that they are the driver of the bus, and to explore the idea that while the passengers may say things like, "If you go out, you'll feel anxious, so you should stay home," clients can choose their own behaviors regardless. With time, all aspects of the ACT model can be explored. Clients further identify their experiences (mindful awareness), name these experiences (which in and of itself can be a distancing or defusing move), examine their responses as either avoiding or approaching their experience (experiential avoidance), relate that to the impact on meaningful living (values), and finally begin a discussion of what choices are available for behavior despite what thoughts and feelings are present (acceptance and defusion, leading to committed actions in line with values).

It may seem a slow process to ask questions or to use experiential exercises as opportunities to assess the client's functioning rather than giving direct instructions about how to approach experiences or direct feedback about distorted thinking. There are many theoretical and clinical reasons not to do so. From a behavioral perspective, all behavior is maintained for some reason. Avoidance is effective at reducing distress in the moment and is only "ineffective" in contexts where approach is more helpful for an individual's goals, or when longer-term functioning would be improved if avoidance was reduced. More important, RFT research suggests that external rules are particularly likely to produce insensitivity. If clients themselves can examine the usefulness of the contexts and the functions that arise in their lives, they are better positioned to generate more flexible responses. Essentially, helping clients become functional analysts of their own behavior is the core work of therapy. Practicing in therapy (via homework and in session) strengthens the client's ability to do self-assessment so that she can evaluate whether later behaviors support meaningful living, even after therapy has terminated.

When to Do Experiential Work

We recommend that clinicians use a stepped approach to implementing deliberate experiential exercises or metaphors, starting with existing examples, and building a repertoire wherein new exercises and metaphors are developed and can be implemented flexibly in session. When learning to use ACT, it may be beneficial to use existing exercises and metaphors for a target process in session for the therapists' first cases. In fact, new therapists may wish to utilize one of the many protocols available in books or other online sources, as they provide detailed accounts of exercises and strategies for developing and implementing theoretically consistent moves from within the ACT therapeutic stance. Also, trying out a few different exercises for each process, even within the same session, can provide both client and clinician with multiple opportunities to explore the process, perhaps from multiple angles, or with particular language that might resonate. This also helps clinicians to develop a deeper sense of the theoretically consistent and intended purpose of any given exercise or metaphor.

Inherent in the model of psychological flexibility is the need for clinicians to also be flexible in how they approach the treatment. Any behavior that promotes flexibility and fosters valued ends can be useful in the therapy room. Once a clinician is clear about an intended function of any activity, exercise, or metaphor, the form that in-session behaviors take is flexible, and ACT therapists often develop and use their own metaphors and exercises and encourage clients themselves to do so as well. This is important, because when clients create their own exercises and metaphors they can make the therapeutic work more genuine, flexible, and hopefully impactful for therapist and client alike.

Parallel Processes and Attending to the Therapeutic Relationship

Just as clients struggle with rigidity and do not live according to their own values, so do clinicians at times. In particular, when considering what is done in therapy and why, clinicians may find themselves being fused with what "should be," may seek paths of avoidance to reduce uncertainty, or may engage in other behaviors that are not in line with their values for being a therapist. Experiential exercises and metaphors can at times be chosen for unhelpful reasons, such as discomfort or uncertainty about what to do or say next. If we look closely, what may underlie these choices? Is it easier to do a scripted or silly exercise than to really "be with the client" and explore the problem in a deeply connected way? Does the therapist notice an urge to "fix the problem" or to expect the client to be more accepting, mindful, or flexible than he is in a given moment?

Although ACT is an active approach, ACT therapists generally don't provide specific linear "how to do it" instructions to improve clients' lives. While there are times when it is useful to take active steps to prevent a client from harming herself or others, for the most part, our client's decisions to live her life are her own and we are mere guides along for the journey. As the old adage goes, "You can lead a horse to water, but you cannot make him drink." We can point the way to successful working by asking questions that may lead the client to assess her behavior, and we may suggest alternatives or help the client generate alternatives, but we must ask ourselves if it is truly in line with our values to pressure someone else to change, no matter how uncomfortable, upsetting, or frustrating it may be to witness another person continue to make decisions we may evaluate as poor or ineffective, or to otherwise continue suffering.

From an ACT perspective, all clients are viewed as whole and perfect; it is human behavior that is useful or not useful, effective or ineffective. This may seem inconsistent with a model that explicitly labels behavioral repertoires indicative of psychopathology, but this stance is vitally important for an ACT therapist. As a contextual behavioral approach, ACT assumes that all clients (barring the most severe cognitive deficits) have a repertoire for *learning*, which in turn allows for the possibility of acquiring new skills or applying old skills in new contexts. What the model does not assume is if clients *should* choose to change behavior to be more in line with meaningful living, only that it is possible. Following from this stance is that an ACT therapist does not work, as a general rule, to directly change feelings, thoughts, or other experiences by advocating or engaging in avoiding, minimizing, reassuring, or soothing the client. Instead, the practice is to support clients in examining their own answers to the four questions discussed earlier and potentially influence clients' responses to be more in line with their chosen values.

However, we may experience frustration when we see clients continuing to behave in ways that lead to suffering when we believe we know other ways of being are possible for the client. Indeed, this experience on the therapist's part is a parallel process to what the client may experience. For example, a therapist may have the thought, "If my client was just [more accepting, more mindful, less fused] she would suffer less and live more meaningfully!" This kind of fusion and nonacceptance move is very similar to how clients often respond to their own experiences—buying into thoughts that they "should" think or feel differently. A therapist can then apply ACT principles to awareness of her own experiences and behavior within the session; notice the fusion with a "should" and practice making space for it so that her behavior is not about trying to make the client "better" or to feel less pain, because from an ACT perspective, direct attempts to remove or reduce unwanted experiences often result in more efforts to control experience and creates less, not more, psychological flexibility.

Conducting therapy from within this ACT stance is not always easy, however. Indeed there has been work published on how therapists can engage in the parallel process of examining their own (in- and out-of-session) behavior within an ACT framework (e.g., Vilardaga & Hayes, 2009). First, the clinician's recognition of her personal struggles in terms of psychological inflexibility can help her to develop a sense of compassion and empathy for the client's struggle to do the difficult work of being in therapy. In the therapy room, if the therapist notices that she is getting caught up in fusion, nonacceptance, or finds herself persisting in nonvalued behavior (such as convincing, arguing, or teaching), it is useful to connect this conduct to old, ineffective patterns that our clients can easily get stuck in. Such recognition in the therapy room may be a cue for engaging in strategic self-disclosure and to modeling the behavior of first noticing unhelpful responses and then making in-the-moment corrections based on the clinician's values for therapy. Consider the following vignette wherein a therapist starts the conversation while being more directive than she intended to be.

CLIENT: I don't know. I guess I just don't have a clear sense of what I really care about. I feel like I should know this, but it's all muddy.

THERAPIST: Well, I think you do have a clear sense. You said you cared about your family, a few sessions ago. That seems to be a good value to have.

CLIENT: I suppose. I mean I care that they are happy, but I'm not sure what my value is for them. They are probably better off without me screwing everything up all the time.

THERAPIST: So, besides your mind telling you that you make things worse, we have a clear value here. You care about your family.

CLIENT: Um, sure. I guess so.

THERAPIST: Hmmm. (*a few-second pause*) You know, I am realizing that I just violated my own value here. You've talked about how others used to tell you what to do all the time, and it seems like I was doing that too; trying to convince you of what you cared about. I'm feeling sad and disappointed about that. What was your experience?

CLIENT: Well, I guess it didn't feel that great for me.

THERAPIST: (*Sighs*) I suppose my mind was chattering away about how I can't possibly know what to do next if a client I am working with doesn't know what they care about. Remember the "Passengers on the Bus" we discussed a few sessions ago? One of my passengers is

"Uncomfortable with Uncertainty" and it tells me to move away from anything unclear really quickly.

CLIENT: Huh. One of your passengers is "Uncomfortable with Uncertainty"? That sounds familiar. I'm surprised that you have passengers like mine.

THERAPIST: Sure, I'm human too! And, I really bought into that chatter that in order for us to move forward I had to convince you of your values so we could do the work! I'm sorry for letting my mind guide us back there; this is your therapy and your time. My value is actually to be present with you and help you explore what matters to you. I'm committing to doing that, even though I know that passenger will probably still yell at me from time to time.

CLIENT: OK. (*playfully*) I'll let you know if I see that one showing up again.

THERAPIST: Great plan!

Several things happened in this exchange. First, the therapist noted the experience of feeling sad and disappointed as cues for something going amiss in session. Then, she took a moment to assess what in her own behavior may have contributed to this experience, and recognized an old behavior of convincing, which she links back to her mind not liking uncertainty. She then shared this experience, as well as the practice of coming back to a valued behavior path. Rather than normalizing the client's experience directly, sharing the therapist's experience in the moment, and walking the client through the antecedents, experiences, responses, and consequences of her own experience allowed the client to generate that idea himself. In addition, his playful response shows that he will also be on the lookout for such passengers in the future, thus increasing his tracking of fusion.

Experiential Work Guided by Clinical Formulation

While the previous example indicates the usefulness of on-the-fly use of experiential work to build the relationship and model the processes, much of the experiential work in ACT can be strategic and aimed at the target processes in the individualized case formulation. There are several ways to do so. One approach is to examine each process and to begin targeting the client's weakest process, aiming most exercises at loosening up rigidity in this target area. Another approach is to explore the client's strengths and use those as a foundation on which the other potential weaknesses are discussed. For instance, if early sessions indicate that the client has a strong sense of values, but has difficulty being present in the room, is easily distracted, and continues to report "I'm fine" when asked what he experiences, it may help to highlight the client's values for a time as a means to gain further traction in the exploration of other domains in which he is less comfortable and less aware of how his behavior is functioning. Yet a third approach is to develop a conceptualization that indicates key linked processes and to use one as a pivot point for targeting another process or other processes. Commonly linked processes are experiential avoidance and cognitive fusion or fusion with self-concept. If the client's greatest weakness is that he appears accepting of very few experiences in his life, what are the thoughts that might maintain this? Perhaps he has rigid rules (fusion) about what constitutes "good" versus "bad" feelings, and engages in behaviors that are avoidant of "bad" feelings, and only approaches situations where he is almost guaranteed to have some kind of "good" feeling. Or, through exploration, he might report that his mind tells him that he is unworthy of having good feelings because of bad things he has done in the past (fusion with self-concept). The therapist may implement exercises and metaphors aimed at reducing fusion prior to working to strengthen acceptance and willingness, as the client's avoidance is likely maintained by these rules.

There is no "right" answer for how to implement therapeutic moves, even when linking them back to a formulation. In the example of the fused client above, the therapist might note that attempting to build willingness and acceptance first feels like a struggle, and the client may respond by talking a lot about his experiences, and perhaps giving the message that there are some experiences he likes and others he absolutely does not like. This is not a failure on the therapist's part, but simply fodder for ongoing conceptualization. If targeting a weak process in the model uncovers other unhelpful behaviors, it may be worth asking questions that might illuminate the relationships between these processes, and trying an intervention from another angle.

Vignette 1: Fusion in the Moment

A 50-year-old male client has been coming to therapy with depression for three sessions. Through assessment and the contingency questions, the therapist believes that the client's weakness is a great amount of cognitive fusion, particularly around self-judgmental thoughts, and the client tends to ruminate at home about them, shutting out the rest of life. However, the client has difficulty contacting the cost of doing so. His fusion is such that he believes if he thinks through his negative thoughts enough, he will figure out the answer and feel better.

THERAPIST: So, you've been noticing the thoughts "I'm a failure" and "Unlovable" showing up for a while.
CLIENT: Yeah.
THERAPIST: And when they show up, what do you tend to do?
CLIENT: I just stay home, thinking about them, trying to analyze them, where they came from. So I can nip them in the bud, maybe, in the future.

THERAPIST: So they kind of dominate what you can see, what you pay attention to?

CLIENT: Yeah.

THERAPIST: Would you be willing to try something with me? Get a little silly?

CLIENT: Sure.

THERAPIST: OK. (*Pulls a chair over to the client.*) I'm going to ask you to stick your head in the chair, like you are inspecting the seat under a microscope.

CLIENT: (*Laughs.*) OK. (*pause*) This is weird.

THERAPIST: Great! So, tell me what you can see with your head in the chair. Really describe it.

CLIENT: Well, I see blue. Fuzzy cloth. A crease in the back. It's kind of gross up close.

THERAPIST: OK, so your mind is having some evaluations. Great, what else do you see?

CLIENT: It's kind of speckled . . . the blue fuzzy cloth.

THERAPIST: Do you see the edges of the chair?

CLIENT: Nope.

THERAPIST: So, now, *without moving your head* . . . can you tell me what is happening outside, through the window?

CLIENT: Uh . . . I have no idea.

THERAPIST: Can't see it.

CLIENT: Yeah. And I'm getting kind of tired looking at this thing.

THERAPIST: OK, so now, pull your head back. What do you see now?

CLIENT: (*Blinks.*) The room, you, the window, stuff outside.

THERAPIST: So, does it ever feel like that with your thoughts? That when they show up, right up close in your face, all loud and demanding attention, that it's kind of like sticking your head in the chair? Like you get an up-close and personal look at them, but you get lost in them. You don't really see the chair as a chair, *or* the room around you.

CLIENT: Yeah.

THERAPIST: And when you pull back a little, give your eyes some perspective, you seem to be able to focus on other things. And the chair is still there. Only now, you can see it as it is: its size, its shape, that it is not an endless blur of blue fuzz. It is just one thing to notice . . . among many. What do you think?

CLIENT: Weird. I never thought about it like that before. But yeah, I do get "stuck in the chair," all the time!

THERAPIST: So, maybe our work could be about practicing that . . . getting enough space to really see what is happening . . . that you are thinking. And if we step back, there are lots of other things around you. Things you may want to pay attention to, things you might want to do. Does that seem like something you may want to try?

This exercise both demonstrates the process and potential cost of cognitive fusion, without directly challenging the belief that the client has to figure out his thoughts. Instead, staying at a process level, this exercise plays out in a physical way what it might be like to simply be consumed with thoughts. From here, the client and therapist may be ready for additional work exploring the impact of previous attempts to control thoughts and feelings.

Vignette 2: Using the Client's Own Metaphors

This therapist has been working with a 25-year-old female client for seven sessions. She has talked about her sadness and feeling disconnected from her family and friends due to her anxiety and fear of failure. Her therapist has rated her moderately low on values, low on committed action, and low on acceptance.

THERAPIST: You have been talking about feeling lonely, and yet you have difficulty putting yourself out there because your mind says you will get hurt. Your mind says it is safer to stay put.

CLIENT: Yes, that's it. It's almost like I'm expecting to become a famous singer by singing in the shower at home. No one can criticize me, but none of the right people are going to hear me either.

THERAPIST: Great metaphor! Let's take this a step further. What do you think matters to the singer? Besides the idea of making a lot of money, of course.

CLIENT: I guess people liking them.

THERAPIST Sure. What else?

CLIENT: Well, I guess when you have a talent, you should share it. It's nice to give something to others.

THERAPIST: Mmm. OK, so maybe sharing something with others. Giving something to others.

CLIENT: Yeah. I guess I want to be able to give something of myself to others. In relationships.

THERAPIST: And does staying home help you live your value of sharing something of yourself with others?

CLIENT: No, not really. But, it's like, I don't know if I can get up and sort of sing some big ballad in front of famous people. That would be super scary.

THERAPIST: So, are there other ways that the singer may be willing to put herself out there . . . in small ways?

CLIENT: Like singing backup or in a small club. Sure. I guess that is what I would tell someone to do.

THERAPIST: What do you think? Is that something you would be willing to take steps toward in service of reaching out, to give to others?

CLIENT: Yeah. I guess I could what . . . go online? Start small, with like a coffee date?

THERAPIST: If it was in service of something important, would practicing willingness to get out there in small ways be worthwhile?

CLIENT: I think so. I'd like to do that. Get out there in small ways.

In this case, the therapist has rolled with the metaphor a client brought in and used a relative strength—values—to bolster another part of the flexibility equation—willingness. Discussing values within the metaphor allowed the client some space to consider the idea of willingness and of doing something in service of her values, without a "how-to" for behavior change, and in a playful way.

Vignette 3: In-Session Moves to Promote Experiential Awareness and Acceptance

A therapist has been seeing a female client for 10 sessions who presents with posttraumatic stress disorder. The therapist has developed a conceptualization in which the client is strongest in the values domain, is weakest in acceptance and defusion, and has relative deficits in flexible present moment awareness and committed action, but demonstrates these repertoires in certain contexts. The following interaction includes the next session discussion (left-hand column) and what the therapist was tracking throughout the interaction (right-hand column).

DISCUSSION	THERAPIST TRACKING
CLIENT: (*breathless and rushed, flopping down in the chair*) Oh my gosh, sorry I'm late. I had an awful ride here on the bus.	
THERAPIST: I'm glad you made it in today.	*Focus on the present.*

CLIENT: (*speaking rapidly*) Yeah, well, I almost didn't make it here. I took a different transfer, and it messed up my schedule so I end up on the bus with a ton of teenagers on their way to a field trip. They were laughing, yelling, standing up, and changing seats, like wild animals. Can you believe that? Like there was no one else on the bus, they're all over, behind me, ahead of me, all around me. I mean, that's super dangerous, I'm amazed that we didn't crash! And their stupid so-called chaperone just sat there! Why she didn't keep them contained I don't know. Ugh. I hate teenagers.

She is responding here and now like she is still on the bus.

THERAPIST: It sounds like a lot is going on for you, both in your mind and in your body.

Point out what is happening in the moment.

CLIENT: Yeah! Of course there is. I hate when I feel trapped like that.

THERAPIST: What do you notice in your body, even as you are telling me this?

Increase awareness of body sensations, focusing on them rather than just on thoughts.

CLIENT: I really don't know. I'm hot. (*Gets up and hangs coat up across the room, and returns to the chair, flopping in it again.*)

THERAPIST: (*slow, calm, and clear*) OK, you notice feeling hot. Where do you notice that?

Continue attention on the body sensations.

CLIENT: (*slightly calmer*) My face. My face is hot.

THERAPIST: Great. What else do you notice in your body as you are sitting in the chair, in this room, on this rainy Tuesday?

Increase awareness of the now and the experiences present in the now.

CLIENT: Uh . . . I guess my shoulders are tense.

THERAPIST: OK, great. So the bus ride is still present for you in this room. Would you be willing to take a moment to settle into this chair in this moment? I'll settle in as well.

CLIENT: Sure.

Reinforce the exploration of experience. Ask permission to conduct a centering exercise to get further into contact with experience.

The therapist conducts a simple centering exercise, drawing the client's attention to the sensations in the places where her body touches the chair, and in her breathing. After 3 minutes, the client and therapist finish the exercise.

DISCUSSION

THERAPIST TRACKING

CLIENT: (*opening her eyes, smiling*) I feel so much better.

THERAPIST: I'm glad to see you here. Your mind seemed to be back on the bus ride when you walked in the room.

Share what the therapist noted earlier in the session.

CLIENT: Yeah. I always feel so relaxed after doing those exercises. I wish I could feel that relaxed when I am like, on the bus, faced with crazy teenagers.

THERAPIST: Hmm, yeah. It seems like your mind is generating that desire to feel better when you are feeling anxious and trapped. Does that fit your experience? (*Client nods.*) What happened before you got on the bus today?

Attend to the process of fusion—noting the thinking mind—rather than exploring the content of the desire.

CLIENT: Before? Well . . . I slept a little later than usual, so I didn't have much time to get ready. I let my dog out but I didn't have time for a walk with her, so she was restless and all over me. I was out of clean shirts, so I threw one in the dryer with a dryer sheet to freshen it up. I was out of coffee, and I still haven't had time to buy some, so I'm exhausted and foggy. Oh, and I couldn't find my keys, so I had go to my creepy landlord's office so I wouldn't get locked out later.

THERAPIST: What are you noticing as you tell me this now?

Bring client back to focus on the in-the-moment experience.

CLIENT: (*Leg is shaking.*) I'm getting amped up—shaky, tense, and stressed out.

THERAPIST: Mmmm. So you had a lot of things happen this morning that threw off your routine, and you are noticing feeling stressed even as you share it with me here and now. How are you reacting, right now, to feeling stressed?

Ask the client about how she responds to her experience (stress, heightened body sensations).

CLIENT: You ask me that a lot. I'm still not sure I know what you mean. But maybe . . . maybe I hate it. I hate myself for getting this stressed out about stupid stuff. I mean I know those kids were just being kids, but I react to it like they're going to slit my throat.

THERAPIST: Yeah, you notice thinking you "hate" it. What does it mean to hate your reaction? What does your mind say?

Reflect the statement from a stance of defusion— reframing as a thinking process.

CLIENT: I feel stupid, and like I'm always going to be a mess. I mean, *my mind says* that I'm stupid and always going to be a mess.

THERAPIST: Great, so you've been able to notice your thinking mind—and even before you've had your coffee! (*Client smiles at therapist.*) And you made it here today, despite starting the day with some anxiety, and feeling quite scared on the bus. There are probably times in your past when you would have gotten off the bus before you made it here. How did you stay on the bus?

Reinforce the client stating her noticing of the thinking mind. Reflect and explore the process of behaving when unwanted experiences are present.

CLIENT: I think I just decided it was worth it. I didn't like it, but it's really important for me to be here and working on me.

THERAPIST: So your values for self-care [that we have talked about before] were really clear to you today. How did you cope with the anxiety around these kids teeming around you?

Restate the previous statement in terms of the therapist's understanding of the client's values. Prompt for an explanation of the process of how the client continued behaving in line with values when anxiety was present.

CLIENT: You know, it's funny. I tried the breathing we do in the mindfulness exercises in here. I know you always say it's not about feeling "better" in the moment. But it was weird. I tried to pay attention to the seat I was in, and the scenery going by outside. It kept me from jumping up out of my seat and screaming at the kids, I think.

THERAPIST: And how did that work for you?

Prompt for the client to track the consequence of using this practice.

CLIENT: Actually kind of well. I mean the kids were still obnoxious, but I got to therapy, which is really all that matters. I still felt anxious and stressed when I came in here, but I'm working on that. Maybe I don't have to listen to my mind telling me I'm always going to be a mess. I think I'm actually doing OK . . .

THERAPIST: Thank your mind for that, right? It seems like it's trying to help you make sense of things . . . and yet your experience is telling you that you are moving toward things that matter. And it sounds like you made some space for the feelings you had on the bus, even if you didn't *like* them.

Join with the client in noting the thinking mind. Identify the difference between thinking/evaluating and direct experience. Reflect the client's choice to accept discomfort.

CLIENT: Yeah, I think so—remember when we talked about my reaction being like saying "OK" or "NOT OK" to my feelings and memories? I would have gotten off the bus if I was really saying "NOT OK" to how I felt today. I definitely felt my heart pounding, but it didn't kill me anymore than those kids did.

THERAPIST: So that practice seems to work well for you. If I've heard you right today, it seems important to you to keep moving toward taking care of yourself, even if you feel anxious on the way. You noticed your mind doing its thing, and made the choice to continue here because it was important. Is that your experience?

Summarize in terms of processes—acceptance linked to valued-action and defusion from the thinking mind.

CLIENT: Yup. Totally.

The therapist's main goal in this interaction was to bring the client's present moment awareness to bear in the room and to help the client develop more contextual control over her experiences. She is *not* still on the bus, but is responding as if she were. On the bus, she responds as if her life is threatened. By asking many questions and tapping into the client's ability to track her in-the-moment experience even if imperfectly, the therapist is helping the client develop a stronger sense of perspective and distance from her distress in the current context, where there are no actual threat cues present.

Debriefing Exercises and Metaphors to Promote ACT Processes

In ACT, the debriefing of experiential exercises is an important opportunity to activate and maintain behavior change. The therapist guides the client in the process of describing the experienced contingencies and drawing functional rules that match these contingencies while still holding rules lightly enough that new learning can take place as other situations are contacted. To this end, the therapist asks questions such as "What did you notice? What did you feel like doing? What did you do? What happened?" and shapes the extraction of rules by evoking statements that summarize the whole sequence with an emphasis on the effectiveness of alternative strategies (e.g., "So in the end, what did you learn from this exercise? So, what would you say is the most effective thing you can do to meet your goals, when you feel your anger get stronger?").

While the therapist always has a particular purpose in mind when choosing a specific exercise, it is important for the therapist to remain open to what actually occurs for the client, and what he observes and learns about his experience. For example, if the therapist suspected that his client's avoidance of emotions got in the way of a valued action, he may chose an exercise such as the Chinese handcuffs (wherein the client puts his fingers in the paper cuffs, but attempts to pull them out only make the bond stronger, and to pull the cuffs off the client must push inward instead; Hayes et al., 1999, pp. 104–105) or a mindfulness exercise consisting of noticing psychological experiences without attempting to change them. However, since the purpose of experiential practice in ACT is to help the client observe and draw useful conclusions, the therapist needs to remain open to a variety of observations. For example, although ACT tends to promote acceptance since this strategy works in many cases, an ACT therapist doesn't promote acceptance as the "best choice" in a rule-governed way, For instance, if a client were to say "Oh, OK, so I should 'push into anxiety' rather than trying to pull out of it, like with the handcuffs," a therapist might encourage the client to explore how this works in the client's life, rather than adopt another rigid rule as the client's use of the word "should" suggests.

When the client seems to misperceive his own experience or is so attached to certain thoughts that he rejects what he directly observed (e.g., "I can't just let my obsessions be there. I have to do something to get rid of it"), the ACT therapist doesn't abandon the aim for building the client's autonomous sense of observation. Instead of trying to convince the client that he should have observed something different or drawn an alternative conclusion, the therapist asks questions orienting the client to unobserved aspects of the situation, and extends his observation to effects in the long term and in other areas. Suppose that when working with a client with relationship issues, using a metaphor designed to show how deliberate control of feelings can backfire (e.g., the *Polygraph Metaphor* [Hayes et al., 1999, pp. 123–124] or the *Feedback Screech* [Hayes et al., 1999, p. 108]), the client responds by claiming that he can avoid feeling anxious in relationships by forceful and focused distraction. Rather than directly challenge that experience, the therapist might explore with him the potential costs in terms of valued activities (e.g., "When you focus your attention on something else other than what makes you anxious with your girlfriend, what impact does it have on your relationship?"). Whether or not an exercise or metaphor has the intended function, there is usually some fruitful information to be learned about the client's difficulties, the client's response to them, or the potential cost of behaving a certain way. Sometimes, it may work well to move on to another metaphor or exercise or to change which process to target. A therapist can come back to that functional idea another time; sometimes the timing is not quite right for that move and may be appropriate later, after other work is done.

Future Directions

For some therapists, particularly those new to the work, it can seem difficult to develop and hone the necessary skills to know when and how to use appropriate exercises with clients. Much like a client's practice of becoming more flexible in their behavior, it can be difficult for clinicians to be patient and flexible when learning and applying a new approach to therapy. The nature of experiential work is that it can be unpredictable. We encourage therapists to think flexibly and to remember that ongoing practice using exercises and metaphors and other in-the-moment experiential work (and having some of the exercises not go as the clinician hoped!) helps develop and strengthen the necessary skills of being present with a client and helping him or her to answer the four questions we outlined earlier. As a result, we have attempted to discuss exercises from a variety of perspectives, including how to debrief exercises, and pointed out that one can reframe an exercise that has gone awry as an opportunity for learning more information about the client's struggles and response repertoires.

As we discussed, there is a growing body of research examining the effectiveness of each of the processes in the ACT model, and researchers are developing new, content-area specific measures of psychological flexibility to better capture changes in the purported mechanisms of change in ACT. Given ACT's focus on understanding and overcoming suffering related to language processes, it may be that ACT is likely to be most effective as a treatment approach for those who are high on ACT problem processes (e.g., fusion, lack of values clarity). Also, given evidence that ACT is often as effective as (and sometimes more effective than) front-line treatments such as traditional CBT, ACT may be most effective for those who have tried other readily-available front-line treatments and who have not found lasting reductions in suffering from them, particularly since evidence suggests that ACT works through different processes of change.

As clinical researchers begin to apply ACT to areas outside of traditional mental health settings, they must take special considerations for doing so. For instance, in a trial applying ACT to prevent suicidality in college freshman (Pistorello et al., 2013), focusing on psychological suffering seemed only to alienate students who had not yet struggled with psychological problems such as anxiety or depression. Instead, researchers advocate for a greater emphasis on building awareness of values and on developing ways to overcome potential barriers toward living these values in these populations. Such discoveries are helpful reminders and point to the importance of tailoring any ACT intervention to the needs of the population at hand. Given mounting evidence that ACT can be a useful intervention for a broad array of populations, further clinical application and rigorous study can help guide practitioners in appropriate applications of the model. We make suggestions for further training and resources below.

Further Resources

Books

- See Hayes, Strosahl, and Wilson (1999, 2011) for a deeper exploration of the ACT model, its theoretical underpinnings, and suggestions for application.
- See Luoma, Walser, and Hayes (2007) for an excellent skills-based book for new ACT therapists that includes a DVD illustrating ACT-consistent and inconsistent moves.
- See Ciarrochi and Bailey (2008) for an explanation of ACT moves from within a primarily traditional CBT perspective.

Online Resources

- The Association for Contextual Behavioral Science website (*www.contextual science.org*) contains many downloadable protocols, measures, suggested books for treating specific populations, and self-help books useful as an adjunct to psychotherapy, targeted suggestions for additional learning, calendars of trainings and workshops available internationally, and a list of smaller chapters and special interest groups available to join for ongoing support. Many resources are available in languages other than English as well.

References

Arch, J. J., Eifert, G. H., Davies, C., Vilardaga, J., Rose, R. D., & Craske, M. G. (2012a). Randomized clinical trial of cognitive behavioral therapy (CBT) versus acceptance and commitment therapy (ACT) for mixed anxiety disorders. *Journal of Consulting and Clinical Psychology, 80,* 750–765.

Arch, J. J., Wolitzky-Taylor, K. B., Eifert, G. H., & Craske, M. G. (2012b). Longitudinal treatment mediation of traditional cognitive behavioral therapy and acceptance and commitment therapy for anxiety disorders. *Behaviour Research and Therapy, 50,* 469–478.

Bohlmeijer, E. T., Fledderus, M., Rokx, T. A., & Pieterse, M. E. (2011). Efficacy of an early intervention based on acceptance and commitment therapy for adults with depressive symptomatology: Evaluation in a randomized controlled trial. *Behaviour Research and Therapy, 49,* 62–67.

Bricker, J. B., Mann, S. L., Marek, P. M., Liu, J. M., & Peterson, A. V. (2010). Telephone-delivered acceptance and commitment therapy for adult smoking cessation: A feasibility study. *Nicotine & Tobacco Research, 12,* 454–458.

Ciarrochi, J., & Bailey, A. (2008). *A CBT practitioner's guide to ACT: How to bridge the gap between cognitive behavioral therapy and acceptance and commitment therapy.* New York: New Harbinger.

Dymond, S., Schlund, M. W., Roche, B., & Whelan, R. (2014). The spread of fear: Symbolic generalization mediates graded threat-avoidance in specific phobia. *Quarterly Journal of Experimental Psychology, 67,* 247–255.

Gaudiano, B. A. (2011). A review of acceptance and commitment therapy (ACT) and recommendations for continued scientific advancement. *Scientific Review of Mental Health Practice, 8,* 5–22.

Gaudiano, B. A., Nowlan, K., Brown, L. A., Epstein-Lubow, G., & Miller, I. W. (2013).

An open trial of a new acceptance-based behavioral treatment for major depression with psychotic features. *Behavior Modification, 37,* 324–355.

Gifford, E. V., Kohlenberg, B., Hayes, S. C., Pierson, H., Piasecki, M., Antonuccio, D., et al. (2011). Does acceptance and relationship focused behavior therapy contribute to bupropion outcomes?: A randomized controlled trial of FAP and ACT for smoking cessation. *Behavior Therapy, 42,* 700–715.

Gregg, J. A., Callaghan, G. M., Hayes, S. C., & Glenn-Lawson, J. L. (2007). Improving diabetes self-management through acceptance, mindfulness, and values: A randomized controlled trial. *Journal of Consulting and Clinical Psychology, 75*(2), 336–343.

Hayes, S. C., Barnes-Holmes, D., & Roche, B. (2001). *Relational frame theory: A post-Skinnerian account of human language and cognition.* New York: Kluwer Academic/Plenum Press.

Hayes, S. C., Brownstein, A. J., Zettle, R. D., Rosenfarb, I., & Korn, Z. (1986). Rule governed behavior and sensitivity to changing consequences of responding. *Journal of the Experimental Analysis of Behavior, 45,* 237–256

Hayes, S. C., Luoma, J., Bond, F., Masuda, A., & Lillis, J. (2006). Acceptance and commitment therapy: Model, processes, and outcomes. *Behaviour Research and Therapy, 44,* 1–25.

Hayes, S. C., Strosahl, K., & Wilson, K. G. (1999). *Acceptance and commitment therapy: An experiential approach to behavior change.* New York: Guilford Press.

Hayes, S. C., Strosahl, K., & Wilson, K. G. (2011). *Acceptance and commitment therapy: The process and practice of mindful change* (2nd ed.). New York: Guilford Press.

Hayes, S. C., Wilson, K. G., Gifford, E. V., Bissett, R., Piasecki, M., Batten, S. V., et al. (2004). A randomized controlled trial of twelve-step facilitation and acceptance and commitment therapy with polysubstance abusing methadone maintained opiate addicts. *Behavior Therapy, 35,* 667–688.

Hooper, N., Saunders, J., & McHugh, L. (2010). The derived generalization of thought suppression. *Learning and Behavior, 38*(2), 160–168.

Juarascio, A. S., Forman, E. M., & Herbert, J. D. (2010). Acceptance and commitment therapy versus cognitive therapy for the treatment of co-morbid eating pathology. *Behavior Modification, 34,* 175–190.

Levin, M. E., Hildebrandt, M. J., Lillis, J., & Hayes, S. C. (2012). The impact of treatment components suggested by the psychological flexibility model: A meta-analysis of laboratory-based component studies. *Behavior Therapy, 43,* 741–756.

Lillis, J., Hayes, S., Bunting, K., & Masuda, A. (2009). Teaching acceptance and mindfulness to improve the lives of the obese: A preliminary test of a theoretical model. *Annals of Behavioral Medicine, 37,* 58–69.

Lundgren, T., Dahl, J., Yardi, N., & Melin, L. (2008). Acceptance and commitment therapy and yoga for drug-refractory epilepsy: A randomized controlled trial. *Epilepsy and Behavior, 13,* 102–108, 118.

Luoma, J. B., Walser, R., & Hayes, S. C. (2007). *Learning ACT: An acceptance and commitment therapy skills-training manual for therapists.* Oakland, CA: New Harbinger.

Pistorello, J., Hayes, S. C., Lillis, J., Long, D. M., Christodoulou, V., & Yadavaia, J. (2013). Acceptance and commitment therapy in classroom settings. In J. Pistorello (Ed.), *Mindfulness and acceptance for counseling college students* (pp. 223–250). Reno, NV: Context Press.

Rost, A. D., Wilson, K. G., Buchanan, E., Hildebrandt, M. J., & Mutch, D. (2012). Improving psychological adjustment among late-stage ovarian cancer patients:

Examining the role of avoidance in treatment. *Cognitive and Behavioral Practice, 19,* 508–517.

Smout, M., Longo, M., Harrison, S., Minniti, R., Wickes, W., & White, J. (2010). Psychosocial treatment for methamphetamine use disorders: A preliminary randomized controlled trial of cognitive behavior therapy and acceptance and commitment therapy. *Substance Abuse, 31*(2), 98–107.

Vilardaga, R., & Hayes, S. C. (2009). Acceptance and commitment therapy and the therapeutic relationship stance. *European Psychotherapy, 9,* 117–139.

Vilardaga, R., Hayes, S. C., Levin, M. E., & Muto, T. (2009). Creating a strategy for progress: A contextual behavioral science approach. *Behavior Analyst, 32,* 105–133.

Villatte, M., Villatte, J. L., & Monestes, J. L. (2014). Understanding and using relational frame theory in experiential clinical practice. In N. Afari & J. Stoddard (Eds.), *Wading through the swamp: The complete guide to ACT metaphors and experiential exercises* (pp. 13–28). Oakland, CA: New Harbinger.

Vowles, K. E., McCracken, L. M., & O'Brien, J. Z. (2011). Acceptance and values-based action in chronic pain: A three-year follow-up analysis of treatment effectiveness and process. *Behaviour Research and Therapy, 49,* 748–755.

Walser, R. D., Karlin, B. E., Trockel, M., Mazina, B., & Taylor, C. B. (2013). Training in implementation of acceptance and commitment therapy for depression in the Veterans Health Administration: Therapist and patient outcomes. *Behaviour Research and Therapy, 51,* 555–563.

Wetherell, J. L., Afari, N., Rutledge, T., Sorrell, J. T., Stoddard, J. A., Petkus, A. J., et al. (2011). A randomized, controlled trial of acceptance and commitment therapy and cognitive-behavioral therapy for chronic pain. *Pain, 152,* 2098–2107.

White, R. G., Gumley, A. I., McTaggart, J., Rattrie, L., McConville, D., Cleare, S., et al. (2011). A feasibility study of acceptance and commitment therapy for emotional dysfunction following psychosis. *Behaviour Research and Therapy, 49,* 901–907.

Wicksell, R. K., Melin, L., Lekander, M., & Olsson, G. L. (2009). Evaluating the effectiveness of exposure and acceptance strategies to improve functioning and quality of life in longstanding pediatric pain—A randomized controlled trial. *Pain, 141,* 248–257.

Zettle, R. D., & Hayes, S. C. (1986). Dysfunctional control by client verbal behavior: The context of reason giving. *Analysis of Verbal Behavior, 4,* 30–38.

CHAPTER 3

Compassion-Focused Therapy

An Introduction to Experiential Interventions for Cultivating Compassion

Dennis Tirch
Paul Gilbert

Introduction and Theory

Compassion-focused therapy (CFT) was developed with and for people who have high levels of shame and self-criticism, elements of client experience that are present transdiagnostically, and are known to be vulnerability factors in a variety of psychopathologies (Gilbert & Irons, 2005; Zuroff, Santor, & Mongrain, 2004). Both shame and self-criticism can seriously interfere with therapeutic progress, regardless of the initial reason for seeking treatment (Rector, Bagby, Segal, Joffe, & Levitte, 2000). Cultivating compassion and affiliative emotion, however, are core processes for addressing shame and self-criticism (Gilbert & Irons, 2005). CFT has now been shown to be helpful for a range of complex and enduring mental health difficulties, including those for people with personality difficulties (Lucre & Corten, 2012), psychosis (Braehler et al., 2013; Mayhew & Gilbert, 2008), eating disorders (Gale, Gilbert, Read, & Ross, 2012) and mixed diagnoses (Judge, Cleghorn, McEwan, & Gilbert, 2012). Indeed, there is increasing evidence that mindfulness and compassion are promising new avenues for therapeutic intervention (Hofmann, Grossman, & Hinton, 2011). This chapter outlines some of the central concepts and interventions of CFT.

Shame and self-criticism often involve a person's preoccupation with thoughts of self-condemnation and emotions of anger, anxiety, or disgust (Gilbert & Irons, 2005). Higher levels of shame and self-criticism (Kannan & Levitt, 2013) and lower levels of self-compassion (Neff, 2009) are correlated with anxiety and depressive symptoms across several diagnoses. Moreover, when a person's experience is dominated by such threat-focused thoughts and threat-based emotions, he or she often has narrowed attention and behavioral repertoires, as well as a reduced capacity for empathy (Wachtel, 1967; Frederickson, 2001). These effects may lead to fewer sources of reward and less availability to a meaningful, purposeful life. Whelton and Greenberg (2005) have shown that the negative effects of self-criticism involve emotions of disappointment, anger, and contempt that accompany self-criticism rather than the content of thoughts alone.

About 20 years ago when using cognitive-behavioral therapy (CBT) to help people reevaluate and reframe their depressed or anxious thinking, one of us (P. G.) found that even when people were trying to generate evidence-based thoughts, the emotional tone of the alternative thoughts was often still hostile or frightened, interfering with progress toward therapy goals (Gilbert, 2009). In turn, helping clients to generate a compassionate emotional experience by stimulating affiliative emotions became one of the central, experiential applications of CFT.

The use of evolutionary insights as a basis for psychoeducation and intervention is a key focus of CFT (Gilbert, 2010). While grounding an applied psychological science in an evolutionary context may seem like a reasonable way to proceed, in and of itself, the roots of this evolutionary perspective have direct clinical implications. By sharing an evolutionary insight into the nature of the human mind with the patient, the CFT therapist aims to help him or her to decenter from the contents and processes of mind, and thus reduce the excessive influence that shame and self-criticism may have upon his or her functioning. CFT shares this emphasis on decentration and compassionate perspective taking as evolutionary processes with acceptance and commitment therapy (ACT; Hayes, Strosahl, & Wilson, 2012). As demonstrated in this book, ACT suggests that people can become overly "fused" and identified with the thoughts and contents of their mind, surrendering their behavioral choices to the control of unhelpful private events rather than their experience of the world in the present moment. Similarly, CFT presents an evolutionary perspective on human suffering that emphasizes mindfulness, decentering, and the primacy of compassion in regulating our responses to shame, self-criticism, and anxiety.

Central to the way CFT engages clients is to contextualize mental events in three domains:

1. The *evolutionary context* that has given rise to our very tricky brain. This brain is full of conflicting motives, emotions and, ways of thinking—rich in potential for suffering.
2. The *context of the individual's unique learning history*. This

context involves how life experiences influence the way our genetic potentials develop. Our learning history, particularly in social contexts, affects development physically, emotionally, and behaviorally. Clinically relevant safety behaviors, self-identification, and patterns of cognition are all shaped by this context.
3. The *present-moment context* of the individual. The third context of CFT includes the multitude of factors giving rise to our moment-by-moment experience, which exert an influence on us. Importantly, CFT involves practicing the stance of mindfully observing the flow of present-moment experience as part of its strategy.

It is easy to recognize that our minds are set up in such a way that they are full of compromises and trade-offs (Brune et al., 2012; Gilbert, 1989). For example, we have evolved with a mind that will treat ambiguous stimuli as though they were dangerous, operating on a "better safe than sorry" system (Barlow, 2004). This might make sense for the preservation of the species, but it can be very tricky when someone is on a first date, flooded with anxiety about social rejection. Importantly, patients involved in CFT learn how they have evolved from the flow of life on this planet with a complex brain, partially based upon the experiences of species that are hundreds of millions of years older than humanity. Patients also learn that their lives have been powerfully determined by a social learning history that they did not choose. So much of what drives our suffering is really not about us at all, not of our choosing, and truly *not our fault*.

The Interaction of Old- and New-Brain Psychology

To show patients how potentially destructive—as well as highly caring and compassionate—the human mind can be we draw with them an outline of the brain and begin to layer it in the way shown in Figure 3.1. First we discuss what for simplicity we call *old-brain psychology*. This involves many behaviors, social motivations, responses, and emotions we share with other animals: being territorial, having conflicts and aggressive interactions, belonging to groups, forming alliances, experiencing sexual desires, looking after offspring—and, crucially, responding to affection and affiliation with calm. So, the idea is to help people gain clear insight into the fact that these motivational and emotional systems have been built for us, *not* by us. We simply "find ourselves here" with a mind that has these kinds of patterns of action (Gilbert, 2009).

Next, we explore the problems humans have that relate to their evolved "new-thinking brain." Indeed, humans have been referred to as *the thinking ape* (Byrne, 1995). Unfortunately, our evolved capacity for "thinking" creates problems as well as benefits. Around 2 million years ago humans began to develop a whole range of cognitive abilities for imagination, reasoning, reflecting, anticipating, and developing a sense of self.

Mindful Brain

New Brain: Imagination, Planning, Rumination, Integration

Old Brain: Emotions, Motives, Relationship Seeking–Creating

Compassion

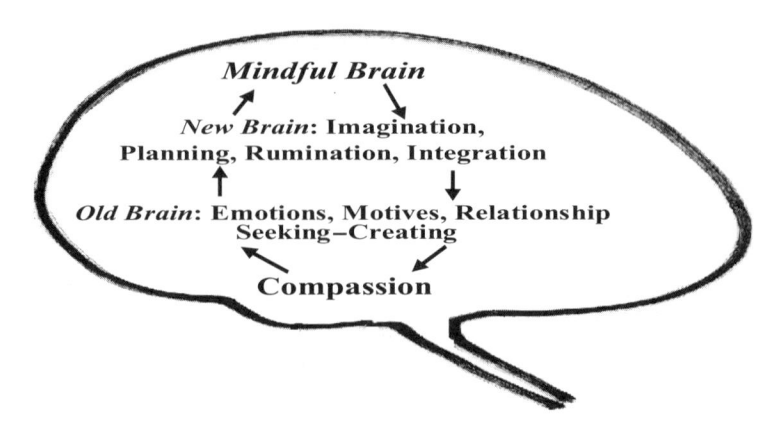

FIGURE 3.1. From Gilbert and Choden (2013). Reprinted with permission from Constable & Robinson Ltd.

Research suggests that these mental abilities may be based on the way that we humans began to derive relations among stimuli in our environment (Torneke, 2010). For humans, a "combination of our genetically evolved capacity and a history of reinforcement by a social community" (Hayes et al., 2012, p. 360) has resulted in the range of what CFT refers to as *new-brain psychology:* capacities for language use, symbolic understanding, problem solving, and elaboration of learning through cognition.

One of the core principles in CFT is understanding the way these new-brain competencies link into, stimulate, and are stimulated by old-brain motivation and emotional systems. While emotions may emerge from preverbal, *old-brain* evolutionary response patterns, the human experience of emotion is expressed and derived from our cognitive and verbal behaviors, which are shaped by social contexts, and involve our *new-brain* capacities. In CFT, we view the interaction of hard-wired, prebirth-determined emotional and motivational responding with *new-brain* cognitive abilities as a part of the source of much human suffering. Take an intelligent mind and fuel it with tribal vengeance and you can end up with horrendous atrocities and nuclear weapons. Equally, take a mind with new-brain competencies and link these into motivational systems that are concerned with caring and helping others and one finds the sources of compassion (Gilbert, 2009).

A Clinical Example of CFT

CFT therapists help clients experience and understand the interaction of *old-brain* and *new-brain* abilities using metaphors and stories such as the one below, which is based on the difference between threat responses in humans and other mammals (Sapolsky, 2004):

"Imagine a zebra running away from a lion. Once the zebra gets away it will calm down very quickly and go back to eating or other zebra things. The zebra's threat based emotions may return to baseline calm within minutes, but this is unlikely for a human, because of our capacity for cognition, predicting events, and creating internal representations of possibilities. A zebra who thought as a human might start to ruminate and imagine, 'What might have happened if . . . the lion had caught me . . . and what might happen tomorrow . . . ?' Our human thinking zebras would then play out intrusive simulations, images and fantasies of being eaten alive; or what might happen if they don't spot the lion tomorrow; or even the disaster of two lions turning up! While the human brain can solve problems and give rise to science and culture, it can also trap us in terrible internal loops, because our thoughts and imaginations, our abilities to run simulations of numerous possibilities in our minds are very stimulating of physiological systems involving evolved motives and emotions."

Evolution, Cognition, and Behavior

In behavioral theory, the term *behavior* is used to represent anything and everything that forms the output of an organism. So a change in heart rate, digestive processes, eye gaze patterns, thought, or emotion, in fact any "output" that is generated by an organism, is termed *behavior* (Torneke, 2010). This is useful because the basic rules of how to predict and influence behaviors have been well studied in experimental psychology, and many of these rules apply to both mental and physical behaviors. Moreover, when we look at our mental behaviors through the lens of learning theory, we find some of the reasons that we get stuck in loops between our *old-brain* and *new-brain* psychologies.

Research has repeatedly demonstrated that humans have a tendency to respond to symbolic, mental events as though they were literal events in the world (Ruiz, 2010), a phenomenon referred to as *fusion* (Hayes et al., 2012). Unpleasant things represented in the mind can put us under aversive control, and imaginary pleasant events can result in appetitive control. So, with the evolutionary emergence of our *new-brain* competencies, human behavior began to be strongly predicted and influenced by the behavior of our thinking and feeling minds. Fusion is of clinical importance because our behavior can be so dominated by the influence of mental events that we are sometimes *more* controlled by our inner representations than by actual factors in the outside world.

When we are under the aversive control of mental events, we tend to try to mentally suppress or avoid such events. It makes sense that we want to run away from feelings, images, and ideas that are unpleasant because running away from dangerous things in the outside world is usually a good strategy, as our zebra discovered in running from the lion. The problem here is that the more we try to push away an unwanted thought or feeling, the more it tends to show up. How many of us have been awake at night trying to avoid thinking about a problem at work or school the next day? Experimental and clinical research has repeatedly established that suppression of thoughts results in their showing up with greater frequency and that attempts at experiential avoidance are what drives a lot of psychological suffering (Wenzlaff & Wegner, 2001; Ruiz, 2010). It is no wonder, then, that our very tricky brains can ensnare us in loops of preoccupation and unhealthy behavioral patterns. Under the dominance of *new-brain* mental events and subsequent *old-brain* emotional responses, we can be hooked into attempts at avoidance and control that can keep us trapped in a cycle of suffering.

Compassionate mind training involves deliberately cultivating mindful attention, acceptance, and other capacities that can help us to be better able to remain in the presence of distressing mental events, without handing our lives and behavioral decisions over to our mental suffering. Beyond mindful acceptance, CFT involves the deliberate activation of specific affect-regulation systems that are designed by evolution to lessen our experience of threat and to broaden our available behavioral repertoires in the face of internal and external challenges. Furthermore, CFT leverages the fusion phenomenon in the service of cultivating compassion, by using specific imagery practices that can train the mind to respond with compassion, courage, and flexibility, by activating emotion regulation systems involved in evolved human caregiver behaviors.

Affect Regulation Processes in CFT

Thus, based on the aforementioned features, CFT is focused on deep, evolved emotional and motivational systems and the stimulation and cultivation of specific affect-regulating systems. CFT follows the psychological scientific view that emotions serve evolved and emergent motives and that emotions also build and strengthen motives. However, motives and emotions follow evolutionary important trajectories such as being part of a group, gaining status, developing friendships, sexual partners, attachment, and caring for offspring (Gilbert, 1989, 2010), and emotions signal how well or poorly we are doing.

Emotions evolved to orient our behaviors, in real time, and it is the anticipation of feeling that often guides motives and behaviors. Evolutionary analysis and affective neuroscience research (DePue & Morrone-Strupinsky, 1995) suggest that there are at least three types of emotional systems that are important for guiding behaviors. These are:

1. *Threat.* Evolved emotions that serve the motives of survival against threat/harm and loss: the defense of self and kinship or friend protection.

These emotions are those such as anger, anxiety, and disgust (Ledoux, 1998).

2. *Seeking/acquiring.* Evolved emotions that serve the motives of acquisition of resources that add to survival and reproductive success. This can sometimes be called "drive systems," and involve "seeking" behaviors (Panksepp, 1994). These are emotions of joy, pleasure, and excitement, and they are associated with achieving winning, succeeding, and acquiring. For example, if an individual won $100 million on the lottery, they would have a mild hypomania linked to the seeking/acquiring system.

3. *Calming/soothing.* Once animals are not under threat or "seeking," they can be quiescent and resting. Hence there have evolved emotions and states that serve the functions of "rest and digest," and offer experience of safeness and peacefulness. For many animals calming can occur simply by the removal of the threat. However, during the evolution of mammalian attachment, adaptations occurred to the rest and digest system such that affiliative signals could also trigger a calming response and signal a state of safeness (Porges, 2007). Thus when an infant is distressed, the presence and physical contact of the parent can down-regulate threat processing and calm the infant.

There is now considerable evidence that as mammals evolved live birth for immature offspring, the attachment system became central to the organization of the emotional regulation between the infant and the parent (Cozolinio, 2007; Mikulincer & Shaver, 2007). In fact, there have been significant modifications to the parasympathetic and sympathetic nervous systems that enables the parasympathetic nervous system to produce a calming response in the context of caring, safe, and affiliative others (Porges, 2007). In addition, a range of specialized brain systems for detecting and responding to affiliative signals that include oxytocin has evolved (Carter, 1998). Oxytocin is involved in trust and affiliative relationships, and it is stimulated in and by affiliative relationships (Uvnäs Moberg, 2013). Moreover, oxytocin exerts direct effects on calming threat processing in the amygdala (Kirsch et al., 2005). So there is now considerable evidence that the experience of affiliative behavior is highly regulating of emotion, and in particular threat emotion (Uvnäs Moberg, 2013). Attachment theorists suggest that the affiliative emotional experiences involved in healthy attachment bonds serve as a "secure base" from which people can begin to explore their world and face challenges (Bowlby, 1969; Mikulincer & Shaver, 2007).

CFT builds on the attachment theorists' approach, with the recognition that internal working models of others as sources for a secure base may be problematic. Many people have experienced abuse, trauma, or neglect by caregivers or in the context of caregiving behaviors. This distorted association can cause the activation of the soothing system to be associated with increased threat, through classical conditioning. This can result in a fear of compassion and difficulty with activation of soothing (Gilbert, 2009). Therefore, CFT seeks to stimulate the affiliative system as an internal point of reference and organizing process, gradually and not overwhelmingly. CFT patients learn to cultivate an inner *compassionate self* and a *compassionate image* that can function as a restorative, parent-like internalized presence.

The Nature of Compassion

In CFT, compassion may be defined as *sensitivity to the presence of suffering in self and others with a commitment to try to alleviate and prevent such suffering*. The definition points to two basic aspects of compassion. The first aspect is *engagement*—involving an opening up to and willingness to work with suffering. The second aspect is alleviation/prevention, which involves working to develop the wisdom and skill necessary to alleviate/prevent the suffering. In CFT these two aspects have a number of components to them, which are illustrated in Figure 3.2. Each of these components represent dimensions of the compassionate mind that can be trained through CFT techniques.

As illustrated in the figure, the psychology of engagement involves identifying and cultivating specific competencies, described in the inner circle as "attributes." These include accessing the motivation to be caring, sensitivity to distress, sympathy, distress tolerance, empathy, and nonjudgment. These qualities of the psychology of engagement are drawn from the research on caregiving behaviors and altruistic behaviors, and they appear to be the foundational elements of a compassionate orientation (Gilbert, 2010).

The psychology of alleviation/prevention involves further competencies for appropriate reflection and action, described in the figure as "skills." CFT uses a systematic approach to train and cultivate these capacities and skills to develop compassion. The specifics of how to work to develop these capacities form a great deal of the wide range of methods found in CFT. We have included some examples in this chapter, as well as a range of resources that you can access, should you wish to take an exploration of CFT further.

Empirical Evidence

The last 10 years have seen a major upsurge in exploring the benefits of cultivating compassion, especially imagery practice (Fehr, Sprecher, & Underwood, 2009). In an early study Rein, Atkinson, and McCraty (1995) found that directing people in compassionate imagery had positive effects on an

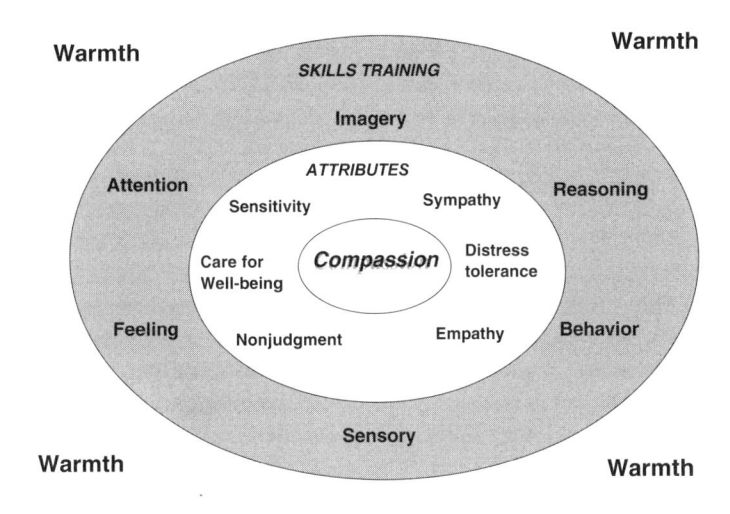

[Diagram: Concentric ovals labeled with "Warmth" at four corners. Outer ring: SKILLS TRAINING — Imagery, Attention, Reasoning, Behavior, Sensory, Feeling. Inner ring: ATTRIBUTES — Sensitivity, Sympathy, Care for Well-being, Distress tolerance, Nonjudgment, Empathy. Center: Compassion.]

FIGURE 3.2. Attributes for engagements and skills for alleviation/prevention. From Gilbert (2009). Reprinted with permission from Constable & Robinson, Ltd.

indicator of immune functioning (S-IgA), while anger imagery had negative effects. Further, neuroscience and imaging research has demonstrated that practices of imagining compassion for others produce changes in the frontal cortex, immune system, and well-being (Lutz, Brefczynski-Lewis, Johnston, & Davidson, 2008). Hutcherson, Seppala, and Gross (2008) found that a brief loving-kindness meditation increased feelings of social connectedness and affiliation toward strangers.

Fredrickson, Cohn, Coffey, Pek, and Finkel (2008) allocated 67 participants to a loving-kindness meditation group and 72 to a wait-list control. They found that six 60-minute weekly group sessions with home practice based on a CD of loving-kindness meditation increased positive emotions, mindfulness, and feelings of purpose in life and social support, and decreased illness symptoms. Pace et al. (2008) found that compassion meditation (for 6 weeks) improved immune function and neuroendocrine and behavioral responses to stress. Also, an exercise as simple as compassionate letter writing to oneself has been found to improve coping with life events and reduce depression (Leary, Tate, Adams, Allen, & Hancock, 2007).

Elements of CFT have been found to enhance psychotherapy outcomes and also to serve as a mediator variable in outcomes. For example, Schanche, Stiles, McCullough, Svartberg, and Nielson (2011) found that self-compassion was an important mediator of reduction in negative emotions associated with Cluster C personality disorders and recommended self-compassion as a target for therapeutic intervention. Beaumont, Galpin, and Jenkins (2012) compared CBT and CBT plus CFT in trauma clients ($N = 32$) and found a nonsignificant trend for greater improvement in the CBT plus CFT. In this study, CFT showed significantly greater improvement in self-compassion, with a large ($d = 0.89$) effect size. This finding led the authors to suggest developing compassion could be an important adjunct to therapy. Ashworth, Gracey, and Gilbert (2011) found CFT to be a helpful addition and focus for people with acquired brian injury. In a study of the effectiveness of mindfulness-based cognitive therapy for depression, Kuyken and colleagues (2010) found that self-compassion was a significant mediator between mindfulness and recovery.

A systematic review of research concerning both clinical and non-clinical settings, compassion-focused interventions have been found to be significantly effective (Hofmann et al., 2011). Research has shown that self-compassion can be distinguished from self-esteem and predicts some aspects of well-being better than self-esteem (Neff & Vonk, 2009). In correlational research using the Self Compassion Scale (SCS; Neff, 2003) self-compassion has been found to offer protection against anxiety and depression, even when controlling for self-criticism. People who report high levels of self-compassion on the SCS also report high levels of many positive psychological traits such as autonomy, competence, and emotional intelligence (Neff, 2003; Neff, Rude, & Kirkpatrick, 2007).

In addition to the growing body of research supporting compassion as a beneficial process in psychotherapy and everyday life, CFT itself is increasingly empirically supported through outcome research. In an early open clinical trial involving a group of people attending a day hospital with chronic mental health problems ($N = 6$), Gilbert and Procter (2006) found that CFT significantly reduced self-criticism, shame, sense of inferiority, depression, and anxiety, with a large effect size for all measures. In a randomized controlled trial using CFT for people with psychotic disorders ($N = 40$), Braehler, Harper, and Gilbert (2012) found significant clinical improvement and increases in compassion, as well as high levels of tolerability and low attrition, as compared to a treatment as usual condition. Pre–post effect sizes in this study were large, with 65% of patients having significant improvement in compassion as compared to 5% of patients in the treatment-as-usual condition. In an uncontrolled clinical trial, Laithwaite and colleagues (2010) found significant effects for depression and self-esteem, and an improvement in "sense of self compared to others," in a sample of patients in recovery from psychosis in a forensic mental health setting. In this study, effect sizes were moderate to large, with a sample of 19 patients. In other outcome research, CFT has been found to be significantly effective for the treatment of personality disorders (Lucre & Corten, 2012), eating disorders (Gale, Gilbert, Read, & Goss, 2012), and heterogeneous mental health problems in people presenting to community mental health teams (Judge et al., 2012). As CFT is more widely disseminated, and a growing number of clinicians and researchers become skilled in their understanding of its philosophy and methods, increasing outcome research is likely to further test the model, leading to innovation and change.

Clinical Application

Rather than being a completely separate "brand" of therapy that requires a therapist to reinvent his or her entire way of working, CFT is designed to be both a stand-alone way of working and a compassionate "approach" that can be applied to the practice of any psychotherapy modality. As a result, CFT applications and techniques range from specific imagery and meditation practices to distinctive forms of psychotherapy methods such as chair-work and compassionate cognitive responding. The techniques included in this chapter are compatible with the aim of the book, being a guide to experiential work with emotions in cognitive and behavioral therapies. Accordingly, a reader can apply these practices, which are grounded in evidence-based processes and procedures, to their CBT treatment plan in an integrative way. For those readers who wish to learn the more finely grained details of the entire CFT approach, a number of resources follow at the end of the chapter, which can establish a road map to more thorough practice. The three following applications represent the way that CFT therapists often introduce the evolutionary model to their patients, an imagery exercise that teaches patients how to use emotional memories and imagery to cultivate compassion, and a central compassionate imagery exercise that is designed to gradually train patients to access the emotional systems involved in compassion for themselves and others.

The Reality Check

Within CFT, a lot of what appears to be "psychoeducation" is actually a fundamental philosophical shift of perspective, which is discussed between the therapist and patient through a process of guided discovery. While the theory and practice of many forms of therapy appear to be separate aspects of the work, engaging with the evolutionary model in CFT is an essential part of cultivating the mindful insight into the nature of being human that can evoke compassion. Adopting an engaged, open, and deliberately emotionally evocative demeanor, CFT practitioners will often begin much of their work in this way to help patients to experientially apply insights from evolutionary psychology regarding the nature of the mind.

The first method presented is a semistructured dialogue known as the "reality check." This is a collaborative discussion, involving stories, metaphors, and guided discovery. Together, the patient and therapist explore the evolutionary context of human suffering by reflecting the fact that "we all are of the same species and share our common humanity." First, the therapist may explain to the patient, "We are all 'built by genes' in more or less in the same way, and this has given rise to our very tricky brain. This brain, and our everyday minds, have common emotions, motives, and ways of thinking. Some of these mental experiences are very helpful, such as problem solving in the face of environmental challenges. Other mental events can be quite painful, such as worrying about events far in the future that we can't have any control over. The patient and therapist may then engage in further guided discovery, wherein the therapist uses Socratic questioning to explore the patient's reaction to his or her role as an emergent being in the flow of life. As the therapist hears the patient's reactions and questions, a CFT practitioner will engage in "affect matching," wherein the client's emotional response is validated through nonverbal communication, affective expressiveness, and depathologizing language. Even at this early stage in the therapy, the therapist may also use "empathic bridging," slowing down the dialogue and deliberately using mindfulness of the therapist's own emotional processes to evoke flexible perspective taking. CFT therapists, from the outset, are aiming to understand the world through the eyes of their patients, while "thinking with the patient and not for them."

Following the introduction of the evolutionary model, the CFT therapist will reflect on the fact that because we are biological beings, life is full of suffering. The therapist will provide a range of examples of this—for example: "There are millions of potential viruses and diseases that can afflict the human condition, and we are quite easy to injure, sometimes with long-term consequences. Our lives are relatively short, about 25,000 to 30,000 days and during this time we will may flourish for a while, but then gradually decay and lose functions." Following this introduction, the CFT therapist will make the social contextual point that anyone is "only one particular version of himself or herself, shaped by his or her social learning history." CFT therapists often use the following example to illustrate the point: "If I had been kidnapped as a 3-day-old baby, and raised by a violent drug gang, what kind of person would I be today? We know that the sons of drug enforcers in cartels most often grow up to conduct violent crimes in the family business. As much as I don't want to think I could be that sort of person, it is possible that with such a learning history, I would be a very different version of myself." We invite the client to reflect on this story in some detail. As he or she gains insight into the fact that the therapist themself might have been aggressive, even murderous, possibly dead or in prison (which is to say, a very different type of person), the shift toward recognizing that *we are all just versions of ourselves*. Indeed, we know that early experiences can even affect genetic expression and the maturation of different brain areas, as that is how powerful social contexts are. So, the next question we pose obviously is, "Is it possible to start to train and choose versions of ourselves that will organize our minds and sense of self in a way that is more conducive to well-being?"

Far from being mere psychoeducation, the shared appreciation of the evolutionary model found in the "reality check" is a first step on the way to helping patients decenter and dis-identify from the contents of mind. They do this while at the same time beginning to take responsibility for cultivating mental states conducive to their well-being, and *taking responsibility* for change processes. Among the range of subsequent in-session techniques for cultivating compassion, experiential imagery methods, practiced in session and as homework, are very important. The following example is a fundamental CFT imagery practice known as the "Compassionate Self" exercise. It is practiced in the greater context of CFT, generally after some psychoeducation, case conceptualization, training in centering/mindfulness, and a relational/experiential introduction to compassion. The example involves many of the processes we have outlined, and engaging with it can begin to impart a sense of what bringing a compassionate focus to your therapy can involve.

The Compassionate Self Exercise

CFT aims to train clients in developing multiple aspects of compassion, including compassionate attention, compassionate thinking, and compassionate behavior (Gilbert, 2009). Imagery-based techniques feature prominently among those employed in this approach. The "compassionate self" visualization is a foundational CFT practice that aims to facilitate a shift from a threat-focused emotional processing system to the activation of a felt sense of safeness that emerges in the soothing, affiliation-focused emotion regulation system. This is accomplished by using the imagination. Just as imagining sexual imagery might activate our sexual response, imagining compassionate imagery can activate our compassion response.

Although such visualization methods are not simply an extension of Buddhist meditation, we can see the antecedents of compassionate imagery in various Buddhist traditions. For example, Tibetan and Japanese Buddhist schools contain a variety of techniques for using the imagination to identify with various symbolic images to stimulate compassion. However, the exercises found in CFT do not depend on religious iconography. In fact, part of the inspiration for the compassionate self exercise was drawn from an adaptation of method acting exercises to mental health interventions, so that clinicians might contact and better relate to the affective states of their patients (Gilbert, 2010). The compassionate self exercise is meant to allow clients to engage in a multisystem form of role play that allows them to guide themselves toward an experiential knowledge of self-compassion.

The following exercise is provided as a script, which you may use to develop your own guidance of this practice with your clients. Some of the language will inevitably be modified to be more in line with your therapeutic style and personal vernacular. However, the essentials of the guided imagery are here in this description, and should be followed as closely as possible. Further audio examples of this and other CFT exercises are available at the websites specified later in the chapter. This practice typically is engaged in once a client has developed a fluency with mindful breathing, and has learned to direct and gather his or her attention. In CFT a form of mindful breathing known as soothing rhythm breathing, which engages the parasympathetic nervous system, is preferred, and can be found at *www.compassionfocusedtherapy.com*. As with other mindfulness- and compassion-based practices, the therapist leading the teaching is advised to have established and maintained his or her own compassionate mind-training program and should be engaging in this exercise with the patient as he or she leads the practice.

Introduction

"This exercise will help you imagine yourself in a very different way than you might be accustomed to, as if you are an actor who is rehearsing a role in a play or a film. The exercise involves the creation of the personification of your compassionate self, whom you will meet and who will be happy to see you."

BUILDING AND BECOMING THE COMPASSIONATE SELF

"Let's take a moment to think about the qualities of our compassionate self by writing down the qualities you would ideally like to have if you were calm, confident, and compassionate. Would you be wise? Strong—and able to tolerate discomfort? Would you have warm feelings toward others, and toward yourself? Would you feel empathy for someone else's suffering, and for his or her behavior? Are you understanding of others' faults and foibles and, as a result, nonjudgemental, accepting, kind, and forgiving? Do you have courage? Ask yourself how you would picture your most compassionate aspect. Perhaps you might imagine yourself older and wiser, or younger and more innocent. This is your exercise, and you are free to embellish and design an image of your compassionate self according to your own desire."

Practice

"To begin, find a place where you will feel safe and may remain uninterrupted for some time. Ideally, this would be a quiet and safe place, such as the one you might use for your mindfulness practice. Allow your eyes to close, bring part of your attention to the soles of your feet as they connect with the floor and to your sitting bones on the chair. Allow your back to be straight and to feel supported. Next, partly direct your attention to the flow of your breath in and out of your body; allow it to find a slow, soothing rhythm and pace. Feel yourself breathe in, and breathe out. Continue this breathing uninterrupted until you've gathered your attention and feel focused on the present moment.

"At this point, recall the qualities of your compassionate self that you wrote down, and now imagine that you already have those qualities. Breathe in as you experience yourself as having wisdom; knowing that you are a part of the flow of life on earth, with a brain and a life history that weren't of your design or your choosing, breathe out. Breathe in and imagine yourself as strong, able to tolerate distress while confronting your fears; breathe out. Experience yourself as committed, with a calm and completely dedicated intention to alleviate the suffering you encounter. As you follow the breath in and out of the body, feel yourself heavy in your chair and rooted to the earth. Your wisdom, strength, and commitment are all present. Imagine yourself as a completely nonjudgemental person who doesn't condemn yourself or others for their faults. Allow yourself to bring to mind the sensory details that you would notice as your compassionate self. What are you wearing? Is your body relaxed and receptive? With body language that signals openness and kindness? Are you smiling? If not, smile now, and at the same time imagine the warmth you feel when you carefully hold an infant. As you breathe in, bring attention into your body, imagine yourself expanding, and welcome your ability to be wise, warm, and resilient.

"For the next few moments, as you are breathing in and out, imagine what the tone of your voice would be if you were this compassionate self. How would you behave? What would the expression on your face be? Allow yourself to take pleasure in your capacity to share kindness with, and care for those around you, and yourself. If your mind wanders, as it so often does for all of us, use your next natural inhale to gently bring the attention back to this image of your compassionate self.

"For the next several minutes continue to give mindful attention, returning and refocusing when needed, to this compassionate self. When you feel ready, and with your next natural exhale, allow any attachment to this exercise to simply melt away. Breathe in again, and with the next natural exhale allow yourself to become aware again of your surroundings and then recognize and acknowledge the effort you have invested in this exercise. As you let go, fully return your attention to your surroundings and carry on with your day."[1]

Compassion Flowing In

Following the guidelines for the compassionate self exercise, the following scripts may be used to walk patients through the "compassion flowing in" practice. This visualization involves the use of emotional memory to stimulate an experience of loving kindness and to activate the soothing system. Therapists are advised to use this with an understanding of the

---
[1] Based on exercises in Tirch (2012) and Gilbert (2009).

developmental history of the client with whom they are working. For some, memories of warmth and affiliation can evoke feelings of anxiety or even reexperiencing of trauma memories. This does not mean that therapists should turn away from exposure to such experiences. The therapeutic work involves compassionate engagement with just such material.

In CFT, we emphasize that the core of compassion is a flow of sensitivity to the presence of suffering in the world, coupled with a heartfelt wish to alleviate this suffering, no matter who or what the object of the sufferer may be. The acceptance that we find in the compassionate mind is nonconditional, and really has nothing to do with evaluation. Just as a parent may feel an outpouring of love and support for his or her child—a love that has nothing to do with how the parent evaluates, ranks, or criticizes his or her child's worth, our compassionate mind is moved by the presence of suffering wherever it is encountered, and a deep motivation is awakened.

"Often, we may find ourselves stuck in self-evaluation, wondering if we are attractive enough, intelligent enough, or successful enough to deserve love and support. Really, compassion and human kindness has nothing to do with these evaluative comparisons. As the science demonstrates, compassion flows from our evolved human caregiver emotions, and, as such, it allows us to feel love and support for every part of the human being. Whether we are met with a disconsolate child screaming in the night, disrupting our sleep, or a gold medal winner at the Olympics, the compassionate mind holds a steadfast warmth, acceptance, and helpful attitude that is separate from social comparisons or criticism.

"Within our hearts and minds, we all contain so many different aspects of ourselves. We can be the petulant child, the raging adolescent, or the neurotic adult—sometimes all at once. If we are to open ourselves to compassion, finding courage and wisdom in the presence of the warmth of the awakening mind, we bring this absolutely unconditional kindness to every part of ourselves, even the dark and distasteful parts of our nature. Metaphorically, compassion is about getting into the mud that brings forth the lotus. It is about loving every part of who we are with acceptance and strength.

"The practice below uses our memories of experiencing the loving-kindness and care of others to help us to connect with the emotions involved in secure attachment and true supportiveness. By recalling those moments when we have been met by unconditional compassion, we may be able to stimulate our experience of loving kindness and support, here and now.

"Begin by bringing attention to your breathing by observing its flow and rhythm for a minute or two. Now, bring part of your attention into your body and feel the strength and compassion that is available to you in your posture. Feel your feet on the floor and your body supported by your cushion or chair. Your posture is grounded and reflects your sense of calm and self-compassion.

Allow your face to form a gentle half-smile, keeping part of your attention on the flow of your breath.

"Using your imagination, remember a pleasant day in your past when someone was compassionate and loving toward you. Aim to remember a person who was nonjudgmental, never condemned you, was empathic, and cared about you and your happiness. As much as you can, remember the sensory details of this experience. Can you remember what you were wearing? Where you were? Was it hot? Or cold? Or raining? Was the wind blowing through the trees or the television on in the background? Now, bring your attention back to the flow of your breath, inhale and exhale, and stay with this image for a while.

"We are now focusing our attention on our experience of loving-kindness and warmth, and we do this by remembering the experience of receiving help and compassion. Whenever your mind is inevitably distracted and wanders away from this memory, gather your attention and make space for whatever is arising. With the in breath, simply return your attention to the image of this compassionate person. As you breathe in again, bring your attention to the facial expression of this person from your past. Allow yourself to remember, as much as you can, his or her body language and movements. What did this person say to you? How did he or she say it? Pay particular attention to the tone and sound of his or her voice.

Stay with this experience for a little while, breathing in and out. Next, bring your attention to the quality of the emotion this person had for you. How did he or she feel toward you? How does this make you feel? Take a few minutes to remain in the presence of this emotion. This is a time to bring attention to the experience of compassion flowing into you. Now, bring your attention back to the flow of your breath, inhale and exhale smoothly, and take a few moments to stay with the way this experience feels. As much as you can, connect with the emotions of appreciation, gratitude, and happiness that arrived with this person's care. For as long as feels right to you, remain in the presence of this memory and this feeling. When it feels right, let this experience go and with your next natural exhale allow the memory and images to fade away. After a few more slow and even breaths, exhale and let go of this entire exercise."[2]

Future Directions

The treatment development strategy that CFT has followed involves grounding interventions in basic science, and methodically and responsibly researching techniques over the course of several years. This gradualist approach, combined with the relatively short period of time that CFT has

---
[2] Based on an exercise in Tirch (2012) and Gilbert (2009).

been in existence means that at the time of this book being published we are only beginning to see the flow of randomized controlled trials of CFT interventions increase. Indeed, the first outcome study of a CFT style group was published only 7 years ago as of this writing (Gilbert & Proctor, 2006). Compared to the hundreds of randomized controlled trials supporting an intervention like Beckian cognitive therapy, CFT has a small outcome evidence base. However, CFT is based on empirically validated processes and principles that are highly likely to prove beneficial in clinical applications and in life. At this point in the development of the technology, most therapists would be advised to integrate CFT as an approach to therapy, adding to their existing repertoires of evidence-based best practices, rather than discarding techniques like exposure and response prevention for anxiety or behavioral activation for acute depression.

The small number of CFT-trained psychologists has resulted in a gradual rate of dissemination as well. The initial expansion of this form of therapy has taken place in the United Kingdom, with the number of therapists, researchers, and trainers growing in North America, Australia, and continental Europe each month. Like any therapy, CFT has a great many subtle techniques and aspects of interpersonal process that are difficult to learn by simply attending a weekend workshop and reading about the modality. As a result, many therapists can come away from a brief CFT training experience looking for more detailed and thorough consultation and supervision than has typically been available to them in their region. Thankfully, Internet-based training, national and international conferences, and an expanding network of CFT trainers can provide supervision opportunities and establish research initiatives more rapidly and effectively than would have been possible in earlier eras of psychotherapy history.

Further Resources

To date, there have been numerous scientific articles and books that outline the theory and practice of CFT. The books are available through a range of online sources, and peer-reviewed publications are widely disseminated online as well. *The Compassionate Mind* (Gilbert, 2009) can serve as a comprehensive introduction to CFT for both clinicians and general readers. For an example of CFT as applied to the treatment of anxiety disorders, *The Compassionate Mind Guide to Overcoming Anxiety* (Tirch, 2012) also can serve as a clear introduction to applied CFT.

The Compassionate Mind Foundation is the primary organization involved in research, development, and dissemination of CFT throughout the world. Through this organization in the United States and United Kingdom, and the Center for Compassion Focused Therapy, readers can access a range of training materials, clinical readings and workbooks, PowerPoint presentations, video tutorials, and free audio recordings of mindfulness and imagery exercises. Training events, peer consultation groups, and access to online and personal consultation and supervision are also available. All of this can be accessed through the following websites, providing a point of entry to a community of compassion-focused clinicians and researchers:

- The Compassionate Mind Foundation: *www.compassionatemind.co.uk*
- The Compassionate Mind Foundation USA: *http://compassionfocusedtherapy.com*
- The Center for Compassion Focused Therapy: *www.mindfulcompassion.com*

References

Ashworth, F., Gracey, F., & Gilbert, P. (2011). Compassion focused therapy after traumatic brain injury: Theoretical foundations and a case illustration. *Brain Impairment, 12*(2), 128–139.

Barlow, D. H. (2004). *Anxiety and its disorders: The nature and treatment of anxiety and panic* (2nd ed.). New York: Guilford Press.

Beaumont, E., Galpin, A., & Jenkins, P. (2012). "Being kinder to myself": A prospective comparative study, exploring post-trauma therapy outcome measures, for two groups of clients, receiving either cognitive behaviour therapy or cognitive behaviour therapy and compassionate mind training. *Counselling Psychology Review, 27*, 31–43.

Bowlby, J. (1969). *Attachment and loss* (3rd ed., vol. 1). New York: Random House.

Braehler, C., Harper, I., & Gilbert, P. (2012). Compassion focused group therapy for recovery after psychosis. In C. Steel (Ed.), *CBT for schizophrenia: Evidence-based interventions and future directions* (pp. 235–266). Chichester, UK: Wiley.

Brune, M., Belsky, J., Fabrega, H., Feierman, J. R., Gilbert, P., Glantz, K., et al. (2012). The crisis of psychiatry— Insights and prospects from evolutionary theory. *World Psychiatry, 11*, 55–57.

Byrne, R. (1995). *The thinking ape: Evolutionary origins of intelligence*. Oxford, UK: Oxford University Press.

Carter, S. C. (1998). Neuroendocrine perspectives on social attachment and love. *Psychoneuroendocrinology, 23*, 779–818.

Cooley, M. (1922). *Human nature and conduct*. New York: Scribners. (Reprinted, 1964, New York: Schocken Books)

Cozolino, L. (2007). *The neuroscience of human relationships: Attachment and the developing brain*. New York: Norton.

Depue, R. A., & Morrone-Strupinsky, J. V. (2005). A neurobehavioral model of affiliative bonding: Implications for conceptualizing a human trait of affiliation. *Behavioral and Brain Sciences, 28*(3), 313–349.

Fehr, B., Sprecher, S., & Underwood, L. G. (Eds.). (2008). *The science of compassionate love: Theory, research, and applications*. Chichester, UK: Wiley.

Fredrickson, B. L. (2001). The role of positive emotions in positive psychology. *American Psychologist, 56*(3), 218–226.

Fredrickson, B. L., Cohn, M. A., Coffey, K. A., Pek, J., & Finkel, S. M. (2008). Open hearts build lives: Positive emotions, induced through loving-kindness meditation, build consequential personal resources. *Journal of Personality and Social Psychology, 95*, 1045–1062.

Gale, C., Gilbert, P., Read, N., & Goss, K. (2012). An evaluation of the impact of introducing compassion focused therapy to a standard treatment programme for people with eating disorders. *Clinical Psychology and Psychotherapy, 21*, 1–12.

Gilbert, P. (1989). *Human nature and suffering*. London: Psychology Press.

Gilbert, P. (2009). *The compassionate mind*. London: Constable & Robinson.

Gilbert, P. (2010). *Compassion focused therapy*. London: Routledge.

Gilbert, P., & Choden. (2013). *Mindful compassion: How the science of compassion can hedlp you understand your emotions, live in the present, and connect deeply with others*. London: Constable & Robinson.

Gilbert, P., & Irons, C. (2005). Focused therapies and compassionate mind training for shame and self-attacking. In P. Gilbert (Ed.), *Compassion: Conceptualisations, research and use in psychotherapy* (pp. 263–325). London: Routledge.

Gilbert, P., & Procter, S. (2006). Compassionate mind training for people with high shame and self-criticism: Overview and pilot study of a group therapy approach. *Clinical Psychology and Psychotherapy, 13*(6), 353–379.

Gumley, A., Braehler, C., Laithwaite, H., MacBeth, A., & Gilbert, P. (2010). A compassion focused model of recovery after psychosis. *International Journal of Cognitive Therapy, 3*(2), 186–201.

Hayes, S. C., Strosahl, K. D., & Wilson, K. G. (2012). *Acceptance and commitment therapy: The process and practice of mindful change*. New York: Guilford Press.

Hofmann, S. G., Grossman, P., & Hinton, D. E. (2011). Loving-kindness and compassion meditation: Potential for psychological interventions. *Clinical Psychology Review, 31*(7), 1126–1132.

Hutcherson, C. A., Seppala, E. M., & Gross, J. J. (2008). Loving-kindness meditation increases social connectedness. *Emotion, 8*(5), 720.

Judge, L., Cleghorn, A., McEwan, K., & Gilbert, P. (2012). An exploration of group-based compassion focused therapy for a heterogeneous range of clients presenting to a community mental health team. *International Journal of Cognitive Therapy, 5*(4), 420–429.

Kannan, D., & Levitt, H. M. (2013). A review of client self-criticism in psychotherapy. *Journal of Psychotherapy Integration, 23*, 166–178.

Kirsch, P., Esslinger, C., Chen, Q., Mier, D., Lis, S., Siddanti, S., et al. (2005). Oxytocin modulates neural circuitry for social cognition and fear in humans. *Journal of Neuroscience, 25*, 11489–11493.

Kuyken, W., Watkins, E., Holden, E., White, K., Taylor, R. S., Byford, S., et al. (2010). How does mindfulness-based cognitive therapy work? *Behaviour Research and Therapy, 48*(11), 1105–1112.

Laithwaite, H., O'Hanlon, M., Collins, P., Doyle, P., Abraham, L., & Porter, S. (2009). Recovery after psychosis (RAP): A compassion focused programme for individuals residing in high security settings. *Behavioural and Cognitive Psychotherapy, 37*, 511–526.

Leary, M. R., Tate, E. B., Adams, C. E., Allen, A. B., & Hancock, J. (2007). Self-compassion and reactions to unpleasant self-relevant events: The implications of treating oneself kindly. *Journal of Personality and Social Psychology, 92*, 887–904.

LeDoux, J. (1998). *The emotional brain: The mysterious underpinnings of emotional life*. New York: Simon & Schuster.

Lucre, K. M., & Corten, N. (2012). An exploration of group compassion-focused therapy for personality disorder. *Psychology and Psychotherapy: Theory, Research and Practice, 86*(4), 387–400.

Lutz, A., Brefczynski-Lewis, J., Johnstone, T., & Davidson, R. J. (2008). Regulation of the neural circuitry of emotion by compassion meditation: Effects of meditative expertise. *PLoS ONE, 3*(3), e1897.

Mayhew, S. L., & Gilbert, P. (2008). Compassionate mind training with people who hear malevolent voices: A case series report. *Clinical Psychology and Psychotherapy, 15*(2), 113–138.

Mikulincer, M., & Shaver, P. R. (2007). Boosting attachment security to promote mental health, prosocial values, and inter-group tolerance. *Psychological Inquiry, 18*(3), 139–156.

Neff, K. D. (2003). Development and validation of a scale to measure self-compassion. *Self and Identity, 2,* 223–250.

Neff, K. D. (2009). Self-compassion. In M. R. Leary & R. H. Hoyle (Eds.), *Handbook of individual differences in social behavior* (pp. 561–573). New York: Guilford Press.

Neff, K. D., Rude, S. S., & Kirkpatrick, K. (2007). An examination of self-compassion in relation to positive psychological functioning and personality traits. *Journal of Research in Personality, 41,* 908–916.

Pace, T. W., Negi, L. T., Adame, D. D., Cole, S. P., Sivilli, T. I., Brown, T. D., et al. (2009). Effect of compassion meditation on neuroendocrine, innate immune and behavioral responses to psychosocial stress. *Psychoneuroendocrinology, 34*(1), 87–98.

Panksepp, J. (1994). The basics of basic emotion. In *The nature of emotion: Fundamental questions* (pp. 237–242). Oxford, UK: Oxford University Press.

Porges, S. W. (2007). The polyvagal perspective. *Biological Psychology, 74*(2), 116–143.

Rector, N. A., Bagby, R. M., Segal, Z. V., Joffe, R. T., & Levitt, A. (2000). Self-criticism and dependency in depressed patients treated with cognitive therapy or pharmacotherapy. *Cognitive Therapy and Research, 24,* 571–584.

Rein, G., Atkinson, M., & McCraty, R. (1995). The physiological and psychological effects of compassion and anger. *Journal of Advancement in Medicine, 8,* 87–105.

Ruiz, F. J. (2010). A review of acceptance and commitment therapy (ACT) empirical evidence: Correlational, experimental psychopathology, component and outcome studies. *International Journal of Psychology and Psychological Therapy, 10*(1), 125–162.

Sapolsky, R. M. (2004). *Why zebras don't get ulcers.* New York: St. Martin's Press.

Schanche, E., Stiles, T. C., McCullough, L., Svartberg, M., & Nielsen, G. H. (2011). The relationship between activating affects, inhibitory affects, and self-compassion in patients with Cluster C personality disorders. *Psychotherapy, 48*(3), 293–303.

Tirch, D. D. (2012). *The compassionate mind guide to overcoming anxiety.* Oakland, CA: New Harbinger.

Torneke, N. (2010). *Learning RFT: An introduction to relational frame theory and its clinical application.* Oakland, CA: New Harbinger.

Uvnäs Moberg, K. (2013). *The hormonal closeness: The role of oxytocin in relationships.* London: Printer and Martin.

Wachtel, P. L. (1967). Conceptions of broad and narrow attention. *Psychological Bulletin, 68*(6), 417.

Wenzlaff, R. M., & Wegner, D. M. (2000). Thought suppression. In S. T. Fiske (Ed.), *Annual review of psychology* (Vol. 51, pp. 59–91). Palo Alto, CA: Annual Reviews.

Whelton, W. J., & Greenberg, L. S. (2005). Emotion in self-criticism. *Personality and Individual Differences, 38,* 1583–1595.

Zuroff, D. C., Santor, D., & Mongrain, M. (2004). Dependency, self-criticism, and maladjustment. In J. S. Auerbach, K. N. Levy, & C. E. Schaffer (Eds.), *Relatedness, self-definition and mental representation: Essays in honour of Sidney J. Blatt* (pp. 75–90). London: Brunner-Routledge.

Part II

Exposure

Evoking and Staying with Difficult Emotions

CHAPTER 4

Exposure in Experiential Context

Imaginal and In Vivo *Approaches*

Dean McKay
Rachel Ojserkis

Exposure therapy is a highly effective method of treating anxiety and associated conditions. The approach has a rich theoretical grounding (Foa & Kozak, 1986) and has been studied extensively in laboratory and applied treatment settings (Eelen & Vervliet, 2006). However, the experiential aspects of exposure have been neglected in the literature, which has instead stressed the technical application of this treatment. In this chapter, we explore the emotional impact of exposure therapy on clients as well as therapists. We then highlight how a specific social psychological theory, terror management theory (Pyszczynski, Greenberg, & Solomon, 1999), can shed light on clinicians' hesitancy to implement exposure and set the stage for alleviating both therapist and client discomfort with this treatment. Finally, we describe the means by which understanding these experiential aspects of exposure therapy can allow clinicians to conduct exposure in a powerful and emotionally salient manner that maximizes client relief.

Defining Experiential Exposure

Theoretical Basis

Exposure therapy is a treatment for anxiety and related disorders in which clinicians help clients to repeatedly and systematically confront anxiety-provoking stimuli in order to decrease clients' symptoms (Richard,

Lauterbach, & Gloster, 2007; Abramowitz, Deacon, & Whiteside, 2011). Exposure therapy was developed based on the behavioral principle of extinction, a learning phenomenon first studied in laboratory animals. R. L. Solomon's classic research with dogs (Solomon, Kamin, & Wynne, 1953) demonstrated that the animals experienced an initial increase in anxiety in response to a feared stimulus, but that this distress eventually decreased the longer the animals stayed in contact with the stimulus. Further, Solomon et al. (1953) found that the dogs' initial spike in anxiety deceased with each subsequent exposure to the feared stimulus so long as adverse consequences were not present. The extinction and acquisition of fear have been extensively studied in laboratory models, which have implicated specific neural networks in these learning processes (for an illustrative discussion of experimental models, see Debiec & LeDoux, 2009).

In the 1970s, psychologists began to apply the principle of extinction to exposure therapy for humans with obsessive–compulsive disorder (OCD; Rachman, Hodgson, & Marks, 1971). Since this time, the fundamental tenets of exposure therapy have been well established: repeated encounters with an anxiety-evoking stimulus in which neither the feared outcome nor avoidance behaviors occur cause individuals to become less afraid of that stimulus (Abramowitz et al., 2011). Over the past several decades, exposure procedures have been developed for the treatment of many anxiety-related conditions in addition to OCD, such as panic disorder, specific phobias, social anxiety disorder (SAD), posttraumatic stress disorder (PTSD), generalized anxiety disorder (GAD), and hypochondriasis (Abramowitz et al., 2011). Exposure has been shown to be approximately 70% effective for these anxiety-related conditions (Richard et al., 2007; see "Evidence in Support of Exposure Procedures", p. 86).

One of the most recent predecessors of exposure treatment for anxiety disorders was implosive therapy, in which clients repeatedly imagined coming into contact with their worst fears in order to reduce their overall level of anxiety (Stampfl & Levis, 1968). Based on Mowrer's two-factor theory of anxiety (Taylor, Cox, & Asmundson, 2009), implosive therapy was predicated on the assumption that anxiety symptoms were generated by an original aversive event that classically conditioned fear, and were subsequently maintained via behaviors that helped an individual reduce or avoid this anxiety. Stampfl and Levis (1968) specified that feared stimuli were "hidden" aspects of behavioral responses, meaning that an individual's internal experience of fear was not visible on its own but became noticeable when avoidance was prevented and anxiety increased. Thus, in implosive therapy, clients were asked to imagine a stimulus associated with a fear-evoking situation (e.g., blood, which was once associated with the pain of injury) in the absence of that actual aversive situation (an injury). It was then assumed that, given the client did not implement any behaviors to reduce or avoid the anxiety caused by the stimulus, extinction would eventually occur (Stampfl & Levis, 1968).

Foa and Kozak's (1986) emotional processing theory offered an alternative theoretical basis for exposure therapy that is widely used in the current conceptualization and delivery of the treatment. Specifically, Foa and Kozak argued that exposure activates an individual's fear structure—an "information structure that serves as a program to escape or avoid danger" (p. 20)—and modifies it with corrective information that ultimately decreases anxiety. Just as Solomon (1953) found with dogs, Foa and Kozak indicated that the reduction of fear resulting from exposure therapy takes place at two levels: within sessions (meaning that initial anxiety responses to stimuli naturally attenuate in the absence of escape, avoidance, and "safety" behaviors) and between sessions (meaning that an individual's overall level of fear decreases with each subsequent exposure).

There are two distinct types of exposure therapy exercises commonly employed by clinicians: *in vivo* (situational) exposure and imaginal (or in imagery) exposure. These techniques can be utilized either separately or in combination, depending on the client's presenting concern. Clinicians who routinely conduct exposure-based treatment refer to individual exercises as "exposures," a term we will adopt from here onward in this chapter. For all exposures, exercises are planned collaboratively by the client and the therapist and are structured in a hierarchy that gradually progresses from least to most anxiety-provoking. Of note, it is important for exposures to have a high degree of specificity. For example, for the case of a client with OCD who avoids driving owing to a fear of hitting pedestrians, an initial exposure may be to imagine driving on a deserted street in broad daylight and to slowly move toward driving in a high-traffic pedestrian area at night. Throughout all exposures, therapists are present to provide support to clients and to monitor their distress via ratings on a Subjective Units of Distress scale (SUDs) ranging from 0 to 100 (see Wolpe, 1990, for a description of developing a SUDs scale).

In vivo exposures specifically help clients to "put their faulty beliefs and assumptions to the test" by confronting approximations of a feared stimulus in person (see also Chapter 5, Behavioral Experiments). Because clients' idiographic symptoms may not always be accessible in the therapist's office, *in vivo* exposures often require conducting portions of sessions outside the office. Using the example of the individual who avoids driving owing to a fear of hitting pedestrians, treatment may be enhanced by incorporating *in vivo* exposures in which the client drives a car with the therapist in the passenger seat. For cases in which the source of anxiety is in anticipation of a delayed consequence rather than an immediately measurable physical event, imaginal exposures may be most appropriate. The main difference between the *in vivo* and imaginal techniques is that imaginal exposure targets feared thoughts, images, or impulses as opposed to immediately present physical stimuli. Imaginal exposures may include writing or speaking about anxiety-provoking mental events, as well as visualizing the feared consequence of the thoughts. In the case of an individual with OCD who engages in ritualized washing for fear of contracting a fatal illness, imaginal exercises may include repeatedly writing, "I am contaminated," as well as visualizing himself coming down with an incurable ailment.

In some cases (especially for clients with OCD; Abramowitz, 1996), imaginal exposure may be used as a precursor or an adjunct to *in vivo* methods in order to optimize treatment. This combined procedure requires the clinician to devise imagery of the catastrophic consequences associated with the *in vivo* exposure. For the above client with contamination fear, an example of successfully combining *in vivo* and imaginal methods may be for the therapist to guide the client through touching a doorknob and not washing his hands, all the while talking to the client about the disease that must be spreading throughout his body and the unfortunate fact that they now may die. Successful *in vivo*/imaginal exposures call for clinicians to exercise creativity, to be attuned and sensitive to clients' reactions to exposures, and often to think on their feet in managing the complexities of this technique. Thus, combined exposure exercises can prove to be particularly difficult for clients and therapists alike (more on this in "Terror Management Theory," p. 91, and "Applications," p. 96). However, the inclusion of imagery serves at least two important functions. One purpose of imaginal exposure is to block the naturally occurring tendency for clients to engage in cognitive avoidance during exposure, a phenomenon that diminishes the value of the corrective experience (Foa & Kozak, 1986). The second is to ensure that fears that are more general than the specific target stimuli are addressed during the *in vivo* exercise. This is in line with the specific aim of implosion (Stampfl & Levis, 1968), whereby learned symbolic processes are targeted, thus allowing clients to generalize their corrective learning experiences to a wider range of anxiety-producing stimuli and situations.

Evidence in Support of Exposure Procedures

Exposure therapy for anxiety is grounded in an extensive body of research. The extant literature spans thousands of investigations across more than 50 years, ranging from small case illustrations to multisite randomized controlled trials. Support for the use of exposure procedures is too extensive to exhaustively detail in this chapter. However, a recent review of the meta-analyses conducted on behavioral interventions for anxiety disorders has suggested that exposure therapy produces robust effect sizes (Olatunji, Cisler, & Deacon, 2010). Disorders with extensive empirical support for the efficacy of exposure approaches include panic disorder, specific phobias, SAD, OCD, PTSD, and GAD (Division 12 (Clinical), American Psychological Association, 2013). Over time, literature on exposure for anxiety disorders has progressed to include refined guidelines for managing complex and refractory cases, which deviate substantially from approaches described in standard protocols (McKay, Abramowitz, & Taylor, 2010).

An important additional point should be raised about the effects of exposure therapy on the cognitive as well as on the behavioral aspects of clients' symptoms. The theoretical basis of exposure emphasizes behavioral change through a mechanism of extinction. However, it has also been noted that exposure produces beneficial cognitive change in clients. In a review of the literature, Hofmann (2008) found that, in experimental trials of exposure, clients showed a decrease in cognitions associated with danger expectations. In a further illustration of the impact of exposure on cognitions, Whittal, Thordarson, and McLean (2005) found that obsessive–compulsive beliefs changed with exposure alone in a manner similar to cognitive therapy. This line of research suggests that exposure is effectively a cognitive therapy as well as a behavioral one, even though cognitive disputation elements are not explicitly present in the treatment.

Experiential Challenges in Exposure Therapy

Despite the sound theoretical basis and extensive empirical support for exposure therapy, clients and therapists alike are often hesitant to engage in it. In fact, some psychologists view exposure therapy as so harmful that they believe that "patients are better off suffering from their anxiety disorder than undergoing this form of treatment" (Olatunji, Deacon, & Abramowitz, 2009, p. 173). Leading exposure therapy researchers have attributed the treatment's "public relations problem" in large part to the interaction between expectations and emotional experiences on the parts of both the client and the therapist (Richard & Gloster, 2007; Olatunji et al., 2009). Specifically, exposure involves a dyadic relationship in which assumptions are made about the client and therapist's inner experiences. Though both parties often expect treatment to alleviate the client's symptoms, exposure therapy increases client's anxiety in the short term rather than ameliorating it. Thus, many have argued that exposure runs counter to basic assumptions about the therapeutic process and even the ethical principle for clinicians to "first, do no harm" (Olatunji et al., 2009). This perceived inconsistency between clients' and therapists' expectations for treatment and the actual experience of exposure leads to challenges in the delivery and receipt of this therapy.

First, much of the public is skeptical about the efficacy and acceptability of exposure therapy. A study of undergraduates and outpatients at a university mental health clinic evaluated vignettes describing exposure therapies for panic disorder, OCD, and PTSD to be unacceptable, unethical, and likely ineffective (Richard & Gloster, 2007). Negative accounts of exposure therapy in the media may help to shape these public attitudes toward the treatment. For example, one *New York Times* article dubbed exposure "the cruelest cure" (Slater, 2003). Such sensationalized press contributes to the general public's opinion of exposure therapy, which in turn may negatively influence individual clients' expectations of the treatment if they personally encounter it.

Second, therapists also are hesitant to utilize exposure therapy, even when treating individuals with anxiety disorders for whom it is highly indicated. One common myth among clinicians that greatly affects dissemination of exposure therapy is that anxiety is intolerable for clients and may lead to severe physical or psychological consequences, such as heart attacks, loss of consciousness, emergence of psychotic processes, and other forms of emotional and behavioral decompensation (Deacon & Farrell, 2013). In addition to therapists' discomfort with initiating temporary anxiety reactions in their clients during exposures, many clinicians choose not to utilize exposure methods owing to a concern that the treatment poses risks to themselves. Some therapists may doubt their capacity to tolerate the anxiety that exposure provokes in their clients (Deacon & Farrell, 2013), and even worry about suffering vicarious traumatization (Zoellner et al., 2011). Still others fear the potential legal ramifications of exposures, which often involve "field trips" outside of the office that reenvision the traditional terms of the therapist–client relationship (Olatunji et al., 2009). Despite research that has uncovered no documented ethical or legal complaints about exposure therapy (Richard & Gloster, 2007) and literature stating that proper training will prepare clinicians for even the most intense sessions (Castro & Marx, 2007), many therapists choose not to conduct exposure for these reasons.

Thus, whether therapists' hesitation to evoke anxiety in session is motivated by a well-intentioned concern for their clients, uncertainty about their own ability to tolerate clients' distress, or fear of litigation, therapists' avoidance of exposure therapy adversely impacts treatment dissemination. Clinicians' impressions of exposure as harmful limit its widespread application in spite of the long-standing and overwhelming empirical support for its efficacy (Olatunji et al., 2009; Becker, Zayfert, & Anderson, 2004). Consequently, many anxiety sufferers do not receive the treatment that they need. In an illustration of the seriousness of this problem with disseminating exposure therapy, the International Obsessive–Compulsive Disorder Foundation sponsors an annual behavior therapy training institute for therapists to learn how to implement exposure for OCD, even though this treatment has been a known efficacious intervention for well over 30 years (Christensen, Hadzi-Pavlovic, Andrews, & Mattick, 1987).

In addition to problems with treatment dissemination, the prominent perception of exposure as potentially dangerous to both clients and therapists also has a profound impact on competent treatment delivery and outcome. Of those clinicians who do report using exposure therapy, many diverge considerably from the treatment procedures studied in randomized controlled trials due to fear of inducing too much anxiety in their clients (Deacon & Farrell, 2013). Specifically, it appears that many community practitioners encourage self-directed rather than therapist-assisted exposures, and implement relaxation and other anxiety-reduction techniques to counteract the intense negative affect that clients experience during exposure exercises (Deacon & Farrell, 2013; Rothbaum & Schwartz, 2002). Yet as Deacon and Farrell (2013) point out, these alterations to exposure protocols may actually hinder clients' long-term improvement, as they interfere with the behavioral principle of extinction on which exposure therapy is based. Deacon and colleagues (2013) recently found that a 21-item scale assessing clinicians' concerns about practicing exposure therapy predicts more cautious and less component delivery of exposure for anxiety disorders. Indeed, therapists' fears of exposure have been linked to suboptimal delivery of this treatment for clients with panic disorder (Deacon, Lickel, Farrell, Kemp, & Hipol, 2013) and OCD (Farrell, Deacon, Kemp, Dixson, & Sy, 2013).

It is worth noting that these highly prevalent fears about exposure on the part of clinicians disregard the reality of exposure treatment done well. First, the increase in anxiety that occurs during a correctly delivered exposure exercise is temporary, takes place within a controlled and supportive environment, and is conducted in the service of decreasing anxiety for clients overall. As Abramowitz et al. (2011) summarize, exposure therapy asks clients to "invest anxiety now for a calmer future" (p. 122). Some critics have also compared the initial increase in negative emotions during exposure therapy to the side effects of medication or physical therapy in which some unpleasant sensations may be tolerated in order to achieve the goal of relieving the primary symptom (Olatunji et al., 2009; Deacon & Farrell, 2013). Finally, clinicians well versed in delivering exposure therapy argue that the anxiety induced in exposure sessions is no different than what clients experience from their anxiety disorders on a daily basis (Olatunji et al., 2009; Deacon & Farrell, 2013). In response to therapist concerns about the harmful effects of exposure, Olatunji et al. (2009) keenly retort that choosing to conduct a less effective therapy in a case for which exposure is indicated because of these fears may be the biggest clinical and ethical violation of all.

Historical Bases and Modern Manifestations of Experiential Exposure

Therapists' and clients' hesitations in exposure therapy have historical roots in philosophical and psychodynamic theories that link anxiety to humans' fear of the ultimate vulnerability: death. One of the first figures to propose this connection between mortality and emotional experiences was Sigmund Freud. In "Beyond the Pleasure Principle," Freud (1920/1952a) retracted his previous assumption that all psychic activity was driven by the motivation to avoid pain or obtain pleasure by introducing Thanatos, or the death instinct. Freud explained the death instinct in the context of the life cycle, arguing that organisms first were created to have very short lifespans, and that even though people have evolved to live longer, humans' destiny is still to return to death. In fact, he went as far as to posit that "the goal of all life is death" (Freud, 1920, p. 652). In a later essay, "Civilization and Its Discontents" (1929/1952b), Freud elaborated on the principle of Thanatos by defining aggression as humans' desire for their own destruction acted out on others.

In his ground-breaking book *The Denial of Death*, cultural anthropologist Ernest Becker (1973) incorporated these psychoanalytic ideas into his own theory of death anxiety. He proposed that humans' higher-order cognitive processes allow our species to have a unique awareness of our own mortality and that this sense of perpetual vulnerability can lead to feelings of terror—or, in psychological terms, anxiety. Becker believed that in order to survive in the face of this overwhelming death anxiety, humans necessarily develop worldviews that systematically repress and deny the ever-present terror of mortality. That is to say, when people have experiences that remind them of their own vulnerability to death (i.e., potentially life-threatening events), automatic processes exist to help individuals avoid that feeling of anxiety. A striking example of Becker's argument for humans' emotional avoidance of morality is the case of molecular biologist James Watson. Even Watson, who mapped out the human genome sequence and published it online in order to encourage a move toward personalized medicine, had great hesitation about studying his own genetics for fear of knowing how his life would end (Bio-IT World, 2007).

If we accept Becker's assertion that anxiety is an indication of increased mortality salience, then exposure therapy can be conceptualized as a treatment that helps clients to better modulate their activations of death anxiety. Indeed, implosive therapy, an earlier version of exposure, had roots in psychodynamic theory in addition to its clear basis in behavioral concepts. Specifically, proponents of implosive therapy argued that anxiety was the symptomatic representation of classic psychodynamic conflicts learned during childhood, including sex, parental hostility, aggression, and, of course, death wishes (Stampfl & Levis, 1968; Abramowitz et al., 2011). Stampfl and Levis (1968) also conceptualized the traditional psychodynamic concept of repression as analogous to avoidance. Thus, a reductionist account of implosive therapy would state that the treatment challenged individuals' repression of death anxiety in order to enact behavioral change. Though modern methods of exposure therapy have moved away from language that explicitly references psychodynamic theory in this way, helping individuals to confront rather than avoid their fears has remained a focal point of successful treatment for anxiety.

In light of the clear ties between mortality salience and anxiety, the classic principles of exposure therapy (Foa & Kozak, 1986) emphasize that symptom reduction requires clients to confront their anxiety when no overtly dangerous elements are actually present. It is thought that aversive emotions are activated during exposures and subsequently decrease when clients stay in contact with these emotions but see that the outcome that they feared did not materialize. This habituation may be induced via cognitive dissonance processes. When individuals' experiences of exposure exercises conflict with their feared outcomes, they must change their previous beliefs in order to achieve consonance with reality. These "corrective emotional experiences" have historically been regarded as the key to behavioral change in exposure therapy and may also account for the aforementioned cognitive change that accompanies this treatment.

Some of the biggest proponents of the therapeutic benefit of "sitting with" negative emotions as is called for in exposure's corrective emotional experiences are the creators of acceptance and commitment therapy (ACT), the so-called "third wave" of cognitive-behavioral therapy (CBT). ACT uses the term "experiential avoidance" to refer to the process of avoiding or modifying aversive private experiences (e.g., thoughts, emotions, bodily sensations, memories) rather than tolerating them (Hayes, Strosahl, & Wilson, 2011). Hayes and colleagues (2011) argue that experiential avoidance is not only ineffective in the ever-changing context of reality, but that it also has the paradoxical effect of intensifying the mood an individual is trying to suppress. Therefore, one of the main tenants of ACT is to help clients accept negative emotional states in a mindful, nonreactive, and nonjudgmental way (Hayes et al., 2011). The experiential pathway to behavioral change promoted in ACT is also highly applicable to exposure therapy,[1] especially in light of the evidence described above suggesting that tolerating rather than reducing anxiety may be the most powerful corrective emotional experience provided by this treatment.

Terror Management Theory and Exposure Therapy

Engaging in exposure therapy is emotionally demanding for both parties in the therapeutic dyad, especially when imaginal and *in vivo* exposures

---

[1] Hofmann and Asmundson (2008) describe the common threads between ACT and CBT generally, with specific reference to exposure. Of note, they state that the philosophical approach of committed action utilized in ACT is most closely related to conducting exposure (p. 6).

are delivered in combination. Exposure requires that clients simultaneously attend to a live fear stimulus, focus on the imagery being provided by the therapist, and tolerate their aversive emotional reactions to these exercises. Conducting exposure also invokes discomfort in many clinicians, particularly those who are new to the treatment. Without adequate understanding of the theoretical basis or empirical support for exposure therapy, the mere notion of guiding clients in confronting the very stimuli that they fear may feel like a violation of clinicians' identities as caring and empathetic people (more on this below). In enduring their mutually unpleasant experiences participating in exposure therapy, the client and therapist are pitted in a joint battle against evolutionary forces that tempt them to escape this distress. In the interests of survival, humans have learned over time to actively avoid unpleasant stimuli that may signal threats to our mortality. In fact, humans avoid experiences and emotions with even remote mortality salience in order to maintain maximal distance from potential danger at all times (Hayes, Schimel, Arndt, & Faucher, 2010). Thus, when clients and therapists confront rather than avoid feared stimuli (even those with low actual mortality threats) and associated anxiety during exposure therapy, they are defying a highly engrained, evolutionarily based behavior.

This human tendency to distance ourselves from potential death reminders, even those that are far removed from actual mortality threats, is described in terror management theory (TMT; Pyszczynski et al., 1999). TMT emerged out of the philosophical and dynamic traditions of Becker and Freud and states that in order to live with the knowledge that death is inevitable, humans create personal and cultural buffers to avoid the terrifying awareness of our own mortality. According to TMT, stimuli with mortality salience are those that challenge our personal esteem, identity, and cultural worldviews, which otherwise serve to protect us from the constant experience of anxiety about our inescapable deaths (Greenberg, Solomon, & Pyszczynski, 1997; Pyszczynski, Solomon, & Greenberg, 1999). TMT explains that humans defend themselves against reminders of mortality via proximal as well as distal processes. Proximal defenses reduce mortality salience in situations that are personally relevant (e.g., the presence of spiders in a person with spider fear), or those that are globally germane but provide immediate, conscious reminders of our individual mortality (Pyscysnski et al., 1999). An example of such a threat may be the fear that persisted among New Yorkers following the attacks of the World Trade Center on September 11, 2001 (Pyszczynski, S. Solomon, & Greenberg, 2003). Distal mortality defenses, in contrast, buffer anxiety produced by thoughts of death at a less conscious level by "providing a sense that one is a valuable contributor to a meaningful, eternal universe" (Pyscysnski et al., 1999, p. 842). An example of a distal morality defense is upholding cultural and personal standards to be kind to others.

TMT has been largely supported in the social psychology arena as a model for explaining avoidance of mortality-salient stimuli. However, TMT is also quite relevant in the application of exposure therapy. While our position is intended as a speculative application of an experiential social psychological model of human behavior, TMT appears to be highly relevant in the experience of exposure for both members of the therapeutic dyad. For clients, the stimuli included in exposures are experienced as immediate and personally relevant threats to survival, as these stimuli have been associated with anxiety via individual learning experiences in which the client was endangered. Thus, there is a natural tendency for clients to exercise proximal mortality defenses against (i.e., avoid) the unpleasant emotions provoked in exposure exercises. Clients' evolutionarily based desire to distance themselves from the proximal morality threats of feared stimuli may take the form of distraction or intellectualization (Hollon, Stewart, & Strunk, 2006) in order to avoid contact with threatening emotions, both of which may compromise the efficacy of exposure therapy (see Foa & Kozak, 1986).

Exposure therapists, on the other hand, exercise distal mortality defenses against the uncomfortable feelings evoked by conducting exposures. Therapists as a group tend to be sensitive to the needs and experiences of others, qualities that are refined and fostered in professional training in order to help clinicians establish effective therapeutic alliances (Castonguay, Constantino, McAleavey, & Goldfried, 2010; see also Safran & Kraus, Chapter 15, this volume). As a result, clinicians form clear personal identities characterized by warmth and empathy and hold professional standards of alleviating clients' symptoms. For clinicians who have not developed identities that include the emotional value of exposure in producing symptom relief, inducing anxiety in clients during treatment may create intense discomfort about whether this therapeutic approach has violated a personal or professional standard (Arndt, Cook, & Routledge, 2004; Greenberg & Arndt, 2012). According to TMT, exposure's threat to the therapist's identity erodes his or her distal buffer against symbolic constructs associated with mortality and activates fear (albeit unconscious) about the inevitability of death (Greenberg, et al., 1997). When exposure promotes mortality salience for therapists in this way, clinicians tend to overlook the clear scientific support for its efficacious outcomes and instead conduct treatment in a manner that may diminish exposure's efficacy in order to uphold their personal and professional identities.

Connecting Exposure and Emotion

Since TMT will dictate the terms of exposure as received by the client and delivered by the therapist, it is important to understand how clinicians may ensure the competent delivery of exposure therapy despite its threats to both proximal and distal defenses against mortality salience. Figure

4.1 depicts a schematic of how therapists' correct application of exposure therapy may attenuate reminders of mortality—and therefore, discomfort with exposure—for themselves and their clients. Before the start of exposure, clinicians can take several steps to reduce clients' mortality salience by implying that death is not anticipated as a consequence of treatment. First, exposure procedures should be developed in a voluntary collaboration between the client and the therapist. Second, the therapist should be clear that they will only attempt exposure exercises that are likely to result in success. Third, the therapist should clearly explain that imagery will regularly be included as part of exposures, and that this imagery is designed to ensure maximal benefit from the hard work in which the client is about to engage. By highlighting the collaborative therapeutic process, an effort that is inherently incompatible with deliberate harm, these measures set the stage for reducing the client's proximal mortality threat, and therefore avoidance in treatment, before exposures even begin.

The distal threats that exposure poses to therapists' identities must also be addressed as a preliminary condition to the successful implementation of exposure treatment. Vail et al. (2012) argue that therapists' direct experience of success in alleviating clients' emotional pain may decrease discomfort for clinicians who are new to exposure by demonstrating that this treatment is less of a threat to their identities and worldviews than initially perceived. Therefore, we recommend that beginning therapists (particularly those trained in nonbehavioral theoretical orientations) should start with cases that are likely to respond well to exposure treatment within a relatively brief timeframe. This initial experience of therapeutic success will lead to a strong emotional response supporting the use of exposure and will allow clinicians to approach future, more difficult cases requiring exposure with less distress from threats to their distal mortality salience buffers.

We propose several additional suggestions for ways that therapists can reduce their own discomfort with exposure procedures owing to activation of mortality threats, thus decreasing the potential for clinicians' avoidance or misapplication of the treatment. First, the extent to which the exposure therapist can successfully convey a supportive and empathic attitude while simultaneously setting the stage for potentially distressing in-session activities will alleviate mortality salience. Next, in addition to seeing the client's distress decline *within* sessions, client reports of *between*-session improvements will bolster the clinician's emotional sense that exposure is safe both for the client and the therapist's professional identity. Finally, therapists' ability to proactively identify potential sources of their own avoidance of exposure practices may help to increase efficacious outcomes.

Here it is appropriate to revisit our discussion of ACT, as the main tenets of this therapeutic modality offer insight into how clients and therapists may overcome the experiential challenges of exposure therapy. First,

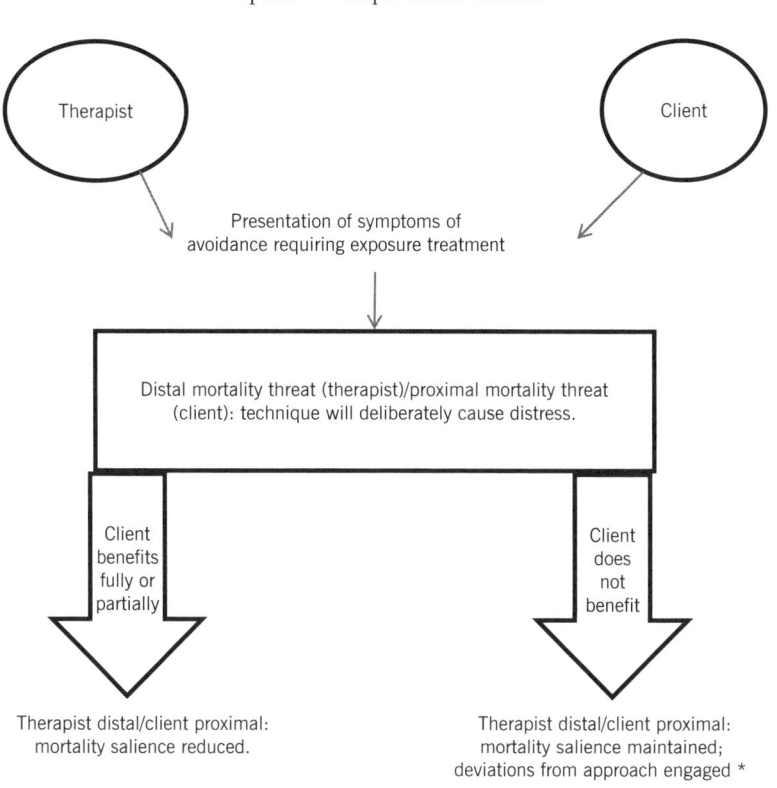

```
                    ┌──────────┐                           ┌──────────┐
                    │ Therapist│                           │  Client  │
                    └────┬─────┘                           └────┬─────┘
                         ↓                                      ↙
                         Presentation of symptoms of
                         avoidance requiring exposure treatment
                                        │
                                        ↓
        ┌───────────────────────────────────────────────────────────────┐
        │ Distal mortality threat (therapist)/proximal mortality threat │
        │ (client): technique will deliberately cause distress.         │
        └──────────────┬────────────────────────────────┬───────────────┘
                       │                                │
              ┌────────┴─────┐                  ┌───────┴─────┐
              │   Client     │                  │   Client    │
              │   benefits   │                  │    does     │
              │   fully or   │                  │    not      │
              │   partially  │                  │   benefit   │
              └──────┬───────┘                  └──────┬──────┘
                     ↓                                 ↓
         Therapist distal/client proximal:   Therapist distal/client proximal:
           mortality salience reduced.         mortality salience maintained;
                                             deviations from approach engaged *
```

FIGURE 4.1. Mechanisms alleviating mortality salience in therapist and client. *If limited success in a first session for therapist, mortality salience may be retained and exposure as a method will be unlikely engaged in future cases. For beginning therapists conducting exposure, best to start with cases with high likelihood of success if original training environment did not endorse exposure methods. Alternate modifications (i.e., relaxation, other cognitive methods) that reduce efficacy likely included.

ACT promotes the acceptance and tolerance of uncomfortable or "dangerous" emotional states, a point that is applicable to exposure therapists and clients alike (Hayes et al., 2011). The ACT process of cognitive defusion (Luoma & Hayes, 2008) may also help both members of the therapeutic dyad to not succumb to the avoidance promoted by mortality threats and feelings of discomfort associated with exposure procedures. For beginner exposure therapists, it may be helpful to decouple exposure's threat of violating their empathetic clinical identities from the marked symptom improvement that many clients experience early in a course of exposure. In other words, therapists must accept that they can induce temporary anxiety in their clients during treatment *and* can still be caring, effective clinicians. Clients are also likely to benefit from cognitive defusion as part of the exposure process. For instance, the emotional experience associated with exposure treatment (i.e., that anxiety can be tolerated without adverse consequences) is typically disconnected from the anxiety experienced spontaneously by the client under everyday circumstances. Thus, through exposure, clients learn new associations between their symptoms and emotional states other than anxiety.

Applications and Illustration of the Experiential Aspects of Exposure

Practicing exposure using a combination of *in vivo* and imaginal methods is a rich and emotionally intense procedure (Dadds, Bovbjerg, Redd, & Cutmore 1997). Clients will feel a strong connection to therapists who can successfully develop and implement these kinds of exercises, which typically significantly reduce symptoms of distress and avoidance both within and between sessions. We would like to highlight that there are many excellent sources that describe the mechanics of developing and conducting exposure (see "Recommended Further Reading"). There is comparably little literature that addresses the emotional change and disposition toward conducting exposure in the therapist, which is what we will focus on for the remainder of our discussion in this chapter.

One of us (D. M.) has conducted many training and supervision sessions with therapists who were new to exposure therapy and often educated in other, non-CBT, psychotherapeutic models. In these supervisory experiences, he has observed how the addition of imagery components to *in vivo* exposures significantly increases mortality salience for therapists in particular. The idea of conducting *in vivo* exposure exercises, while viewed with hesitancy, was something that most beginning exposure clinicians could tolerate. However, the prospect of being responsible for providing additional anxiety-inducing imagery was the point that caused extreme discomfort for therapists, countering expectations for their own professional conduct. Consider the following illustration from a supervision session in which a new therapist was being trained in interoceptive exposure (hyperventilation, using a brown paper bag) for panic disorder:

SUPERVISOR: How long did your client indicate she could hyperventilate during the session?

THERAPIST: She said she could tolerate it at a SUDs of 6 if we hyperventilated for 1½ minutes.

SUPERVISOR: What did you say to her immediately after she completed the hyperventilation?

THERAPIST: I didn't say anything. We just stayed quiet and waited for the aversive sensations to pass.

SUPERVISOR: OK. That is a good start. Now in the next session, consider including some imagery. I recall you indicated that this client was afraid of dying if she had the physical sensations from panic.

THERAPIST: What are you suggesting?

SUPERVISOR: I am suggesting you include imagery of her dying immediately after the hyperventilation.

THERAPIST: I don't see how I could possibly do that! She is far too fragile for that kind of thing. And besides, what if she has a panic attack? I don't think I could handle that, and then she will drop out of treatment.

In this instance, the therapist is expressing her own reluctance to potentially induce increased distress in her client. Yet prior to this supervisory exchange, the therapist accepted the notion of conducting *in vivo* exposure. The inclusion of imagery was what caused the distress and a range of justifications for avoidance on the part of the therapist.

The next illustration is from supervision provided by one of us (D. M.) with an established doctoral-level psychologist who was beginning to apply exposure methods after practicing for over 20 years as a psychodynamically oriented practitioner. The therapist's client exhibited symptoms of contamination fear associated with OCD. The specific nature of the client's symptoms revolved around potentially contracting hepatitis from surfaces in his work environment, as well as a number of other medically related fears. The client engaged in extensive washing rituals, avoided pharmacies (as her client stated, "where sick people shop") and hospitals, and monitored his coworkers for signs of colds or other ailments. The following illustration depicts portions of supervision for the therapist's treatment of this client over the course of three supervisory sessions.

FIRST SUPERVISION: CLIENT AT SESSION 6

SUPERVISOR: Tell me about how the exposures have been going for your client.

THERAPIST: I am finding it difficult. I understand the concept of going through the hierarchy with him, but he reports feeling hesitant about doing the exercises that we agreed to when we began treatment.

SUPERVISOR: So you mean he is hesitant about doing something that he has come to therapy to overcome?

THERAPIST: I see. Yes, he is hesitant to do something that he fears. When we discussed this at the training session, it seemed so easy to persuade someone to do these things. Now I am finding myself feeling very uneasy about this. What if I go too far?

SUPERVISOR: Well, first, tell me what things you have successfully done that is in line with exposure methods.

THERAPIST: OK. We have practiced touching countertops and phones at work. I have been on the phone with him guiding him through the process. He says he experiences distress at a SUDs of 45 to 55 for this. It is lower than what he predicted on the hierarchy.

SUPERVISOR: What are you saying to him when he does these exercises?

THERAPIST: I am encouraging him.

SUPERVISOR: Recall during the training session when we reviewed the development of imagery to accompany the *in vivo* exercises. Have you been able to do this as well?

THERAPIST: I am afraid he will not be able to tolerate it. When we have tried to do things that are higher on the hierarchy, such as eat food while his hands are contaminated, he complains that he will be frightened.

SUPERVISOR: Yes, this will be difficult. Do you recall the discussion we had at the training? Specifically, when the topic came up about the dangers of conducting exposure involving imagery?

THERAPIST: We all concluded that this was the most effective method of ensuring good treatment outcome.

SUPERVISOR: Yes, that is right. Try to keep in mind this important fact—the first time you conduct imagery with the client, you will feel uneasy about the exercise. It will feel terribly wrong. It will actually defy all you have done professionally to this point. In order to help *you* feel comfortable with the work you will need to do, practice the imagery you would develop for your client with me now.

At this point, the therapist practiced guiding the supervisor through the process of exposure with her client and included the imagery necessary to produce a good outcome. This process required feedback to ensure that it was done without undue hesitation or with trepidation about the intensity of the content.

SECOND SUPERVISION: CLIENT AT SESSION 9

SUPERVISOR: Tell me how you have been doing now that we practiced developing imagery to accompany *in vivo* exposure.

THERAPIST: Well, he has been improving a great deal, about a 40% reduction in symptoms based on the symptom measure we used from the training session.

SUPERVISOR: That is great! What areas are still difficult for your client?

THERAPIST: Well, he is having trouble with a coworker now, one who he indicated has come down with a curable form of cancer.

SUPERVISOR: So his symptoms now cause him to feel that he may contract the same form of cancer, correct?

THERAPIST: Yes, only if he comes in contact with anything his coworker has touched. It is a problem now, since they work on a project together.

SUPERVISOR: Can he, without it being intrusive or in any way obvious, get a pen or paper that belongs to his coworker?

THERAPIST: Oh, yes, easily. In fact, he regularly attempts to avoid these things.

SUPERVISOR: Let's practice the kind of imagery you would need to develop with him during *in vivo* exposure.

THERAPIST: OK, so let's use paper as our example since he just tossed out paper from this coworker and it was the topic of some discussion in my last session with him. Once he touches the paper, I would tell him that he is going to contract this form of cancer. He would begin to feel a small tumor develop on his skin, like a melanoma, and it will bother him mildly, maybe sting slightly. He'll notice the tumor metastasizing . . . are you sure I should do this?

SUPERVISOR: How different are the things you are saying from the things he is already likely thinking? How much damage are you doing when he is doing this already? I know this is hard for you, but consider how much you will be helping him, particularly given how much he has already gained. And remember, I am available to help *you* as you help him.

THERAPIST: OK, thanks, that helps. It is just that this is so contrary to how I've practiced before. I know intellectually this will be helpful, but it feels wrong somehow to me.

The therapist proceeded to get more comfortable with encouragement from the supervisor. This was a difficult process, but one that was worthwhile since delivering the imagery activated fears in the therapist that she was behaving contrary to her personal identity as a clinician. Following this supervision session, the therapist contacted the supervisor after she met with the client in Session 8. She felt uneasy after conducting the imagery as discussed in supervision, expressing that she felt she may have gone too far and that she was worried about the client's symptoms worsening. After some discussion about how this is a normal concern among therapists when they first practice exposure, and exploring all of the ways in which the client may or may not worsen, it was agreed that an emergency supervision session would be held in the event the client had an adverse reaction to the combined imaginal/*in vivo* exposure. The therapist later indicated via e-mail that no emergency follow-up was necessary and that the client continued to show improvement when he arrived for Session 9.

THIRD SUPERVISION: CLIENT AT SESSION 15

SUPERVISOR: How is your client doing now? And how have you been feeling as you've pursued this form of treatment with him?

THERAPIST: He is doing markedly better. The session I had with him after our last supervision was very difficult. I really had my doubts about whether this was a good idea, whether I was cut out for this kind of therapy. But my client is doing great. He says he feels much calmer now, is not fearful of going to work, and has begun to do many things he has not done in years. Last week I guided him through the act of going to a pharmacy for the first time in several years. His symptom reduction is over 80% from when he started.

SUPERVISOR: Let's do an exercise now. I would like you to conjure an image for yourself, that you now have to treat a different client with similar symptoms, but this time it is a parent fearful of harming his children. Can you walk me through the imagery necessary for our hypothetical client?

The aim of this final supervision session was to bolster the therapist's sense of efficacy in conducting exposure for other clients. Additionally, helping the therapist to integrate exposure procedures into her professional identity was essential so that she would not experience undue discomfort in treating future clients who would rightly benefit from exposure.

Future Directions

Exposure therapy is an intense curative intervention that has extensive data supporting its use, as well as a rich history in the psychotherapeutic literature (Olatunji et al., 2010). However, it has been difficult for the field to achieve widespread dissemination of empirically supported interventions, including exposure (McHugh & Barlow, 2010). TMT may help to explain reluctance to engage in exposure therapy on the part of both clients and therapists. When viewed through the lens of TMT, exposure therapy necessarily activates clients' proximal mortality threats and thus causes initial distress during treatment. Exposure procedures may activate distal mortality threats in therapists by raising concerns about upholding their professional identities and the inherent risks of exposure for therapists and clients alike. These concerns are especially prominent for clinicians trained in therapeutic traditions that do not emphasize direct contact with aversive emotions (Pyszczynski et al., 1999). We assert here that exposure, when conducted properly, cultivates a strong sense of emotional satisfaction for therapists and bolsters their professional identity as caring and empathic individuals. Moreover, correctly implemented exposure therapy should reduce proximal mortality salience, and therefore symptoms, in clients who present to treatment for anxiety-related disorders.

More work is needed to demonstrate the principles necessary to train therapists in the experiential aspects of exposure therapy. Supervision that explicitly addresses the emotional concerns of beginner exposure therapists will ensure the successful application of this treatment. Thus, training for therapists who are new to exposure may require clinicians to change emotionally and cognitively, rather than simply to learn new techniques. It is only through emotional growth on the part of exposure therapists that emotional and behavioral change in clients may be achieved through the use of this powerful treatment.

Further Resources

Articles

- For a recent discussion of theoretical issues in the application of exposure, see Abramowitz (2013).
- Coverage of cross-theoretically relevant imagery components of exposure are described in Levis (1995).

Books

- For a detailed theoretical and practical discussion of exposure methods, see Abramowitz, Deacon, and Whiteside (2011).
- For an excellent review of exposure for a wide range of psychological conditions as well as impediments to implementation and dissemination, see Richard and Lauterbach (2007).

Videos

- The American Psychological Association has a series of videos that illustrate the application of exposure for different psychological conditions. Of note are:
- Tomkins, M. A. (2012). *Cognitive-behavior therapy for specific phobias* [DVD]. Washington, DC: American Psychological Association.
- Olatunji, B. O. (2011). *Cognitive-behavior therapy for clients with anxiety and panic* [DVD]. Washington, DC: American Psychological Association.

References

Abramowitz, J. S. (1996). Variants of exposure with response prevention in the treatment of obsessive–compulsive disorder: A meta-analysis. *Behavior Therapy, 27*, 583–600.

Abramowitz, J. S. (2013). The practice of exposure therapy: Relevance of cognitive behavior theory and extinction theory. *Behavior Therapy, 44*, 548–558.

Abramowitz, J. S., Deacon, B. J., & Whiteside, S. P. (2011). *Exposure therapy for anxiety: Principles and practice.* New York: Guilford Press.

Arndt, J., Cook, A., & Routledge, C. (2004). The blueprint of terror management: Understanding the cognitive architecture of psychological defense against the awareness of death. In J. Greenberg, S. L. Koole, & T. Pyszynski (Eds.), *Handbook of experimental existential psychology* (pp. 35–53). New York: Guilford Press.

Becker, C. B., Zayfert, C., & Anderson, E. (2004). A survey of psychologists' attitudes towards and utilization of exposure therapy for PTSD. *Behaviour Research and Therapy, 42,* 277–292.

Becker, E. (1973). *The denial of death.* New York: Free Press.

Bio-IT World. (2007). Project Jim: Watson's personal genome goes public. Available at *www.bioitworld.com/newsitems/2007/may/05-31-07-watson-genome.*

Castonguay, L. G., Constantino, M. J., McAleavey, A. A., & Goldfried, M. R. (2010). The therapeutic alliance in cognitive-behavioral therapy. In J. C. Muran & J. P. Barber (Eds.), *The therapeutic alliance: An evidence-based guide to practice* (pp. 150–171). New York: Guilford Press.

Castro, F., & Marx, B. P. (2007). Exposure therapy with adult survivors of childhood sexual abuse. In D. C. S. Richard & D. Lauterbach (Eds.), *Comprehensive handbook of the exposure therapies* (pp. 153–168). New York: Academic Press.

Christensen, H., Hadzi-Pavlovic, D., Andrews, G., & Mattick, R. (1987). Behavior therapy and tricyclic medication in the treatment of obsessive–compulsive disorder: A quantitative review. *Journal of Clinical and Consulting Psychology, 55,* 701–711.

Dadds, M. R., Bovbjerg, D. H., Redd, W. H., & Cutmore, T. R. H. (1997). Imagery in human classical conditioning. *Psychological Bulletin, 122,* 89–103.

Deacon, B. J., & Farrell, N. R. (2013). Therapist barriers to the dissemination of exposure therapy. In E. A. Storch & D. McKay (Eds.), *Handbook of treating variants and complications in anxiety disorders* (pp. 363–373). New York: Springer.

Deacon, B. J., Farrell, N. R., Kemp, J. J., Dixon, L. J., Sy, J. T., Zhang, A. R., et al. (in press). Assessing therapist reservations about exposure therapy for anxiety disorders: The Therapist Beliefs about Exposure Scale. *Journal of Anxiety Disorders, 27,* 772–780.

Deacon, B. J., Lickel J. J., Farrell, N. R., Kemp, J. J., & Hipol, L. J. (2013). Therapist perceptions and delivery of interoceptive exposure for panic disorder. *Journal of Anxiety Disorders, 27,* 259–264.

Debiec, J., & LeDoux, J. (2009). The amygdala networks of fear: From animal models to human psychopathology. In D. McKay, J. S. Abramowitz, S. Taylor, & G. J. G. Asmundson (Eds.), *Current perspectives on the anxiety disorders: Implications for DSM-5 and beyond* (pp. 107–126). New York: Springer.

Division 12 (Clinical), American Psychological Association. (2013). A guide to beneficial therapy. Available at *www.apa.org/divisions/div12/cppi.html.*

Eelen, P., & Vervliet, B. (2006). Fear conditioning and clinical implications: What can we learn from the past? In M. G. Craske, D. Hermans, & D. Vansteenwegen (Eds.), *Fear and learning: From basic processes to clinical implications* (pp. 17–35). Washington, DC: American Psychological Association Press.

Farrell, N. R., Deacon, B. D., Kemp, J. J., Dixon, L. D., & Sy, J. T. (2013). Do negative beliefs about exposure therapy cause its cautious delivery?: An experimental investigation. *Journal of Anxiety Disorders, 27,* 763–771.

Foa, E. B., & Kozak, M. J. (1986). Emotional processing of fear: Exposure to corrective information. *Psychological Bulletin, 99,* 20–35.

Freud, S. (1952a). Beyond the pleasure principle. (C. J. M. Hubback, Trans.) In R. M.

Hutchins (Ed.), *Great books of the Western world: Freud* (Vol. 54, pp. 639–663). Chicago: Encyclopedia Britannica. (Original work published 1920)

Freud, S. (1952b). Civilization and its discontents (J. Riviere, Trans.) In R. M. Hutchins (Ed.), *Great books of the Western world: Freud* (Vol. 54, pp. 767–802). Chicago: Encyclopedia Britannica. (Original work published 1929)

Greenberg, J., & Arndt, J. (2012). Terror management theory. In P. A. M. van Lange, A. W. Kruglanski, & E. T. Higgins (Eds.), *Handbook of theories of social psychology* (Vol. 1, pp. 398–415). Los Angeles: Sage.

Greenberg, J., Solomon, S., & Pyszczynski, T. (1997). Terror management theory of self-esteem and cultural worldviews: Empirical assessments and conceptual refinements. *Advances in Experimental Social Psychology, 29*, 61–139.

Hayes, J., Schimel, J., Arndt, J., & Faucher, E. H. (2010). A theoretical and empirical review of the death-thought accessibility concept in terror management research. *Psychological Bulletin, 136*, 699–739.

Hayes, S. C., Strosahl, K. D., & Wilson, K. G. (2011). *Acceptance and commitment therapy: An experiential approach to behavior change* (2nd ed.). New York: Guilford Press.

Hofmann, S. G. (2008). Cognitive processes during fear acquisition and extinction in animals and humans: Implications for exposure therapy of anxiety disorders. *Clinical Psychology Review, 28*, 199–210.

Hofmann, S. G., & Asmundson, G. J. G. (2008). Acceptance and mindfulness-based therapy: New wave or old hat? *Clinical Psychology Review, 28*, 1–16.

Hollon, S. D., Stewart, M. O., & Strunk, D. (2006). Enduring effects for cognitive behavior therapy in the treatment of depression and anxiety. *Annual Review of Psychology, 57*, 285–315.

Levis, D. J. (1995). Decoding traumatic memory: Implosive theory of psychopathology. In W. T. O'Donohue & L. Krasner (Eds.), *Theories of behavior therapy: Exploring behavior change* (pp. 173–207). Washington, DC: American Psychological Association Press.

Luoma, J. B., & Hayes, S. C. (2008). Cognitive defusion. In W. O'Donohue, J. E. Fisher, & S. C. Hayes (Eds.), *Cognitive behavior therapy: Applying empirically supported techniques in your practice* (pp. 71–78). Hoboken, NJ: Wiley.

McHugh, R. K., & Barlow, D. H. (2010). The dissemination and implementation of evidence-based psychological treatments: A review of current efforts. *American Psychologist, 65*, 73–84.

McKay, D., Abramowitz, J. S., & Taylor, S. (2010). *Cognitive behavior therapy for refractory cases: Turning failure into success*. Washington, DC: American Psychological Association Press.

Olatunji, B. O., Cisler, J. M., & Deacon, B. J. (2010). Efficacy of cognitive behavioral therapy for anxiety disorders: A review of meta-analytic findings. *Psychiatric Clinics of North America, 33*, 557–577.

Olatunji, B. O., Deacon, B. J., & Abramowitz, J. S. (2009). The cruelest cure?: Ethical issues in the implementation of exposure-based treatments. *Cognitive and Behavioral Practice, 16*, 172–180.

Pyszczynski, T., Greenberg, J., & Solomon, S. (1999). A dual process model of defense against conscious and unconscious death-related thoughts: An extension of terror management theory. *Psychological Review, 106*, 835–845.

Pyszczynski, T., Solomon, S., & Greenberg, J. (2003). *In the wake of 9/11: The psychology of terror*. Washington, DC: American Psychological Association Press.

Rachman, S., Hodgson, R., & Marks, I. M. (1971). The treatment of chronic obsessive–compulsive neurosis. *Behaviour Research and Therapy, 9*, 237–247.

Richard, D. C. S., & Gloster, A. T. (2007). Exposure therapy has a public relations problem: A dearth of litigation amid a wealth of concern. In D. C. S. Richard & D. Lauterbach (Eds.), *Comprehensive handbook of the exposure therapies* (pp. 409–425). New York: Academic Press.

Richard, D. C. S., & Lauterbach, D. (Eds.). (2007). *Comprehensive handbook of the exposure therapies.* San Diego, CA: Academic Press.

Richard, D. C. S., Lauterbach, D., & Gloster, A. T. (2007). Description, mechanisms of action, and assessment. In D. C. S. Richard & D. Lauterbach (Eds.), *Comprehensive handbook of the exposure therapies* (pp. 1–28). New York: Academic Press.

Rothbaum, B. O., & Schwartz, A. C. (2002). Exposure therapy for posttraumatic stress disorder. *American Journal of Psychotherapy, 56,* 59–75.

Slater, L. (2003, November 2). The cruelest cure. *The New York Times.* Retrieved June 14, 2013, from *www.nytimes.com.*

Solomon, R. L., Kamin, L. J., & Wynne, L. C. (1953). Traumatic avoidance learning: The outcomes of several extinction procedures with dogs. *Journal of Abnormal Psychology, 48,* 291–302.

Stampfl, T. G., & Levis, D. J. (1968). Implosive therapy—A behavioral therapy? *Behaviour Research and Therapy, 6,* 31–36.

Taylor, S., Cox, B. J., & Asmundson, G. J. G. (2009). Anxiety disorders: Panic and phobias. In P. H. Blaney & T. Millon (Eds.), *Oxford textbook of psychopathology* (pp. 119–145). New York: Oxford University Press.

Vail, K. E., Juhl, J., Arndt, J., Vess, M., Routledge, C., & Rutjens, B. T. (2012). When death is good for life: Considering the positive trajectories of terror management. *Personality and Social Psychology Bulletin, 16,* 303–329.

Whittal, M. L., Thordarson, D. S., & McLean, P. D. (2005). Treatment of obsessive-compulsive disorder: Cognitive behavior therapy versus exposure with response prevention. *Behaviour Research and Therapy, 43,* 1559–1576.

Wolpe, J. (1990). *The practice of behavior therapy* (4th ed). Elmsford, NY: Pergamon Press.

Zoellner, L. A., Feeny, N. C., Bittinger, J. N., Bedard-Gilligan, M. A., Slagle, D. M., Post, L. M., et al. (2011). Teaching trauma-focused exposure therapy for PTSD: Critical clinical lessons for novice exposure therapists. *Psychological Trauma: Theory, Research, Practice, and Policy, 3,* 300–308.

CHAPTER 5

Behavioral Experiments

Using Experiences to Test Beliefs

Susan Daflos
Rachael Lunt
Maureen Whittal

Theoretical Basis

The purpose of the behavioral experiment (BE) is to engage in behavioral exercises that induce emotional arousal and cognitive change. In order to define and understand the essence of BEs, it is necessary first to understand the cognitive theory of psychopathology from which they are derived.

Since they were first introduced in Beck's early work (Beck, 1967, 1976), cognitive models have repeatedly been demonstrated to be effective in the treatment of a wide range of disorders including depression (Beck, 1967), anxiety disorders (Clark & Beck, 2010), eating disorders (Cooper, 2012), and personality disorders (Beck, Freeman, Davis, & Associates, 2003; Linehan, 1993). Regardless of the disorder, cognitive theory suggests that problems arise not from specific events or triggers themselves (e.g., a car accident; the loss of a relationship), but rather from the meaning given to these events and the way in which they are interpreted (e.g., The world is dangerous; I'm unlovable). These misinterpretations affect physiology and emotion, which often are dealt with through maladaptive behavioral coping responses. Although in the short term these coping responses may appear effective by removing the perceived threat and decreasing emotional arousal, they paradoxically maintain the problem by preventing the disconfirmation of key cognitions.

Cognitive models for each disorder differ in the specification of the *kinds* of key cognitions that are hypothesized to maintain the disorder. For example, whereas catastrophic misinterpretations of physical sensations are central to the development and maintenance of panic disorder (e.g., "I'm having a heart attack"), a catastrophic misinterpretation of intrusive thoughts (Rachman, 2003) is central to obsessive-compulsive disorder with primary obsessions (e.g., "If I have the thought of stabbing my husband, that must mean I'm an evil person capable of doing so"). Subsequent behaviors designed to avert the feared catastrophe (e.g., staying away from crowds to avoid further panic attacks; hiding all knives in the house to avoid images of stabbing one's spouse) temporarily decrease emotional arousal, although they reinforce this reaction and these beliefs over the long term. To break or weaken this cycle, the validity of the key beliefs must be tested.

A number of strategies are used to assist the client in identifying and testing maladaptive cognitions that underlie negative patterns of emotions and behavior. One strategy suggested by the cognitive model is the use of methods such as diary cards and Socratic questioning to achieve propositional learning. Allowing individuals to identify their own faulty and maladaptive beliefs (e.g., "I might die from having a panic attack") and behavioral patterns (e.g., "I'm avoiding going to the grocery store because of fear I might have a panic attack") can set the stage for the elimination of maladaptive coping behaviors (e.g., going to the grocery store). However, clients often state that even though they are cognitively aware that their beliefs are flawed, they continue to act as if they are correct because they "feel real in the moment." This concern is consistent with research showing that techniques that facilitate affective changes produce more powerful changes than those targeted solely at the cognitive level (Castonguay, Goldfried, Wiser, Raue, & Hayes, 1996; Watson & Rennie, 1994), and may even be necessary for assimilating new information (Goldfried, 2003). As a result, cognitive models suggest that an experiential learning component may be necessary for emotional change to take place (Teasdale & Barnard, 1993).

BEs are collaboratively planned experiential activities that may be designed either as an experiment or as an observation that directly tests specific client beliefs derived from a cognitive formulation of the client's problem. Rather than the clinician providing the client with information, the client is able to use the experience gained through the BE to discover new information cognitively, physically, and emotionally. By obtaining new information, clients may:

- Test the validity of their existing beliefs.
- Develop or test new more adaptive beliefs.
- Verify or contribute to the cognitive case formulation.

BEs are similar to the behavioral technique of *exposure*, in which an individual purposefully seeks contact with an emotion-inducing trigger, such as uncomfortable physical sensations, situations, thoughts, or images. While the goal of exposure is to extinguish the emotional response (e.g., fear, guilt, shame, anger) through habituation, without explicitly testing cognition, the primary goal of a BE is to test the validity of appraisals through the engagement of emotional learning. As described by Beck and his colleagues, "For the behavior therapist, the modification of behavior is an end in itself; for the cognitive therapist it is a means to an end—namely cognitive change" (Beck, Rush, Shaw, & Emery, 1979, p. 119).

Taking anxiety as an example, a cognitive model of anxiety assumes that difficulties with anxiety begin with the perception of danger or threat. The nature of the threat varies according to the specific focus of the anxiety (e.g., fear of dying from a panic attack; fear of harming someone else from unwanted intrusive thoughts of stabbing others; fear of uncertain situations when worrying uncontrollably). As one might expect of someone who truly believes that she is in danger, anxious individuals engage in an array of "safety behaviors" that are perceived to (at least temporarily) prevent the feared catastrophe from occurring. For example, a socially anxious client who believes that she will be fired for doing a horrible job of presenting her department's updates at a staff meeting may ask a coworker to present the updates for her. By avoiding delivery of the presentation, the client's anxiety and fear will decrease because she believes she has avoided looking incompetent, which would have resulted in the loss of her job. However, her behaviors will have prevented her from observing the more likely outcome that she would not have been fired, even if her presentation was poor, preventing possible disconfirmation of her belief. In fact, engaging in "safety-seeking behavior" (Salkovskis, 1991; often simply called "safety behaviors") not only reinforces beliefs, but may exacerbate the problem by appearing to confirm the predictions. For instance, the socially anxious client who has avoided speaking at several meetings experiences shaking hands, severe perspiration, and stuttering when finally being forced to present at her staff meeting, resulting in several coworkers commenting on how nervous she appeared. The client is so focused on how severe her anxiety felt at the time, as well as the comments from her coworkers, that she fails to notice that her primary feared outcome—being fired—did not occur.

In contrast to simply enduring distressing experiences as they typically have in the past, clients engaging in a BE approach the situation like scientists testing a hypothesis. Clients begin by identifying a specific belief that is stated in the form of a clear prediction that they will be testing. Once a specific prediction has been selected, the client and therapist work together to identify all unnecessary precautions or safety behaviors the client typically engages in to prevent the feared outcome. The BE is designed to obtain empirical evidence that can be used against or in support of the belief. These experiments may involve manipulation of key variables or changing the client's behavior (e.g., going to the supermarket alone vs. with a spouse to test the belief that the client will pass out due to panic if he or she goes alone). In situations in which manipulation is not possible, observation may be used to gather relevant information that may support or weaken key beliefs (e.g., observing a busy intersection and counting the number of accidents or dangerous driving behaviors to test the belief that the intersection is too dangerous for the client to drive through). There may also be situations, such as those wherein core beliefs are being tested (e.g., "I am unlovable"), when the client is unable to identify an alternate belief to test. In these situations, the client may be guided in the direction of BEs designed toward discovery (e.g., "How might a loveable person act in this situation?") to gather data that may shape a more adaptive belief. However, just like scientific experiments, BEs and their impact may be affected by extraneous variables that may make the interpretation of results more difficult, and even ambiguous. The therapist must pay careful attention to detail to control as many variables as possible in each BE, increasing the chances the client will be able to gain more realistic beliefs.

Evidence Supporting the Use of BEs

Many clinicians find that not only are BEs useful methods for producing cognitive change, they "offer the most powerful means to cognitive change in cognitive therapy" (Wells, 1997, p. 78). According to cognitive theory, they are effective because they provide the client with hard evidence relevant to his or her beliefs. Yet, although BEs are essential to cognitive therapy (Beck et al., 1979; Clark, 1989; Wells, 1997), there has been little focus on BEs in the research literature since they are used and evaluated as part of a treatment package, rather than as isolated strategies. Since 2000, however, a number of researchers have created novel ways of testing the effectiveness of BEs by comparing them to exposure.

Cognitive or Extinction Rationales?

Since there is an abundance of research showing that exposure is an effective treatment for a wide variety of disorders, clinicians commonly question what the benefit is to presenting an exercise in a cognitive versus an extinction framework. A recent meta-analysis conducted by McMillan and Lee (2010) reviewed studies across a number of anxiety disorders examining the effects of BEs versus exposure alone. They found support that BEs result in greater reduction in subjective ratings of anxiety, maladaptive cognitions, and specific anxiety symptoms than exposure alone. Fisher and Wells (2005) examined this effect in application to OCD using a single-case experimental design ($N = 4$). Results indicated that presenting exposure as a behavioral experiment resulted in decreased anxiety, believability of cognitions, and urges to neutralize obsessions in comparison to the traditional exposure condition. Salkovskis, Hackmann, Wells, Gelder, and Clark (2007) similarly randomly assigned 16 individuals with panic disorder and agoraphobia to participate in either habituation-based exposure therapy or exposure therapy planned as a belief disconfirmation strategy. Clients in the belief disconfirmation condition showed significantly greater improvements in self-report measures of anxiety, panic, and situational avoidance, with large effect sizes ranging from $d = 1.7–2.7$. These results hold promise that exposure therapies may be more effective by slightly altering their presentation in such a way as to support cognitive reappraisal.

Cognitive Mediation

Both Sloan and Telch (2002) and Kamphuis and Telch (2000) conducted exposure exercises with students suffering from claustrophobic fears endorsed via self-report questionnaires. In the first study, 51 students were randomly assigned to complete traditional exposure tasks or exposure tasks with guided threat reappraisal, similar to instructions that may be given during a BE. The addition of guided threat reappraisal resulted in the greatest level of fear reduction and the lowest level of return of fear. Additionally, Kamphuis and Telch (2000) found that when 58 randomly assigned students were given a distraction task to increase their cognitive load, they achieved lower levels of fear reduction, regardless of the focus of their available attention. These results suggest that cognitive appraisal may be a crucial factor in the efficacy of both exposure and BEs. Kim (2005) provided further support for the importance of disconfirming false beliefs by randomly assigning 45 undergraduate psychology students who were clinically assessed to meet criteria for social phobia to engage in exposure with or without the use of safety behaviors or exposure and either an extinction or cognitive rationale. Individuals who had a cognitive rationale produced significantly greater reductions in anxiety and belief ratings for feared outcomes than individuals in the other conditions, suggesting that the cognitive process of disconfirmation of negative thoughts is a critical element in determining the effectiveness of decreased safety behaviors. In an attempt to explicitly examine whether the effects of exposure and behavioral experiments are mediated by a change in cognitions, Raes, Koster, Loeys, and De Raedt (2011) randomly assigned 31 individuals recruited from the community who met criteria for spider phobia to one session of either behavioral exposure or exposure as a test for maladaptive cognitions. Both exposure and BE formats showed large treatment effects ($d = 2.23–2.81$) and strong cognitive mediation of these effects ($p \leq .005$) with no between-group differences, suggesting that exposure effects are cognitively mediated, even if cognitions are not specifically targeted. Thus the majority of the studies examining cognitive mediation in experiments that directly compare exposure and BEs show that both exposure and BEs achieve their effects through cognitive change.

Using BEs in Clinical Practice

BEs Used in Different Stages of Treatment

BEs have three main purposes that generally correspond to the three stages of treatment in which their use may be most helpful: (1) elaborating the case formulation, (2) testing negative cognitions or maladaptive beliefs, and (3) constructing and testing new adaptive beliefs and perspectives.

Elaborating the Case Formulation

Early in cognitive-behavioral therapy, various tools such as assessments and thought records are often employed to obtain information needed for a case formulation. However, there are times when significant information is missing, either because the client is unable to access it through standard memory-based verbal reports (e.g., "I don't know why I have to wash my hands 10 times after touching a pen someone else was using. I just automatically do it"), or because the behaviors are unobservable to the client and therefore not reported in session. By having the client complete a BE in session, the therapist can witness subtle thinking or behaviors that are invisible to the client, while also teaching and encouraging her to make these observations for herself.

For example, a client experiencing unwanted intrusive thoughts of stabbing her husband and children reports that while she does attempt to ignore the thoughts and distract herself with some activity, she does not engage in any compulsive avoidance of sharp or dangerous objects, and her behaviors are not observable to others. After collaboratively discussing with the therapist various ways in which this fear could be induced in the room with the therapist, the client agreed to have the therapist place a pair of scissors in a desk drawer near the client. The therapist observed the client sit on her hands and inch her chair away from the desk, all while avoiding eye contact with the therapist. The client had been unaware that she was engaging in physical avoidance of dangerous objects when around others, and this behavior was added to her cognitive case conceptualization as a maintaining factor that contributes to her belief that she is an evil and dangerous person.

Testing Negative Cognitions or Maladaptive Beliefs

Once a case formulation has been created and core beliefs, unhelpful assumptions, and negative automatic thoughts have been identified, their credibility can be tested using BEs. Old unrealistic assumptions and beliefs are phrased in a clear, explicit way that can be confirmed or questioned based on the evidence collected. For example, to test the belief that only evil people have thoughts of harming others, a client suffering from unwanted intrusive thoughts of stabbing her family members asks her close friends and family to review a list of common intrusive thoughts experienced by individuals without OCD (Rachman & de Silva, 1978) and anonymously endorse which thoughts they have experienced. She discovers that nearly all of her friends and family, whom she believes are not evil, dangerous people, endorsed at some point experiencing strange unwanted thoughts that included harming themselves or others, and that most people thought that these are "just thoughts" and do not mean anything about them as people. In this situation, the client used observation of other's reactions to test the validity of her own thoughts, which resulted in the weakening of her own beliefs.

Manipulation of a client's behavior or environment may also be used to challenge the validity of beliefs. For example, to test the belief that having a "bad thought," such as "What if my husband gets into a car accident on the way home?", makes it more likely for the imagined event to happen, the client thought and wrote down several bad and good thoughts (e.g., "What if my husband gets into a car accident on the way to work today?"; "What if I won the lottery?"). The evidence obtained through this BE, that having a thought does not make it more likely that the imagined event will happen, may weaken the previously held beliefs, or it may even lead to the creation of new alternative perspectives that need to be tested. It is important to note that, while recently acquired appraisals may be fairly easy to disprove, beliefs that are held longer or more deeply will likely take a considerable amount of evidence to weaken and disprove. Following disconfirmation of threat, it is typical that this positive outcome will be negated (e.g., "That was lucky; What if next time I'm not so lucky?"). To build confidence in alternate appraisals it may entail repeating the same BE several times during and in between sessions. It also may mean testing the same hypothesis in multiple ways to ensure that ambiguity is not impacting the interpretation of the results. Testing negative cognitions may be done at any point in therapy and will likely facilitate the construction of new adaptive beliefs.

Constructing and Testing New Adaptive Beliefs

In the middle and last stages of treatment, once negative thoughts have been challenged, it often becomes necessary for clients to formulate and test new, more adaptive beliefs. Although the disconfirmation of negative beliefs may result in symptom reduction, it does not necessarily lead to the adoption of more adaptive beliefs, which is beneficial for long-term treatment gains and to avoid relapse. For example, a client with panic attacks who has learned, through a series of BEs, that panic attacks will not result in her passing out in the grocery store may not believe that it is safe and natural to experience dramatic spikes in her anxiety levels. She will likely need to create a new belief (e.g., "I can experience panic attacks and/or high anxiety and still continue with my daily tasks") and obtain evidence to support this belief through a series of BEs. This process is helpful for two reasons: instead of just disproving maladaptive beliefs, clients are able to replace these beliefs with ones that endorse effective coping behaviors, and by doing so they learn how to adopt and adapt belief systems based on evidence collected through experience, rather than on strong emotional reactions.

Setting Up the Experiment

Although it is possible to directly test the validity of core beliefs (e.g., "I am a failure"), it is often more effective to begin challenging beliefs associated with safety behaviors, as they are often more specific and easily tested. Safety behaviors should be identified in the earliest therapy sessions and then be incorporated into the cognitive case conceptualization. To build a strong therapeutic alliance and maintain the client as an active participant, the therapist and client should collaborate together to decide which belief and safety behavior, as identified in the case conceptualization, will be challenged first. The therapist may then ask the client questions such as "If this belief were true, what would you expect to happen in this situation? How would you cope with that outcome?" or "If the opposite outcome happened, what would that mean?" It is often useful to spend an entire session identifying a belief that will be tested, discussing what each possible result may mean, and discussing the specific details of carrying out the experiment, including when it will take place, in what specific location, which parts of the experiment the client will attend to in order to collect evidence, and whether the use of safety behaviors will be permitted. Experiments may be conducted in or out of session, depending on the nature of the experiment.

Clinical Example

A male client, Steve, is suffering from posttraumatic symptoms following a motor vehicle accident. The accident occurred at night, when Steve was driving in the right-hand lane and a truck from the left lane tried to merge into the right lane without seeing Steve. Although Steve was driving his vehicle at the time of the accident, his fears have generalized beyond driving or even being a passenger in a car, to crossing busy streets as a pedestrian. When preparing to cross a street, Steve has the thought "A driver will not see me and hit me," as well as images of himself being hit by a car while he is crossing the road. Steve has also recently begun intently watching the cars as he crosses the road to decrease his anxiety to a manageable level. Steve and his therapist have agreed that his hypervigilant observance of cars while crossing the road is contributing to his belief that he is unsafe crossing the road. Below is an example of Steve and his therapist creating a BE based on this conceptualization:

THERAPIST: Steve, you've done a really great job of noticing your need to stare at the cars around you until you've completed crossing the street in order to decrease your anxiety. What are you afraid will happen if you don't stare at the cars?

STEVE: Well, I'm pretty sure that if I don't watch the cars, one of them will hit me.

THERAPIST: Are you crossing the road at a crosswalk when you have these fears?

STEVE: Yes, but it doesn't really matter if there's a crosswalk with a stop sign or not. There are so many times drivers just aren't paying attention, and the only way I can guarantee they won't hit me is by looking out for them so I can jump out of the way if they don't stop for me.

THERAPIST: How likely do you think it is that you would be hit when crossing the street and *not* staring at the cars, but looking at the sign telling you to walk instead?

STEVE: Um, pretty likely. Maybe 75%?

THERAPIST: Okay, 75% is quite high. That's three out of every four times you cross the road. Do you think that you need to stare at every car stopped at the crosswalk, or is it okay to skip some of them?

STEVE: Every car—if I miss one then there's still a 75% chance I could get hit.

THERAPIST: So, what is your evidence supporting this? How many times have you been hit when crossing the street?

STEVE: Well, none. But I was hit while I was driving and the other driver didn't pay attention. So I know it happens. Drivers don't pay attention.

THERAPIST: I remember, and that was a very scary situation when it happened to you. But it seems like you don't actually have any experience of being hit at crosswalks. Have you seen someone else hit by a car while crossing the street?

STEVE: No.

THERAPIST: And have you ever crossed the street without staring at every car you pass?

STEVE: Yes, and I wasn't hit those times either. But it feels different now. It feels like it's more likely to happen.

THERAPIST: Yes, when you experience so much fear crossing the street it definitely feels like there should be something to be afraid of. And you have a lot of evidence showing you that staring at the cars you walk by helps keep you safe. But it seems like you haven't recently tested what would happen if you crossed the street without staring at the cars.

STEVE: No, not recently. I know nothing's happened in the past, so I guess I *could* try again and see what happens.

THERAPIST: I'm glad to hear that! Let's talk about when and where you can do this.

Steve and his therapist decide on a street with heavy pedestrian traffic that Steve will cross four times during the next week. He will only attend to the crosswalk light and other pedestrians, purposefully turning his attention away from the cars once the crosswalk light turns green. After each experiment, he will write down the outcome of the experiment, including any accidents or injuries he or any other pedestrian experienced while crossing the street.

THERAPIST: Wow, it looks like you completed the experiment for all 4 days you committed to. How did it go?

STEVE: Really well, I think. I was really scared the entire time I was crossing the street, but I just kept staring at the crosswalk sign the entire time. And nothing happened!

THERAPIST: So what do you think that means about your belief that you are very likely to get hit by a car if you don't watch all the surrounding cars when crossing the street?

STEVE: I think maybe that's not so true. Although, I did the experiment in sunny weather at an intersection with lots of pedestrians [example of negating positive outcome]. I think it's only 10% likely I would be hit at that intersection, but I do still think I could be hit at another intersection that's not as busy in rainy weather.

After only one session, Steve has already experienced a weakening of his beliefs, although this belief change has not generalized to other settings. Since the initial BE was successful, a similar processing model can be used during the following session, with Steve completing a similar BE at various crosswalks at different times of day and with different weather conditions. Often—with such strong beliefs—it is helpful to ask clients to practice the exercise several times between sessions to strengthen the impact of the BE and gather as much experiential evidence as possible.

Using BEs to Identify Beliefs and Assumptions

There may be times when belief change is difficult because the client has had little real experience relevant to proving or disproving that belief or assumption. An example of this can be found in an exercise completed with clients with OCD who have ego-dystonic intrusions of physically or sexually harming others. A typical belief associated with this type of obsession is that if an individual is not careful, he will act on his thoughts, that the intrusion is a reflection of what he desires, and that it is his true self bubbling to the surface. For individuals who have intrusive sexual thoughts that coincide with genital awareness that is interpreted as arousal, it is taken as a further sign of desire. In such cases, clients are unaware of the difference between true desire and fear of desire. BEs can help to separate these two constructs. Designing such an experiment can be tricky, as what is typically construed as a reflection of desire, something sexual, cannot be used because of the interference from OCD intrusions.

Clinical Example

Jenny, a heterosexual female client, has been experiencing unwanted intrusive sexual thoughts about her female employer. The thoughts are distressing to Jenny because she believes that she is heterosexual and questions why she would have such thoughts if she was not a lesbian. Whenever she experiences one of these thoughts, Jenny's attention immediately shifts to her genitals, an attentional shift that she believes means she must secretly be sexually attracted to women. Jenny is not upset by the thought that she may be gay. In fact she states that she has many gay friends and at one point considered the possibility that she could be sexually attracted to women before deciding that she was only attracted to males. The thoughts bother Jenny because she believes that they mean she is not able to consciously identify her desires.

THERAPIST: Jenny, what is your favorite meal to eat? It could be a main course, junk food, dessert, anything that you look forward to no matter what is going on in your life?

JENNY: Um, that's easy, lasagna. I could eat it every day of the week and not be sick of it!

THERAPIST: OK, I'm wondering if you can try something out for me. Would you be willing to skip lunch next Tuesday, the day before our next session, and have lasagna for dinner?

JENNY: Yeah, I guess I could do that. That's it?

THERAPIST: I want you to make sure you don't have any snacks in between.

You need to be quite hungry when you sit down for dinner. And before you eat, I want you to write down a paragraph about what it feels like to experience the thoughts of the lasagna. Specifically, so you indulge in these thoughts or images? Do you let yourself fantasize about them or push them away? Do you like them, are they pleasurable, or do you dislike them?

JENNY: I guess I can do that. What does this have to do with the sexual thoughts we've been talking about?

THERAPIST: I'd actually like to talk about that next week. I know it may seem like it's unrelated to our discussion, but I'd really like you to just try out this exercise and report on your experience, without my influencing it in any way.

JENNY: OK, I'll give it a try.

As much as possible the intention behind the exercise prior to engaging in it is not discussed as it might take away from the experiential component of it. Jenny's therapist has also purposefully set up an experiment that will involve Jenny identifying her true desire for her favorite food, which can then be compared to the fear of desire she experiences during her intrusive sexual thoughts. Food has been used as the desired object to ensure that misinterpretation of physical sensations does not interfere with any interpretations Jenny may have after her experience.

THERAPIST: So, how did your lasagna dinner go last night? What did you notice before you started eating?

JENNY: Well, I had a lot of thoughts about the lasagna. Not only verbal thoughts like "I really want to eat this now," but I also saw all sorts of pictures dancing in my brain about different lasagna I've had that's been delicious. I swear I could taste it.

THERAPIST: When you had those thoughts, did you like them or dislike them?

JENNY: They were great. I loved them; I couldn't stop thinking about them. I started really getting into them, imagining all sorts of details like the steam rising off the dishes, the consistency of the cheese and sauce. I'm drooling now just thinking of it.

THERAPIST: It sounds like you really enjoyed those thoughts, almost as much as the lasagna.

JENNY: I did.

THERAPIST: Did you push the thoughts away at all? Did you feel disgusted or fearful in response to experiencing the thoughts?

JENNY: No, not at all.

THERAPIST: How similar or different are they from the unwanted sexual thoughts you have about your employer?

JENNY: They are nothing like those thoughts. The sexual thoughts are upsetting to me because I don't think I like women. I definitely don't fantasize about them like I did about the lasagna. They totally make me want to think of something else.

THERAPIST: So which experience do you think is more representative of you really desiring something, your reaction to the sexual intrusive thoughts, or your reaction to the lasagna?

JENNY: Definitely the lasagna.

Typically there is little overlap between true desire for something like food and fear of desire resulting from unwanted sexual or physical harm intrusions. An additional advantage of this exercise is that the type of meal or food can be referred to in a shorthand fashion in subsequent sessions to remind clients about the extensive differences between true desire and fear of desire (e.g., the lasagna experiment, the steak homework).

Difficulties with Implementation

The purpose of conducting BEs is to create an emotional response that can take over for a previously experienced response associated with anxiety, guilt, anger, or shame. Therefore, it is imperative that the experiment be closely tied to the client's symptoms and history. It is also important to avoid situations that will evoke little to no emotional response from the client.

Situations in which there is a high likelihood that a maladaptive belief will be reinforced, such as having Steve cross the middle of a busy street instead of crossing at a crosswalk with a functioning sign, should be avoided. Therapists should work with their clients to ensure that there is a high likelihood that they will be successful in their experiment, and will obtain evidence disconfirming their maladaptive beliefs, and confirming more effective interpretations. However, the purpose of the experiments is to provide clients with an accurate assessment of their beliefs. This means that there will likely be times when, despite the therapist's best efforts to guard against it, a BE results in evidence supporting a maladaptive belief. In such cases, it may be useful for the therapist to further explore the outcome with the client by asking questions such as: Was the feared/expected outcome as awful as the client expected? Was there any additional evidence suggesting that an alternate belief may have also been supported? How many times has the participant engaged in such an experiment and received a similar outcome? Every time? Infrequently? Such questions can help the client see that even though his feared outcome may occur, it likely does not occur at the frequency and severity he believes it will, and he is often much better able to cope with the feared outcome than he predicted.

If clients are not succeeding with their planned BEs, therapists should spend time examining any safety behaviors the client may voluntarily or involuntarily be engaging in, as well as any other extraneous factors that may be confounding the results. If the client is not completing a BE, it is possible that the experiment was either too difficult for the client, inducing higher levels of emotional arousal than the client was willing to tolerate, or that the client did not fully agree with the proposed cognitive model or rationale for the BE. In either case, further collaboration with the client may be necessary to fully engage him in treatment and have treatment progress at a pace with which he is comfortable.

Future Directions

Like most cognitive therapy techniques, BEs should only be used with individuals who have the cognitive ability and insight to identify and challenge their maladaptive thought and behavior patterns. Individuals who are unwilling to monitor and identify maladaptive thoughts or those not willing to engage in potentially anxiety- or distress-provoking situations would not likely benefit from BEs. Likewise, clients who present with emotional concerns that therapists, despite good efforts, are not able to connect to clearly defined maladaptive beliefs may not be good candidates for the use of BEs.

Although there has been an increase in the number of studies in the past 15 years indicating that cognitive framing of exposure is more effective than extinction framing in symptom reduction, more evidence is needed to support this claim. Studies that compare the specific techniques of cognitive versus extinction framing of exposure exercises, rather than the techniques as part of a treatment package are necessary. In particular, studies examining whether the mediating effects of cognitive change are necessary to achieve therapeutic benefits using BEs will further illuminate how BEs work as well as how to further enhance their implementation.

Further Resources

Articles

- For an excellent summary and analysis of 14 studies comparing exposure therapy to BEs in the treatment of anxiety disorders, see McMillan and Lee (2010).

Books

- See Bennett-Levy et al. (2004) for an excellent text on BEs in cognitive therapy.

References

Beck, A. T. (1967). *Depression.* New York: Harper & Row.
Beck, A. T. (1976). *Cognitive therapy and the emotional disorders.* Oxford, UK: International Universities Press.
Beck, A. T., Freeman, A., Davis, D. D., & Associates. (2003). *Cognitive therapy of personality disorders* (2nd ed.). New York: Guilford Press.
Beck, A. T., Rush, A. J., Shaw, B. F., & Emery, G. (1979). *Cognitive therapy of depression.* New York: Guilford Press.
Bennett-Levy, J., Butler, G., Fennell, M. J. V., Hackmann, A., Mueller, M., & Westbrook, D. (Eds.). (2004). *The Oxford guide to behavioural experiments in cognitive therapy.* Oxford, UK: Oxford University Press.
Castonguay, L. G., Goldfried, M. R., Wiser, S., Raue, P. J., & Hayes, A. M. (1996). Predicting the effect of cognitive therapy for depression: A study of unique and common factors. *Journal of Consulting and Clinical Psychology, 64*(3), 497–504.
Clark, D. A., & Beck, A. T. (2010). *Cognitive therapy of anxiety disorders: Science and practice.* New York: Guilford Press.
Clark, D. M. (1989). Anxiety states: Panic and generalized anxiety. In K. Hawton, P. M. Salkovskis, J. Kirk, & D. M. Clark (Eds.), *Cognitive behavior therapy for psychiatric problems: A practical guide* (pp. 52–96). New York: Oxford University Press.
Cooper, M. (2012). Cognitive behavioural models in eating disorders. In J. Fox & K. Goss (Eds.), *Eating and its disorders* (pp. 204–224). Chichester, UK: Wiley-Blackwell.
Fisher, P. L., & Wells, A. (2005). Experimental modification of beliefs in obsessive–compulsive disorder: A test of the metacognitive model. *Behaviour Research and Therapy, 43*(6), 821–829.
Goldfried, M. R. (2003). Cognitive-behavior therapy: Reflections on the evolution of a therapeutic orientation. *Cognitive Therapy and Research, 27*(1), 53–69.
Kamphuis, J. H., & Telch, M. J. (2000). Effects of distraction and guided threat reappraisal on fear reduction during exposure-based treatments for specific fears. *Behaviour Research and Therapy, 38*(12), 1163–1181.
Kim, E.-J. (2005). The effect of the decreased safety behaviors on anxiety and negative thoughts in social phobics. *Journal of Anxiety Disorders, 19*(1), 69–86.
Linehan, M. M. (1993). *Cognitive-behavioral treatment of borderline personality disorder.* New York: Guilford Press.
McMillan, D., & Lee, R. (2010). A systematic review of behavioral experiments vs. exposure alone in the treatment of anxiety disorders: A case of exposure while wearing the emperor's new clothes? *Clinical Psychology Review, 30*(5), 467–478.
Rachman, S. J. (2003). *The treatment of obsessions.* New York: Oxford University Press.
Rachman, S. J., & de Silva, P. (1978). Abnormal and normal obsessions. *Behaviour Research and Therapy, 16*(4), 233–248.
Raes, A. K., Koster, E. H. W., Loeys, T., & De Raedt, R. (2011). Pathways to change in one-session exposure with and without cognitive intervention: An exploratory study in spider phobia. *Journal of Anxiety Disorders, 25*(7), 964–971.
Salkovskis, P. M. (1991). The importance of behaviour in the maintenance of anxiety and panic: A cognitive account. *Behavioural Psychotherapy, 19*(1), 6–19.
Salkovskis, P. M., Hackmann, A., Wells, A., Gelder, M. G., & Clark, D. M. (2007). Belief disconfirmation versus habituation approaches to situational exposure in panic disorder with agoraphobia: A pilot study. *Behaviour Research and Therapy, 45*(5), 877–885.

Sloan, T., & Telch, M. J. (2002). The effects of safety-seeking behavior and guided threat reappraisal on fear reduction during exposure: An experimental investigation. *Behaviour Research and Therapy, 40*(3), 235–251.

Teasdale, J. D., & Barnard, P. J. (1993). *Affect, cognition, and change: Re-modelling depressive thought.* Hillsdale, NJ: Erlbaum.

Watson, J. C., & Rennie, D. L. (1994). Qualitative analysis of clients' subjective experience of significant moments during the exploration of problematic reactions. *Journal of Counseling Psychology, 41*(4), 500–509.

Wells, A. (1997). *Cognitive therapy of anxiety disorders: A practice manual and conceptual guide.* Hoboken, NJ: Wiley.

CHAPTER 6

Application of Exposure and Emotional Processing Theory to Depression
Exposure-Based Cognitive Therapy

Adele M. Hayes
C. Beth Ready
Carly Yasinski

In a comprehensive review of randomized controlled trials of current treatments for major depressive disorder (MDD), Hollon and Ponniah (2010) report that pharmacological and psychosocial treatments for depression have efficacy rates of approximately 60%. Cognitive therapy, behavioral therapy, and interpersonal therapy are as effective as medication in treating acute MDD, and the rates of relapse after psychotherapy are significantly lower with psychotherapy. Although these findings are promising, relapse rates are still high across treatments, and the risk increases dramatically with each subsequent episode. These data highlight the need to improve treatments for depression and reduce the substantial risk of relapse.

Exposure-based cognitive therapy (EBCT; Hayes, Beevers, Feldman, Laurenceau, & Perlman, 2005; Hayes et al., 2007) is a multimodal approach that integrates components of current psychotherapies for depression, principles of therapeutic change from the treatment of anxiety disorders, and principles of wellness and resilience. Within this framework, EBCT aims to reduce relapse by targeting specific risk factors:

1. The *avoidance–intrusion–rumination cycle*, which involves avoidance of emotions, a rebound or flood of the avoided material, chronic unproductive processing of emotional experiences, hopelessness, and further avoidance (Brewin, Gregory, Lipton, & Burgess, 2010).
2. *Depressive attentional biases*, which are characterized by an orientation toward and difficulty disengaging from negative emotion stimuli (Gotlib & Joormann, 2010).
3. A *positive blockade* (Disner, Beevers, Haigh, & Beck, 2012), which includes an attentional bias away from positive emotion stimuli, a tendency to dampen or avoid positive emotion, and decreased sensitivity to reward.

Targeted changes in these attentional and processing dysfunctions can increase flexibility, openness to new information and experiences, and healthy processing of emotional experiences. EBCT also teaches skills to build personal resources and increase resilience (Garland et al., 2010). The treatment is a cognitive therapy that adds principles of exposure and emotional processing from treatments for anxiety disorders.

Principles of Exposure and Emotional Processing in the Treatment of Anxiety Disorders

Exposure-based therapies are among the most effective treatments for anxiety disorders. Exposure therapy involves decreasing the pathological avoidance that maintains anxiety disorders and activating the fear structure related to a given disorder. The fear structure is an associative network of cognitions, behaviors, affect, and somatic functioning (Foa & Kozak, 1986; Lang, 1977). It is important to activate the different nodes of the network, and, in this context, to expose clients to novel information that challenges and destabilizes the pathological network. This dissonance between the old learning and new information creates the opportunity for *emotional processing*, which is indicated by new emotional responses to the feared stimuli and shifts in perspectives and meaning (Foa, Huppert, & Cahill, 2006). Exposure therapy also teaches clients to distance (or decenter) from conditioned fear responses and increase their tolerance for distress (Arch, Wolitzky-Taylor, Eifert, & Craske, 2012). In addition, it involves affect labeling, or putting words (written or verbal) to emotions, which has been demonstrated to be associated with less distress (Pennebaker & Chung, 2007; Lieberman et al., 2007) and to facilitate the effects of exposure (Tabibnia, Lieberman, & Craske, 2008).

Recent developments in human and animal learning research have further informed emotional processing theory. Consistent with Foa and colleagues' (1986, 2006) assertion that affective engagement is a critical condition of exposure and therapeutic change, both human and animal research suggests that the amygdala plays a central role in the acquisition, consolidation, and modification of memories of emotional experiences (McGaugh, 2004). Also consistent with exposure principles, research on the neuroscience of memory suggests that reactivating old learning makes it more labile and plastic. With reactivation, old learning can be reconsolidated and strengthened, or if novel and unexpected information is presented at this time, the old memory can be updated in a process called "updated consolidation" (Nadel, Hupbach, Gomez, & Newman-Smith, 2012). When new learning is strengthened over time and contexts, it can be used to inhibit or compete with the previous learning of the anxiety network (Bouton, 2002). Traditional exposure therapies have focused on weakening the pathological fear structure. Until recently, less emphasis was placed on developing a healthier associative network to inhibit or challenge the old learning.

Application of the Principles of Exposure and Emotional Processing to Depression

Moses and Barlow (2006) highlight important points of overlap in the psychopathology and treatment of anxiety disorders and depression. Some common processes that maintain these disorders include (1) avoidance of thoughts, emotions, and other internal stimuli (experiential avoidance; Hayes, Wilson, Gifford, Follette, & Strosahl, 1996); (2) maladaptive beliefs; and (3) repetitive, unproductive processing such as rumination, worry, and venting. These are the targets of exposure therapy, which might be a common intervention strategy. EBCT (Hayes et al., 2005, 2007) applies the principles of emotional-processing theory (Foa et al., 2006) and related principles of learning to the treatment of depression, a disorder with high rates of relapse and recurrence. A particular emphasis is placed on developing and strengthening a new, positive network to minimize the recurrence of depression symptoms. The application of exposure to depression requires some adaptation.

As with anxiety disorders, depression can be associated with avoidant emotion regulation styles such as experiential avoidance, disengagement, emotional blunting, thought suppression, and hopelessness (Hayes et al., 1996; Trew, 2011). Chronic avoidance of disturbing material is associated with a rebound effect, whereby the avoided material intrudes, overgeneralizes to memories that are thematically related (e.g., failure, defectiveness, helplessness), and feeds rumination and hopelessness (Brewin et al., 2010; Nolen-Hoeksema, 2010). Brewin et al. (2010) contend that this cycle maintains depression and, as in posttraumatic stress disorder (PTSD), reflects the presence of "unprocessed" experiences. From an experiential–humanistic perspective, Greenberg and Paivio (1997) also conceptualize depression as a disorder of avoidance and incomplete processing of emotional experiences. Worry, rumination, and other unproductive processing also focus attention away from other negative emotions and prevent the processing of difficult experiences (e.g., Borkovec, 2002; Watkins & Teasdale, 2004). Thus, both avoidance and rumination inhibit learning and must be addressed so that exposure does not inadvertently induce more hopelessness and depression.

Another set of processes that must be considered when applying exposure principles to depression are the depressive attentional bias and dysfunction in the positive emotion system (Gotlib & Joorman, 2010). The bias toward negative emotions and stimuli prolongs negative mood, heightens stress reactivity (Tran, Seimer, & Joormann, 2011), and can make it difficult for depressed individuals to benefit from new information, which too easily can be assimilated into existing depressive schemata.

The positive emotion system requires more direct intervention than with most anxiety disorders because of what Disner et al. (2011) call a neural "positive blockade." They review neuroimaging studies that demonstrate an attentional bias away from positive stimuli, decreased reward sensitivity, and decreased capacity to recognize, process, and sustain positive emotion. In addition, those who are depressed tend to actively avoid positive emotions and experiences and dampen those that are activated (Gotlib & Joormann, 2010; Joormann, 2010). This combination of problems interferes with the processing of new and potentially corrective information. In addition, it is difficult to capitalize on the benefits of positive emotions, which can spark "upward spirals" of physical and psychological wellness and resilience (Garland et al., 2010).

Together, these findings suggest that depression might be a disorder of inhibited processing due to the chronic vacillation between avoidance and rumination and the biases toward negative emotion and away from positive emotion (Brewin et al., 2010; Joormann, 2010). A central goal of treatment, then, is to facilitate healthy emotional processing, which has been proposed as a key mechanism of change in exposure-based therapies for anxiety disorders (Foa et al., 2006). A number of theorists have proposed that exposure and emotional processing might be relevant to the treatment of depression. For instance, Rachman (1980; Taylor & Rachman, 1991) introduced the concept of fear of sadness, akin to the fear of fear construct in anxiety disorders, and speculated that exposure might be useful to process this fear and address the avoidance cycles in depression. Behavioral activation therapy (Martell, Addis, & Jacobson, 2001) assigns graded tasks, which is similar to exposure, to reengage depressed clients and combat the tendency to withdraw and avoid. Teasdale (1999) proposed that cognitive therapy might produce its effects by moving clients from "mindless emoting" and "conceptual processing" (or intellectual analysis) to "experiential processing," which involves the engagement of emotion together with reflection and analysis. He further contends that having clients "decenter," or take a step back from their thoughts and feelings, is a key component of processing, as this allows clients to take a wider perspective and engage new information. Brewin et al. (2010) add that therapeutic processing involves verbalizing and contextualizing depressive memories, modifying maladaptive associations with this contextual information, and improving inhibitory control of old, maladaptive memories. Pascual-Leone and Greenberg (2007) also propose that emotional processing is a key mechanism of change in emotion-focused therapy for depression. Although explicit exposure techniques are not included in these treatments for depression, the emphasis on affective engagement, processing of emotional material, and decentering is strikingly similar to modern emotional processing theory in anxiety disorders (Craske et al., 2008; Foa et al., 2006).

EBCT for Depression: General Overview

EBCT applies the principles of exposure and emotional processing theory in anxiety disorders (Foa et al., 2006) to a cognitive therapy foundation for treating depression. We distill and integrate components from behavioral activation (Martell et al., 2001), mindfulness-based (Segal, Williams, & Teasdale, 2002), schema-focused (Beck, Rush, Shaw, & Emery, 1979; Young, Klosko, & Weishaar, 2003), and emotion-focused (Greenberg & Watson, 2006) therapies for depression. We also include strategies to promote wellness and resilience (Garland et al., 2010). Together, these techniques help clients reduce experiential avoidance, consider corrective information, process fragmented memories related to defectiveness and worthlessness, and develop healthier associative networks. It is important to be clear that EBCT applies the *principles* of exposure, but the techniques differ somewhat from those used to treat anxiety disorders, as they are adapted to treat depression.

Exposure in the treatment of anxiety disorders targets feared stimuli, such as spiders in spider phobia, internal cues in panic disorder, and traumatic memories in PTSD. In depression, we view fear and avoidance as related to emotions in general (positive and negative) and to deeply held negative views of the self, which center around themes of defectiveness and worthlessness. The depressive belief system is well elaborated and evokes strong negative emotions that lock into painful cycles of avoidance, intrusion, and rumination, and, at times, suicidality. These powerful inhibitory processes receive more emphasis in EBCT than in exposure for anxiety disorders. In addition, positive emotions and memories can be frightening because they can quickly convert into feelings of loss, dashed hopes, missed opportunities, and a view of the future as dismal and hopeless (Joormann, 2010). Emotions and one's negative view of self are the targets of exposure in EBCT.

The theme of exposure is infused in the entire course of EBCT, although it receives most emphasis in the middle phase of treatment. Exposure is applied in four ways: (1) weekly narratives that clients write about their depression to activate emotions and put them into words; (2) mindfulness meditation exercises to teach clients to decenter from and tolerate difficult emotions without judgment, avoidance, and rumination; (3) the activation and processing of memories related to clients' view of themselves as defectiveness and worthlessness; and (4) exercise of the positive emotion system, which activates fear, a sense of dread, and bracing for loss. Throughout the treatment, clients learn to acknowledge fears and emotions, use them as information, and become less overwhelmed by them. The final phase of EBCT aims to elaborate and strengthen the network of healthy cognitive, affective, behavioral, and somatic patterns that emerge in treatment.

Evidence for Outcome and Mechanisms of Change

Outcome

We have begun a program of research to examine the utility of applying the principles of exposure and emotional processing to the treatment of depression and the role of emotional processing in the change process. In the first open trial of EBCT (Hayes et al., 2005) with 29 patients diagnosed with MDD, the treatment was associated with a significant reduction in depressive symptoms and large effect sizes (Beck Depression Inventory–II [BDI-II; Beck, Steer, & Brown, 1996]: d intent-to-treat [ITT] = 1.73; d completers [comp] = 2.32). In another open trial conducted in Switzerland (Holtforth et al., 2012), EBCT was again associated with significant reductions in depressive symptoms (BDI-II: d [ITT] = 1.85; completers, d[comp] = 2.14). In a randomized controlled trial (RCT; Grosse Holtforth et al., 2014), both EBCT (N = 73) and cognitive-behavioral therapy (CBT; N = 71; Hautzinger, 2003) showed large between-group effect sizes on the BDI-II (EBCT d[ITT] = 1.52; CBT d[ITT] = 1.54; EBCT d[comp] = 1.87; CBT d[comp] = 1.82), and outcomes of two treatments were comparable. The effect sizes across these three studies were in the range of the benchmark effect sizes in a meta-analysis of 35 RCTs of psychotherapies for depression (Minami, Wampold, Serlin, Kircher, & Brown, 2007). Thus, the initial findings on the efficacy of EBCT are quite promising.

The Process of Change

Empirical research seems to converge on the notion that the combination of emotional arousal and the cognitive reflection of its meaning, rather than the mere activation of emotion, is associated with lasting changes

(Whelton, 2004). As in exposure therapy for anxiety disorders, the exposure phase of EBCT is associated with affective arousal, but in the form of transient spikes in depressive symptoms rather than spikes in anxiety. We have found a cubic pattern of symptom change in each of the three clinical trials (Hayes et al., 2007; Grosse Holtforth et al., 2014; Holtforth et al., 2012). This pattern is characterized by a decrease in depression symptoms in the first phase of treatment, an increase in depression as the depression network is activated, and a subsequent decrease in symptoms. Ratings of clients' weekly narratives revealed that more emotional processing occurred during the exposure phase, and only emotional processing during this phase (and not earlier) predicted improvement in depression. In contrast, avoidance was associated with less processing and worse outcomes (Hayes et al., 2005, 2007). This pattern of findings was replicated using self-report measures in the two Swiss trials of EBCT (Holtforth et al., 2012; Grosse Holtforth, 2014). In the RCT, more emotional processing in the exposure phase of EBCT predicted improvement in depression, whereas this was not the case in CBT. Affective arousal and emotional processing have also been reported to be significant predictors of outcome in emotion-focused therapy (Pascual-Leone & Greenberg, 2007; Pos, Greenberg, Goldman, & Korman, 2003).

We next examined whether the process of change in EBCT might involve destabilization of the depressive network and the development of a more adaptive associative network, as proposed in modern emotional processing theory for anxiety disorders (Craske et al., 2008; Foa et al., 2006). Raters coded the content of clients' weekly narratives for cognitive, affective, and behavioral components of a depressive network and for a positive network (Hayes, Yasinski, Ready, & Laurenceau, 2014). As would be predicted by emotional processing theory, more processing during the second phase of EBCT was indeed associated with destabilization of the depressive network and with more activation of the positive network, which in turn predicted depression at the 3-month follow-up. Putting words to feelings in therapy and in the between-session narratives is also likely to be an important aspect of processing (Arch et al., 2012; Pennebaker & Chung, 2007). These findings are consistent with research showing that the interconnectedness and strength of positive and negative cognitive self-schemas change with cognitive therapy (Dozois et al., 2009).

Application: Implementation on a Practical Level

EBCT consists of 21 weekly sessions of individual therapy delivered in three phases (Stress Management, Exposure and Processing, and Positive Growth and Consolidation) and three monthly continuation sessions. Clients write essays about their depression each week throughout the course of treatment. These essays help them to identify depressive patterns, engage in affect labeling and emotional processing between sessions, and become aware of stuck points and positive changes. The treatment occurs in phases but is flexible, as clients might need more or less emphasis on the components in a given phase of EBCT.

Stress Management Phase (Phase I: Sessions 1–8)

Goals of Phase I

- Decrease patterns that inhibit change: rumination, avoidance, hopelessness.
- Increase coping and problem-solving skills to decrease stress generation.
- Build personal resources for change and general wellness: mindfulness meditation, healthy eating, sleeping, and exercise habits.

Depression is maintained by a number of inhibitors that can interfere with engagement in exposure exercises, block access to new information, and interfere with the mood repair benefits of positive emotion. The default avoidance–intrusion–rumination cycle, the attentional biases toward negative stimuli and away from positive stimuli, and the dysfunction in the positive emotion system are inhibitory processes that must be addressed to ready the person for change. This is the focus of Phase I.

Approach and acceptance-based coping skills and mindfulness meditation are taught to counter the tendency to avoid and ruminate. Clients keep avoidance and rumination logs between sessions to identify the triggers for these response styles and the early warning signs that they are overusing them. Therapists also use the weekly essays as an additional source of information on avoidance and rumination and can illustrate the effects of these strategies on functioning. Coping and problem-solving skills and mindfulness meditation are taught as healthy alternatives to these default depressive responses. Mindfulness meditation teaches clients to engage with emotions (both positive and negative) in a healthy way, increase distress tolerance, unhook from the depressive cascade, and decrease critical judgment of self and others. This stress management phase of EBCT also teaches healthy lifestyle habits related to eating, sleeping, and exercise to counter the physical depletion that so often accompanies depression. The skills taught in this phase help reduce stress generation and mood reactivity, two significant predictors of depression relapse (Hammen, 2012; van Rijsbergen et al., 2013).

In this phase of treatment, clients learn the adaptive functions of negative and positive emotion and how they tend to respond to both types of emotion. They learn about the tendencies to dismiss, dampen, or miss altogether positive emotions and experiences, and how such problems with positive emotion feed the disorder. Behavioral activation exercises jumpstart and exercise the positive emotion system and tune clients to detect, encode, and elaborate positives. They learn that the depressive network of cognitions, emotions, behaviors, and somatic functioning is easily activated, difficult to disengage, and densely interconnected. In contrast, the positive, more healthy network is difficult to activate and sustain and sparsely interconnected. A graphic representation of these networks helps to make this concept more concrete. This metaphor is revisited in the next phase of treatment.

Exposure and Processing Phase (Phase II: Sessions 9–17)

Goals of Phase II

- Identify the "depressive network" (cognitive, affective, behavioral, somatic components).
- Identify what sets off or triggers the depressive network.
- Identify early experiences that contributed to the development of the network (learning history).
- Identify core themes related to defectiveness, worthlessness, and hopelessness.
- Help the client explore and make sense of depressive memories and core themes, question assumptions, see new perspectives, and integrate all this into a more healthy perspective.
- Start to develop a healthier network.

This phase of treatment involves going into the core of the depression and exploring one's most negative view of self, without avoiding, ruminating, and overgeneralizing. Clients gradually face what is most feared and overwhelming and do so from a healthy distance. This is difficult and disturbing. As clients explore their view of themselves as defective, a failure, and fundamentally flawed, they apply the principles of mindful curiosity and nonjudgment, and the emotions are less overwhelming. They can then explore more differentiated facets of themselves and break out of the narrow focus on the defective and worthless self.

General Principles

PREPARATION

The exposure phase of therapy induces a temporary increase in distress, so it is important to assess readiness to undergo this process. This phase of treatment is not recommended for those in the midst of destabilizing life events, such as a death in the family, divorce, or bankruptcy. However, if the problems are ongoing and under control, most clients can tolerate the distress associated with this phase. The intensity of the work can be modulated each week, if the stressor becomes more critical on a given week. This more intense exposure work is also not recommended for clients with borderline personality disorder, psychotic symptoms, ongoing substance abuse, suicidality, or homicidality. Indicators of readiness by the end of Phase I include some reduction in depression, avoidance, and rumination, and evidence that distress tolerance and emotion regulation skills are being applied to ongoing life events. If the client is not yet ready to begin Phase II, Phase I can be continued to help stabilize him or her and improve coping and distress tolerance as needed. It is also possible to move forward with the exposure exercises with lower levels of emotional engagement that the person can tolerate.

EMOTIONAL ENGAGEMENT

In order to facilitate processing in EBCT, therapists activate the depressive network, and clients process the experiences without avoiding and ruminating. If emotional engagement is too low, the depressive network is not fully activated, and there is usually some avoidance. If emotional engagement is too high, the client can begin ruminating, overgeneralizing, and become highly emotional. Such conditions are not optimal for processing and can reinforce emotional avoidance. It is therefore important to maintain a moderate level of engagement and affective arousal. As with exposure for anxiety disorders, therapists assess the levels of distress throughout the exercises to get a sense of how disturbing the material is for that person. Hembree, Rauch, and Foa (2003) provide a useful guide of indicators of underengagement and overengagement and strategies to modulate level of engagement.

Low levels of engagement can be marked by flat or blunted emotion, overly intellectualized or detailed responses, distraction or lack of focus, as well as inappropriate humor, venting, or blaming of others. Therapists can help clients understand why the avoidance is occurring and how it maintains depression. They can also ask for more detail and emotion words. Reflective listening skills can be used to highlight and amplify the client's affect, as can focusing attention on multiple modalities (thoughts, feelings, emotions, and somatic responses). Tuning into somatic responses can be especially evocative. Excessive levels of emotion can be indicated by high ratings of distress that continue with little change, high levels of rumination, and spreading across time frames, past to future (overgeneralization). Feelings of sadness, loneliness, abandonment, guilt, and shame are expected, but panic and fear can indicate that the feelings are becoming overwhelming. Emotion can be contained by redirecting attention to less threatening aspects of the experience; using mindfulness and breathing; interrupting rumination, worry, and venting; and moving the person from overgeneral to more concrete and specific thinking (Watkins & Teasdale, 2004).

EMOTIONAL PROCESSING

The goal of this phase of EBCT is to help clients identify their depressive network and recall key experiences that contributed to its development. Because depression is characterized by chronic unproductive processing such as rumination and worry, doing this without therapist guidance typically ends in hopelessness, avoidance, and disengagement. Now that clients have some control over their attentional biases, better emotion regulation skills and distress tolerance, and more engagement with positive emotions, therapy focuses on activating the depressive associative network and helping the client approach the disturbing material. The therapist helps the client to maintain a moderate level of emotional engagement and recount the experiences by taking a step back to get perspective. From here, he or she identifies core emotions and themes and make sense of fragmented and unprocessed experiences related to these themes. As the goal of this phase of treatment is to facilitate emotional processing, the therapist should look for indicators of processing, such as:

- Affective engagement: temporary increase in depression and related emotions
- Ability to stay with the memories without avoiding and ruminating
- Reflection and insights on how fragments of memory and experiences fit together
- Ability to see nuance and start to integrate information
- Depressive material becomes less disturbing (a decrease in distress)
- New perspectives emerge
- Positive, healthier aspects of self emerge
- Client engages in new, more adaptive behaviors and takes growth-oriented risks

How to Activate the Depressive Network and Facilitate Processing

The exposure exercises in this phase of treatment involve activating and identifying the depressive network, working through the fear and overwhelming emotion associated with it, and examining core depressive beliefs without avoiding, ruminating, or overgeneralizing across time frames and facets of the self.

THE DEPRESSIVE NETWORK (TWO SESSIONS)

In this exercise, clients are reminded of the concept of a depressive network learned in Phase I. The focus now is on identifying the cognitive, affective, behavioral, and somatic components of this network; what triggers it; and its history. Clients learn that understanding the depression network can reduce its ability to blindside or overpower them. They are asked to think about a time that captures what depression is like for them and to describe the experience as if they are reliving it. They should choose a recent example when they felt particularly depressed. The essays from the early weeks of treatment can be useful to stimulate ideas. Historical memories that capture more general themes are not used until the next exercise, when the exposure is more emotionally evocative. As in exposure exercises for anxiety disorders, therapists focus clients' attention on multiple domains of functioning. They are asked to describe the depressive thoughts about the self (related to themes of defectiveness, worthlessness, and hopelessness), and the associated emotions, behaviors (coping responses, compensatory strategies), and somatic responses that they experienced during this time. They are also asked about their views of others, how they respond to others, and how others respond to them to provide interpersonal context. Finally, clients identify the historical experiences that might have contributed to their beliefs. A time perspective is added by having clients present a timeline of each previous depressive episode and the precipitants of each episode to show the fluctuation of the depressive network, high-risk situations, and network triggers. Therapists should check-in with clients regarding their level of distress throughout this exercise to guide the intensity of the experience. Markers of affective engagement and strategies for modulating the intensity of exercises are presented in the earlier "Emotional Engagement" section.

This exercise makes explicit and concrete the pattern of responses that characterize one's depression. Clients are told that because this network has been activated and examined in therapy, they are likely to feel particularly sensitive and raw between sessions. Unlike exposure treatments for anxiety disorders, clients are not instructed to repeat exposures between sessions. The work of exposure is done in session with the therapist because of the difficulty controlling rumination and hopelessness. Clients are reminded that the tendencies to ruminate and avoid will be strong, but they are to practice the skills that they learned in Phase I to disengage from these maladaptive strategies and use more adaptive coping.

CASE EXAMPLE. Jemma is an African American woman in her early 30s who identified as a lesbian and had been in a long-term relationship for 2 years. She had three previous depressive episodes, each preceded by an interpersonal loss or rejection. She was on no psychiatric medication and had been in supportive therapy once after the first episode of depression.

On occasion, she had panic attacks, although she did not meet criteria for panic disorder. Her parents were from Africa, where she had lived when she was younger. The cultural values of that country and Catholicism were the foundation of the family's values.

In this context, Jemma was viewed as a source of shame for the family because of her sexual orientation. She also received the message to temper her dreams because she is female and therefore limited. Her lifestyle was viewed as defying the cultural norms and bringing shame to the family. This left her feeling defective, unlovable, and disconnected from family, religion, and country. These cognitions were associated with feeling sad, lonely, alienated, ashamed, and angry. Her attempts to regulate these feelings included being a "super coper," trying to be perfect and please others (especially her family), self-sacrificing, suppressing her emotions, keeping a distance from others, and at times lashing out. The tension of emotional suppression took its toll physically in the form of panic attacks, gastrointestinal distress, and muscle tension. These feelings of inadequacy and vulnerability were associated with an avoidant style of interacting with others and compulsive self-reliance. She was guarded because relationships meant more burden and responsibility to bear. She vacillated between what she called "total emotional control and distance" to "child-like vulnerability." In the latter state, she would have "meltdowns" with long periods of depressed mood and trouble engaging with others, talking, or even getting out of bed. It was difficult for her to be there for her partner and to receive help. Offers of help and support would make her feel more weak and like a failure, which in turn would trigger fears of abandonment. The network was triggered by perceived interpersonal criticism and rejection, particularly from her partner and family. The historical roots of the core sense of defectiveness related to messages from her parents that family needs should be put above her own needs and that she was inadequate because she is female and gay. In other words, she started out early in life with two strikes against her and no way out. After gathering this information, the therapist created a graphic representation of the cognitive (defective, unlovable, disconnected), affective (sad, lonely, alienated, ashamed, and angry), behavioral (suppress emotions, self-sacrifice, please others, lash out, keep a distance), and somatic (panic attacks, gastrointestinal distress, and muscle tension) components of Jemma's depressive network. This helps the client to concretely understand the patterns and vicious cycles that get activated, as well as what sets off this depressive reaction.

THE DEPRESSIVE NETWORK: GOING INTO THE CORE
(TWO TO THREE SESSIONS)

Clients are next told that therapy will involve going into the core negative beliefs about the self now that they are less depressed. The first exercise is more descriptive, and therapists explain that in this second exposure exercise, clients will access memories and emotions that are more painful and fundamental. Clients are oriented by the therapist to take a stance of openness, curiosity, and nonjudgment about the depressive material, as they learned in the mindfulness exercises. The therapist also takes this stance and must not fear the deep emotions and disturbance that arise or try to fix or quell the distress prematurely. As our data on the process of change suggest (Hayes et al., 2014), this disturbance can reflect a loosening of the client's negative perspectives of self and world, which is an opportunity for new ways of thinking, feeling, and behaving to emerge. Although it is difficult to sit with pain, it is critical for both client and therapist to do so. As with exposure for anxiety disorders, it is at times counterintuitive that such raw pain can be therapeutic. The work in this phase of EBCT involves not simply venting and catharsis, but rather trying to understand what is so fundamentally flawed about the person and looking at this sense of defectiveness and worthlessness with curiosity, rather than with the harsh lens of criticism and self-loathing that is so characteristic of depression. Therapists help clients to connect this negative view of self with experiences associated with its development and to process those experiences.

Clients work through at least two memories that epitomize their feelings of defectiveness and worthlessness. Therapists can begin by helping clients identify a memory that is particularly evocative or representative of their negative view of the self. For some, this may be a childhood memory involving a salient experience with an early caregiver, while for others it may be an experience that occurred during the teenage or adulthood years, such as experiences related to suicidal periods or relationship dissolutions. Once a memory is chosen, clients are guided to describe the experience in detail and to involve multiple modalities, much like exposure exercises in PTSD (Foa & Rothbaum, 1998). Therapists may ask clients to close their eyes if they feel that this will contribute to an optimal level of emotional engagement. They may leave their eyes open if they appear to be fully engaged, or if they have a tendency toward overengagement. Clients recall the event in the initial part of this exercise with little interruption from the therapist, and this is followed by more processing of the memory than is often the case when treating anxiety disorders. Imagery and rescripting therapy (Wheatley et al., 2007) involves a similar recall of traumatic memories related to depression, but EBCT focuses on examining and processing these memories as they relate to one's view of self and does not involve rewriting or changing the outcome of the memory.

The therapist should adopt an open-ended and reflective style that is characteristic of emotion-focused therapy (Greenberg & Watson, 2006) and other client-centered approaches, rather than a more traditional cognitive therapy style. Questions and reflections should be used to increase activation and awareness of emotion and to aid the client in making connections and gaining insight into the origin of his or her negative self-schemas and how its components interconnect. It is especially important to assess distress levels during these exercises and to use this information at the end of the exercise to illustrate how the client was able to tolerate what was considered intolerable.

Clients are then asked to describe how they view themselves when they are most depressed, how they put themselves down, and the possible sources of these feelings. The therapist has the client attend to subtle nuances and work through the depressive tendency to focus on negative aspects and ignore or minimize positive aspects of their experiences. Using mindfulness skills to engage emotional content without ruminating, avoiding, or becoming overwhelmed, they are able to understand how messages from others and experiences shaped this depressive view of self and to consider the context relevant at that time. They are taught to stay with the specific experience and not to overgeneralize to multiple examples of defectiveness and failure that span past, present, and future time frames. As in exposure therapy for PTSD (Foa & Rothbaum, 1998), clients' perspectives begin to broaden, they can consider more information, and their memories of the experiences become less fragmented and more coherent. The essay writing during this period can facilitate this process.

This exercise should be completed with at least two separate memories. This section of therapy can be increased by a few sessions if clients are having difficulty with avoidance or putting words to feelings. The therapeutic alliance is particularly important during this exercise, as is the therapist's willingness to experience or "sit with" emotion in session. The despair and hopelessness associated with the depressive core can be a powerful mood induction for the therapist. Therapists should be aware of their own tendency to downplay or avoid their emotions, as this can give the wrong signal to their clients and reduce the impact of this exercise.

CASE EXAMPLE. Jemma recalled two experiences in which she felt defective, shameful, and profoundly alienated from her family, religion, and country of origin. The memories included early messages from her father that she should give up her dreams because she is a female and that she must do well in school or she would end up as a prostitute. She was told that she was a sinner in the eyes of God and a shame to the family because she was a lesbian. Her parents, however, expected her to take care of the family and handle all of the family emergencies. She described feeling like the family servant and mediator, but not loved. She was an efficient machine and was supposed to handle everything, with no emotions or needs of her own. Jemma also feared coming out as gay because of the response of her family. When recounting these memories, she became visibly anxious and tried to get control over her emotions by minimizing the problems and apologizing to the therapist for her distress. The therapist asked Jenna to take a mindful stance and lean into, instead of away from, the emotions. She sobbed through much of the session and accessed her core view of her defectiveness, as a little girl who was never good enough and was hungry for attention and affection all of the time. She could not escape the prison of her gender and sexual orientation. Jemma did not trust anyone with these feelings and always kept a distance in romantic relationships. She feared being consumed, further burdened with self-sacrifice, and devastated if relationships ended. This was not unreasonable, given that each of her episodes of depression was preceded by an interpersonal loss.

After the description of her memories, Jemma reported during the processing part of the exercise that she felt weak and self-indulgent and that this was a good example of the weakness that interferes with her ability to be a good daughter and partner. She reported that she was damaged, incompetent, a failure, and stuck forever. Yet, she also saw a beauty in that child-like vulnerability that she felt in the session. It revealed a potential for real human connection, even if frightening. As she recounted the memories, she also realized she had a very strong side that maintained her identity against formidable forces of family, religion, and culture. Over the week, she reported feeling sensitive and out of sorts, and she had somatic symptoms of distress and was somewhat numb at times. Yet, she also felt some relief and lightness. The therapist let her know that this was the destabilization that comes from examining one's foundational views and the experiences that contributed to them. During this turbulent period, Jemma's interpersonal sensitivity, vulnerability, and fears of abandonment played out in her relationship with her partner. She felt urges to distance and lash out, both of which she did in moderation. Avoidance and rumination came back on line, as they often do, but clients have learned to recognize these strategies and to unhook from them.

FACETS OF THE SELF (TWO SESSIONS)

The processing of the defectiveness memories and experiences reveals multiple facets of the self beyond the defective self that is so prominent when depressed. When processing the memories with clients, therapists look for different sides of the self that contribute to depression and those that try to protect them from feelings of defectiveness. This exercise is not included in exposure therapy for anxiety disorders, but we consider this work essential because the self is so fractured and damaged in depression. Exploring the maladaptive and destructive sides of the self can also be conceptualized as a form of exposure, as this exercise activates a range of strong negative emotions that block processing. Some common facets of the self reported in depression include: (1) a hurt and beaten-down side, (2) a harsh and relentless critic, (3) a side that compensates for the defectiveness, and (4) a side that sees a different way and is more healthy. This healthy side is often difficult to access and is underdeveloped. Therapists help clients to identify the different facets of the self, their function, and how strong a role each facet plays in their lives (percentage of time active; these sides co-occur, so the percentage does not total 100%). The learning history of each facet is also discussed.

CASE EXAMPLE. Jemma had a weak and incompetent defective side. She viewed this part of herself as needy and scared. This side was at the core of her depression and was active about 80% of the time. She viewed this side as pitiful and embarrassing. However, when examining the function of this side, she realized that her basic needs for connection were felt and expressed by this side. Her critical side was active about 90% of the time and maintained the depression by constantly reminding her of all that was wrong with her, that her need for affection was disgusting, and that it was hopeless to think that things could get better. In exploring this side, she realized how harsh and insensitive it was. The critic's function was to drive her to succeed in life but, like her father, it had gone overboard. This motivational function was important but could be done in a more healthy way. The "super coper" side of herself, which was active about 80% of the time, developed strong coping and problem-solving skills to control her emotions and keep her ready to serve others. Depression was unacceptable from this perspective. This side also held unrealistic expectations of selflessness and perfection, but it also drove her to help others and connect with something larger than herself. Through these discussions, she realized that she likes to give and volunteer and that she could do this without going to the point of destructive self-sacrifice. The therapist put the spotlight on another facet of herself revealed in the previous exercises on the core of her depression. Jemma described a side that was very strong and saw a very different life than what her parents, religion, and culture described for her. This side allowed her to pursue the life that she wanted, even if it meant feeling alienated. However, she estimated that it was only active about 20% of the time and mostly came out under duress.

Even with this work, the defective view of self is often so entrenched that more work must be done to dislodge it. Therapists have the client examine the core sense of defectiveness using more traditional cognitive therapy techniques, such as Socratic questioning and cognitive restructuring, that involve having him or her generate experiences and examples that are not consistent with this view. Clients then go through the negative view of self and examine what parts of this perception might be accurate and need acceptance, what can be viewed as a self-improvement project that they can change, and what is better accepted as unchangeable and out of their control. Therapists may use the traditional cognitive technique of examining evidence for and against specific aspects of the client's negative view of self, if necessary.

PUTTING IT TOGETHER AND MOVING INTO ACTION (ONE SESSION)

With an understanding of multiple, interacting facets of the self and how they developed, the client can build on the strengths and adaptive components of each facet and apply these in concrete ways in daily life.

CASE EXAMPLE. Jemma learned that her vulnerable side protected her from becoming hardened to the positive benefits of human connection. She decided to allow that side more expression, but in a mature way and without shame. She and her partner began couples therapy, and she learned to be more open and expressive in her relationship with her partner. Although Jemma recognized that the function of her critical side was to motivate her, her self-evaluation was unrealistically severe and harsh. The therapist helped Jemma use her motivation and positive coping skills to contain her self-criticism and engage constructive feedback. The super coper had excellent coping, problem-solving, and mediation skills, and Jemma learned to balance these abilities with her ability to be open, vulnerable, and engage with her emotions. She applied this side of herself in a new job helping underserved and impoverished children and in supporting her friends and family, but without self-sacrificing and ignoring her own emotions. In one of her weekly essays, Jemma noted that she was quite upset by a series of family events but that "I realize today that I am human, and that is OK." She began engaging in life from her healthy self. She was able to see how strong and competent that side of herself was and how open she could be in relationships. She came out as gay at work and in her community and reported a real sense of support and relief. In a stroke of good timing, gay marriage became legal in her state. She proposed to her partner and received a very positive response. Jemma also talked with her father in an open and curious way about his criticism of her. He explained that his motivation was to push her so that she could have the best life possible and avoid the limits placed on many African American women. He made clear that he was very proud of the person that she had become and that he was trying to accept her partner, although he had many cultural and religious issues that made that difficult.

Positive Growth Phase (Phase III: Sessions 18–21)

Goals of Phase III

- Identify and elaborate components of the "positive network."
- Exercise and strengthen this network.
- Practice self-compassion and solidify healthy lifestyle habits.

- Identify core values and begin setting goals to orient life toward these goals.
- Review the course of change, identify risk factors, and review strategies to disengage from the avoidance–intrusion–rumination response and engage the positive emotion system.

After working through the negative emotions that interfere with processing and deconstructing the deeply engrained core negative beliefs about the self, this phase of EBCT focuses on solidifying treatment gains and working on areas that need improvement so that the client can move closer to his or her goals. The focus of this phase of treatment is to develop and strengthen more adaptive patterns of behavior across the cognitive, affective, behavioral, and somatic domains of the positive network. This new learning can then compete with, and over time perhaps alter, the depressive patterns and help prevent relapse when the client encounters situations akin to those associated with depressed mood (Bouton, 2002). Therapists again remind clients of their tendencies to disengage from positive experiences and the importance of positive emotion in maintaining health, buffering the impact of negative life events, and generating upward spirals of positive emotions and personal resources (Garland et al., 2010). This phase of EBCT involves working with current strengths and also sketching out directions in which the healthy self can grow. This focus on positive aspects of one's self and on future growth orientation can be conceptualized as another form of exposure in that the exercises in this phase often evoke another wave of fear related to hope and the possibility of failure. One depressed client captured this well: "Things are so good that I am filled with fear. I know I'm going in the right direction—away from a harmful person and toward a more enriching life—but there are so many disconnects and unknowns. Depression, being so familiar, almost seems like a place where I can feel comfortable. I am anxious with my new life, waiting for the other shoe to drop." Therapists help clients to apply the principles that they learned when working with negative emotions in the other phases of EBCT. They apply the breathing and openness from mindfulness and learn to allow the positive emotions and hope and to savor such experiences.

The Positive Network (One Session)

In this exercise, clients are asked to build on what they learned about their healthier, integrated sense of self from the exercises in Phase II. They are also asked to describe what they like about themselves and to do so in as much detail as possible. They are asked to write about this positive self at home to elaborate this and to provide them with material to activate this view of self when the depressive network is strongly activated. They also describe how they want to develop this positive self. Similar to discussions of the depressive network, the cognitive, affective, behavioral, and somatic elements of the positive network are identified. The therapist can use a white board or flipchart to help clients visualize and integrate the information being discussed. The graphic of the positive network is shown again to illustrate how weak and underdeveloped this network is relative to the densely connected depressive network. Clients are asked to describe role models who might be helpful in developing this more healthy self. These can include figures in the media, characters in books, or people from their current or past environments. In a sense, this exercise involves creating a fantasy or potential self, which includes using imagination and creativity. Clients are encouraged to adopt a growth orientation and view this as a lifelong process rather than as an opportunity to disappoint and fail. They are then asked which people or activities in their lives could support this healthy self, who might discourage it, and how they can exercise it. They are encouraged to interact with their environment from this place, even if it feels awkward. Therapists check each week to see how these interactions went and give feedback.

Self-Acceptance and Compassion (One Session)

In this exercise, therapists bring forward material that clients learned in Phase I on mindfulness and self-care. Depression is associated with self-loathing, withdrawal from others, and often very little self-care and soothing. Clients are taught the importance of kindness to the self, even if flawed, and the ability to give a break to, calm, and pamper the self, especially in stressful circumstances. They learn how to release the narrow self-focus of depression and think about activities and strategies to encourage them to connect with something larger. They also note the areas of self-care that they neglect when depressed, such as sleep, diet, exercise, and leisure, and how to recognize when they are slipping into bad habits. Clients generate ways that they can soothe and nurture themselves when they are distressed or suffering. Therapists give feedback on their attempts to apply these skills between sessions. Mindfulness skills and behavioral activation are used to increase the client's purposeful engagement with self-care activities, which can increase the person's sense of worth and self-compassion. Initially, self-care can activate fears and feelings that they do not deserve this positive treatment, that taking time for oneself is a sign of laziness, or an urgency to attend to other chores or work. These activities often require that the client use mindfulness skills to accept feelings of discomfort associated with caring for the self.

Moving toward Goals (Two Sessions)

This exercise helps to sharpen what the client wants out of life and what has held him or her back from reaching those goals. Clients are asked to rate the importance of different domains of life, how satisfied they are with each area, and how they want to expand in those areas of most importance. The domains have been adapted from quality of life measures and are similar to the values worksheet in acceptance and commitment therapy (Hayes, Pankey, Gifford, Batten, & Quiñones, 2002). The domains include health, self-esteem, religion or spirituality, money, work/school, hobbies, helping others, romantic love, family, friends, home, and neighborhood/community. This exercise is also an exposure of sorts because it can evoke a fear response, as hope and dreaming are associated with potential loss and failure. Clients again learn to tolerate this distress and work through their urges to disengage from positive emotions. Behavioral activation activities are used to increase the client's movement toward these goals and values and can reinforce positive views of the self.

The therapist also reviews with clients the concepts of the depressive and healthy networks and notes that the depressive network is still in memory and will make appearances for a while. However, clients are now aware of this and can take steps to disengage and to activate the healthier network. They are reminded of the factors that can increase the risk of relapse—the avoidance–intrusion–rumination cycle, the attentional biases of depression, and their urges to disengage from positive experiences. The benefits of active engagement with positive emotion and experiences is reiterated. The client is asked to think about what circumstances could trigger his or her depression in the future. The therapist and the client work together to review lessons and skills from therapy and to plan possible responses to such high-risk circumstances.

Continuation Sessions (Two to Three Monthly Sessions)

Two to three monthly continuation sessions are provided so that clients can receive feedback on their use of therapeutic skills in their everyday life. These sessions are less change-oriented and more aimed at increasing generalization, stabilization, and further growth.

Future Directions

EBCT is based on a foundation of research on the psychopathology of depression, principles of change from treatment research, and principles of wellness and resilience promotion. The treatment is built on a strong foundation, and its efficacy seems promising in initial clinical trials. EBCT applies exposure-based techniques within a cognitive framework, and the process of change is similar to that in the treatment of anxiety disorders. An important next test is to examine the prophylactic effects of EBCT, as the rates of relapse and recurrence in depression are significant, and each episode worsens the course of the disorder.

Given the problem of maintaining the gains of treatment, another area of development is to facilitate the transfer of skills from therapy to the daily lives of clients. Our treatment team is developing a smartphone application (app) that can monitor and give feedback on the risk and protective factors that influence the course of depression. This app will be used to monitor the use of skills that clients are learning and then for 1 year after treatment coach them to apply the skills and provide information on risk and health. Such use of technology might have a significant impact on the generalization of treatment effects.

Another task is to identify concrete indicators of readiness to undergo the exposure and processing phase of EBCT, which is associated with turbulence and a transient spike in depression symptoms. A key principle of the treatment is that the person must be stable enough to destabilize. The loosening of old pathological patterns creates conditions ripe for change, but this same opening can also lead to a reinforcement of the old learning, a worsening in functioning, or to decompensation (Hayes et al., 2007). The list of possible indicators presented earlier in this chapter can provide guidelines for assessing readiness and could be examined empirically.

With the recognition of the chronicity of depression and the moderate efficacy of current treatments, researchers are moving toward more integrative and transdiagnostic approaches to treatment. Such movement suggests the increasing sophistication of an area of science. The overlap of the treatment approaches in this section of the book point to common themes across the various theoretical orientations, and exposure and emotional processing principles represent one such point of convergence. It is for this reason that these principles are at the heart of EBCT for depression.

Further Resources

- For a general overview of emotional processing theory, see Foa, Huppert, and Cahill (2006) and Whelton (2004).
- For helpful guidelines on exposure-based treatments, see Hembree, Rauch, and Foa (2003).
- For initial data on outcome and the process of change in EBCT, see Holtforth et al. (2012); Hayes, Beevers, Feldman, Laurenceau, and Perlman (2005); and Hayes et al. (2007).

References

Arch, J. J., Wolitzky-Taylor, K. B., Eifert, G. H., & Craske, M. G. (2012). Longitudinal treatment mediation of traditional cognitive behavioral therapy and acceptance and commitment therapy for anxiety disorders. *Behaviour Research and Therapy, 50*(7–8), 469–478.

Beck, A. T., Rush, A. J., Shaw, B. F., & Emery, G. (1979). *Cognitive therapy of depression.* New York: Guilford Press.

Beck, A. T., Steer, R. A., & Brown, G. K. (1996). *BDI-II, Beck Depression Inventory: Manual*. San Antonio, TX: Psychological Corporation.

Borkovec, T. D. (2002). Life in the future versus life in the present. *Clinical Psychology: Science and Practice, 9*(1), 76–80.

Bouton, M. E. (2002). Context, ambiguity, and unlearning: Sources of relapse after behavioral extinction. *Biological Psychiatry, 52*(10), 976–986.

Brewin, C. R., Gregory, J. D., Lipton, M., & Burgess, N. (2010). Intrusive images in psychological disorders: Characteristics, neural mechanisms, and treatment implications. *Psychological Review, 117*(1), 210–232.

Craske, M. G., Kircanski, K., Zelikowsky, M., Mystkowski, J., Chowdhury, N., & Baker, A. (2008). Optimizing inhibitory learning during exposure therapy. *Behaviour Research and Therapy, 46*(1), 5–27.

Disner, S. G., Beevers, C. G., Haigh, E. A. P., & Beck, A. T. (2011). Neural mechanisms of the cognitive model of depression. *Nature Reviews Neuroscience, 12*(8), 467–477.

Dozois, D. J. A., Bieling, P. J., Patelis-Siotis, I., Hoar, L., Chudzik, S., McCabe, K., et al. (2009). Changes in self-schema structure in cognitive therapy for major depressive disorder: A randomized clinical trial. *Journal of Consulting and Clinical Psychology, 77*(6), 1078–1088.

Foa, E. B., Huppert, J. D., & Cahill, S. P. (2006). Emotional processing theory: An update. In B. O. Rothbaum (Ed.), *Pathological anxiety: Emotional processing in etiology and treatment* (pp. 3–24). New York: Guilford Press.

Foa, E. B., & Kozak, M. J. (1986). Emotional processing of fear: Exposure to corrective information. *Psychological Bulletin, 99*(1), 20–35.

Foa, E. B., & Rothbaum, B. O. (1998). *Treating the trauma of rape: Cognitive-behavioral therapy for PTSD*. New York: Guilford Press.

Garland, E. L., Fredrickson, B., Kring, A. M., Johnson, D. P., Meyer, P. S., & Penn, D. L. (2010). Upward spirals of positive emotions counter downward spirals of negativity: Insights from the broaden-and-build theory and affective neuroscience on the treatment of emotion dysfunctions and deficits in psychopathology. *Clinical Psychology Review, 30*(7), 849–864.

Gotlib, I. H., & Joormann, J. (2010). Cognition and depression: Current status and future directions. *Annual Review of Clinical Psychology, 6*, 285–312.

Greenberg, L. S., & Paivio, S. C. (1997). *Working with emotions in psychotherapy*. New York: Guilford Press.

Greenberg, L. S., & Watson, J. C. (2006). *Emotion-focused therapy for depression*. Washington, DC: American Psychological Association Press.

Grosse Holtforth, M., Krieger, T., Altenstein, D., Dörig, N., Meisch, L., & Hayes, A. M. (2014). *Exposure-based cognitive therapy as an intervention to foster emotional processing in depression: A randomized comparison with cognitive-behavioral therapy*. Manuscript submitted for publication.

Hammen, C. (2012). The social context of adolescent depression: Vulnerabilities and consequences. *Journal of Experimental Psychopathology, 3*(5), 739–749.

Hautzinger, M. (2003). *Kognitive verhaltensthreapie bei depressionen: Behandlungsanleitungen und materialien* (Vol. 6, überar. Aufl.). Weinheim: Beltz PVU.

Hayes, A. M., Beevers, C. G., Feldman, G. C., Laurenceau, J., & Perlman, C. (2005). Avoidance and processing as predictors of symptom change and positive growth in an integrative therapy for depression. *International Journal of Behavioral Medicine, 12*(2), 111–122.

Hayes, A. M., Feldman, G. C., Beevers, C. G., Laurenceau, J., Cardaciotto, L., & Lewis-Smith, J. (2007). Discontinuities and cognitive changes in an exposure-based cognitive therapy for depression. *Journal of Consulting and Clinical Psychology, 75*(3), 409–421.

Hayes, A. M., Yasinski, C. W., Ready, C. B., & Laurenceau, J. (2014). *A method for *studying change in psychotherapy from a dynamical systems perspective: Emotional processing, associative networks, and state space grids.* Manuscript submitted for publication.

Hayes, S. C., Pankey, J., Gifford, E. V., Batten, S. V., & Quiñones, R. (2002). Acceptance and commitment therapy in experiential avoidance disorders. *Comprehensive handbook of psychotherapy: Cognitive-behavioral approaches* (Vol. 2, pp. 319–351). Hoboken, NJ: Wiley.

Hayes, S. C., Wilson, K. G., Gifford, E. V., Follette, V. M., & Strosahl, K. (1996). Experiential avoidance and behavioral disorders: A functional dimensional approach to diagnosis and treatment. *Journal of Consulting and Clinical Psychology*, 64(6), 1152–1168.

Hembree, E. A., Rauch, S. A. M., & Foa, E. B. (2003). Beyond the manual: The insider's guide to prolonged exposure therapy for PTSD. *Cognitive and Behavioral Practice*, 10, 22–30.

Hollon, S. D., & Ponniah, K. (2010). A review of empirically supported psychological therapies for mood disorders in adults. *Depression and Anxiety*, 27, 891–932.

Holtforth, M. G., Hayes, A. M., Sutter, M., Wilm, K., Schmied, E., Laurenceau, J., & Caspar, F. (2012). Fostering cognitive-emotional processing in the treatment of depression: A preliminary investigation in exposure-based cognitive therapy. *Psychotherapy and Psychosomatics*, 81(4), 259–260.

Joormann, J. (2010). Cognitive inhibition and emotion regulation in depression. *Current Directions in Psychological Science*, 19(3), 161–166.

Lang, P. J. (1977). Imagery in therapy: An information processing analysis of fear. *Behavior Therapy*, 8(5), 862–886.

Lieberman, M. D., Eisenberger, N. I., Crockett, M. J., Tom, S. M., Pfeifer, J. H., & Way, B. M. (2007). Putting feelings into words: Affect labeling disrupts amygdala activity in response to affective stimuli. *Psychological Science*, 18(5), 421–428.

Martell, C. R., Addis, M. E., & Jacobson, N. S. (2001). *Depression in context: Strategies for guided action.* New York: Norton.

McGaugh, J. L. (2004). The amygdala modulates the consolidation of memories of emotionally arousing experiences. *Annual Review of Neuroscience*, 27, 1–28.

Minami, T., Wampold, B. E., Serlin, R. C., Kircher, J. C., & Brown, G. S. (2007). Benchmarks for psychotherapy efficacy in adult major depression. *Journal of Consulting and Clinical Psychology*, 75(2), 232–243.

Moses, E. B., & Barlow, D. H. (2006). A new unified treatment approach for emotional disorders based on emotion science. *Current Directions in Psychological Science*, 15(3), 146–150.

Nadel, L., Hupbach, A., Gomez, R., & Newman-Smith, K. (2012). Memory formation, consolidation and transformation. *Neuroscience and Biobehavioral Reviews*, 36(7), 1640–1645.

Nolen-Hoeksema, S. (2011). Lost in thought: The perils of rumination. In *Psychology and the real world: Essays illustrating fundamental contributions to society* (pp. 189–195). New York: Worth.

Pascual-Leone, A., & Greenberg, L. S. (2007). Emotional processing in experiential therapy: Why "the only way out is through." *Journal of Consulting and Clinical Psychology*, 75(6), 875–887.

Pennebaker, J. W., & Chung, C. K. (2007). Expressive writing, emotional upheavals, and health. In H. Friedman & R. Silver (Eds.), *Foundations of health psychology* (pp. 263–284). New York: Oxford University Press.

Pos, A. E., Greenberg, L. S., Goldman, R. N., & Korman, L. M. (2003). Emotional processing during experiential treatment of depression. *Journal of Consulting and Clinical Psychology*, 71(6), 1007–1016.

Rachman, S. (1980). Emotional processing. *Behaviour Research and Therapy, 18*(1), 51–60.

Segal, Z. V., Williams, J. M. G., & Teasdale, J. D. (2002). *Mindfulness-based cognitive therapy for depression: A new approach to preventing relapse.* New York: Guilford Press.

Tabibnia, G., Lieberman, M. D., & Craske, M. G. (2008). The lasting effect of words on feelings: Words may facilitate exposure effects to threatening images. *Emotion, 8*(3), 307–317.

Taylor, S., & Rachman, S. J. (1991). Fear of sadness. *Journal of Anxiety Disorders, 5*(4), 375–381.

Teasdale, J. D. (1999). Emotional processing, three modes of mind and the prevention of relapse in depression. *Behaviour Research and Therapy, 37*(Suppl. 1), S53–S77.

Tran, T. B., Siemer, M., & Joormann, J. (2011). Implicit interpretation biases affect emotional vulnerability: A training study. *Cognition and Emotion, 25*(3), 546–558.

Trew, J. L. (2011). Exploring the roles of approach and avoidance in depression: An integrative model. *Clinical Psychology Review, 31*(7), 1156–1168.

van Rijsbergen, G. D., Bockting, C. L. H., Burger, H., Spinhoven, P., Koeter, M. W. J., Ruhé, H. G., et al. (2013). Mood reactivity rather than cognitive reactivity is predictive of depressive relapse: A randomized study with 5.5-year follow-up. *Journal of Consulting and Clinical Psychology, 81,* 508–517.

Watkins, E., & Teasdale, J. D. (2004). Adaptive and maladaptive self-focus in depression. *Journal of Affective Disorders, 82*(1), 1–8.

Wheatley, J., Brewin, C. R., Patel, T., Hackmann, A., Wells, A., Fisher, P., et al. (2007). "I'll believe it when I can see it": Imagery rescripting of intrusive sensory memories in depression. *Journal of Behavior Therapy and Experimental Psychiatry, 38*(4), 371–385.

Whelton, W. J. (2004). Emotional processes in psychotherapy: Evidence across therapeutic modalities. *Clinical Psychology and Psychotherapy, 11*(1), 58–71.

Young, J. E., Klosko, J. S., & Weishaar, M. E. (2003). *Schema therapy: A practitioner's guide.* New York: Guilford Press.

CHAPTER 7

Creating Change through Focusing on Affect
Affect Phobia Therapy

Kristin A. R. Osborn
Pål G. Ulvenes
Bruce E. Wampold
Leigh McCullough

Theoretical Introduction

Affect phobia therapy (APT) is an integrative psychodynamic therapy that seeks to help patients function better by resolving emotional conflict through reducing their avoidance of adaptive, activating emotions. The focus on emotion in APT is important for several reasons. According to Fridja (1986), emotions are the means and measure of a person's engagement with the world. Tomkins (1995) stressed that affects are biological motivating mechanisms that can be understood as having primacy in human agency. Maladaptive use of emotions has therefore been suggested as central to psychopathology (see, e.g., Gross, 1998, 1999; Gross & Muñoz, 1995; Schore, 2003; Southam Gerow & Kendall, 2002). Indeed, Post (2003) stated, "It is not surprising that emotional dysfunction lies at the core of a variety of psychopathological conditions" (p. 899).

The central goal of APT is therefore to help people experience and express their emotions in an adaptive way. Aristotle (as quoted in Leonard, Miles, & Van der Kar, 1944) said that anybody can become angry—but "to be angry at the right person and to the right degree and at the right time and for the right purpose and in the right way—that is not within everybody's power and is not easy" (p. 203). Essentially Aristotle was alluding to the idea that affect is important for social relations, an idea that is central to current theory and research on emotion (see, e.g., Fischer & Manstead, 2008).

APT is an integrative model of psychotherapy. The framework originated in psychodynamic theory and important concepts included from this tradition are conflict, defenses, and insight. However, the traditional psychodynamic concept of unconscious conflict between the id and the superego is replaced by a focus on the experience of emotional conflict, based on the theory of Tomkins (1995), and relies on the motivational function of affect. The conflict in APT is conceptualized as the tension between activating and inhibiting affects. The model integrates learning theory when describing how associations between affects are formed, how affects are experienced, and how affects are expressed. In APT, therapeutic change relies on an integration of principles from dynamic therapy (i.e., transference and countertransference, self and object relations), cognitive therapy (utilizing the time between sessions, psychoeducation, testing assumptions), emotion-focused therapy (focusing on and experiencing affect), and behavior therapy (exposure for warded-off affect).

Central to APT is the concept of affect phobia. APT defines an *affect phobia* as a phobia for experiencing or expressing emotions. Just like people can have phobic reactions to external stimuli—for instance, spiders, needles, or elevators—people can have phobic reactions to internal stimuli, importantly, their feelings. A person with a spider phobia will be fearful when in proximity of spiders and will avoid situations where he or she might come in contact with a spider. Similarly, patients may find various emotions aversive and engage in a variety of strategies to avoid them. The concept of phobias refers to an irrational *fear*, but APT uses the word *phobia* in a broader, more metaphorical sense, as APT recognizes that fear is not the only cause of avoidance of certain affects. A person with a phobia against experiencing and expressing anger might feel guilt and anxiety when anger is activated and might try to avoid the discomfort of experiencing this conflict between aggression and guilt by intellectualizing that there was no reason to set limits for herself, and she might try to avoid situations where setting limits will be important for her (McCullough et al., 2004; McCullough Vaillant, 1997). Although some of the symptoms and consequences of affect phobia may resemble alexithymia, an affect phobia typically is specific to certain feelings and has very specific dynamics involving relationships among feelings.

APT postulates that there are two broad categories of affects: inhibitory affects and activating affects. This distinction stems from the early writings of William James (1890/2011). James postulated that if affect is motivational there must be at least two types of affect: affect that motivates approach behavior and affect that motivates avoidance. Significantly, in APT one does not separate affects into categories without looking at the function they serve for a person in a specific context. Anger is a prime example. Anger can be maladaptive if it leads to aggression in the workplace, in intimate relations, or when driving a car, or is used to avoid intimacy or grief. As well, anger can be maladaptive if a person aggressively attacks herself, which prevents the person from experiencing positive affects toward herself. But anger can also function as an adaptive activating affect when it motivates the person to set limits with others, to resolve conflicts, and to express displeasure with others' inappropriate behavior. On the whole, anger, sadness/grief, closeness, and self-compassion tend to be activating and important for the person to experience and express appropriately, whereas anxiety, guilt, shame, emotional pain, disgust, contempt, and fear tend to be inhibitory affects because they tend to inhibit other emotional responses. Typically patients seeking therapy, who do not have problems with impulsivity, will need help to experience more of the activating affects and less of the inhibitory affects (McCullough et al., 2004; McCullough Vaillant, 1997).

An affect phobia is a maladaptive pattern that occurs involuntarily. An activating affect is aroused (e.g., sadness, anger, or joy) and an opposing, inhibitory affect (e.g., anxiety, guilt, shame, pain) is aroused simultaneously. If the inhibiting affect is so strong that it prevents or distorts the experience of the activating affect, the capacity to experience and express the activating adaptive affect becomes inhibited or blocked. It is not uncommon for any one activating affect to have more than one inhibitory affect associated with it. Feelings of guilt and shame might for instance be activated when a person is in a situation where it would be adaptive to experience anger. This conflict between the affects is uncomfortable for the person, and in order to avoid the discomfort the person uses defenses such as intellectualization or repression, or coping strategies such as avoiding situations where the discomfort will be elicited, or by ruminating obsessively. Even though defenses and coping strategies are different phenomena, they function similarly. Defenses tend to be unconscious efforts to ward off conflicted affects, whereas coping strategies often are conscious behaviors to achieve the same goal (Cramer, 1998). The end result is that this maladaptive affect pattern, the affect phobia, prevents the person from experiencing and expressing her natural reactions to events in her life in an adaptive manner. The relationships between activating affects, inhibitory affects, and defenses are summarized in what is referred to as the "triangle of conflict," one of two triangles in affect phobia that schematically summarizes important concepts in the model (see Figure 7.1; Malan, 1979; Menninger & Holzman, 1958).

The triangle has activating affects at the bottom corner, indicating that these affects are underlying phenomena in affect phobias. These affects

```
         Defense           Inhibitory
                            affects
              SELF


              Activating
               affects
```

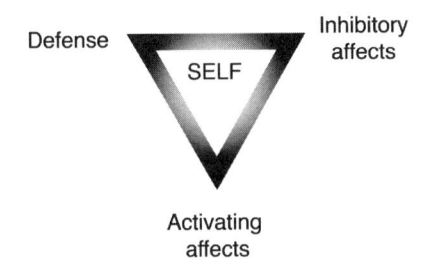

FIGURE 7.1. The conflict triangle.

are aroused, but through experiences the person has learned an association between these affects and inhibitory affects. The right corner of the triangle represents the inhibitory affects. In a well-functioning person the inhibitory affects modulate and adapt the activating affects to fit the situation in which the person finds herself, and the person is able to function well in a variety of situations needed to have a functional life (i.e., does not avoid situations where the conflict may arise). Shame might regulate grief so that a person will not sob while at the store, but allow the grief to come to the surface in the presence of supportive friends. But in an affect phobia the inhibitory reactions associated with the activating affects are too strong. The experience and expression is either strongly reduced or blocked. In order to ward off these conflicted feelings, the person resorts to defenses, represented by the top left corner of the triangle (McCullough et al., 2004; McCullough Vaillant, 1997).

Working with restructuring this maladaptive pattern is one of the treatment objectives of APT. Even if affects are basic motivational processes (Tomkins, 1995), maladaptive emotional patterns are learned, often very early in life (McCullough Vaillant, 1997). A typical example can be a young boy experiencing grief. He is told that men don't cry and his father shames him every time he feels sad. At the same time he might receive reinforcement from his father every time he is able to suppress his sadness, and consequently he avoids his uncomfortable reactions and seeks his father's approval by suppressing sadness. The boy learns that shame is associated with grief, and as a grown man the feelings of shame may prevent him from experiencing grief in his current relationships, thus sacrificing the intimacy necessary for close relationships. He is not able to experience and express emotions related to his losses, and might well then avoid situations where grief can be elicited. This pattern may also be present in the interaction with the therapist when the person comes to therapy. This patient's pattern of developing an affect phobia can be formulated in the second triangle used in APT, the "person triangle" (see Figure 7.2). At the bottom corner is the earlier relationship wherein the phobia originated, at the right corner

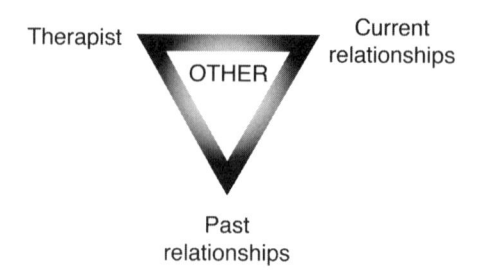

```
        Therapist  ╲▼▼╱  Current
                ╲OTHER╱   relationships
                 ╲   ╱
                  ╲ ╱
                   ▼
                  Past
               relationships
```

FIGURE 7.2. The person triangle.

is the current relationships wherein the patterns are experienced presently, and at the left corner is the therapist. Understanding the development and function of the maladaptive pattern in this triangle is a second treatment objective in APT. This is sometimes also referred to as "insight into maladaptive patterns" or "insight into defenses" (McCullough et al., 2004; McCullough Vaillant, 1997).

The patient's sense of self is an important concept in APT, and has implications for how one understands the patient's affect phobia. The renowned cognitive researchers Neisser and Jopling (1997) described an interpersonal self as an agent in social exchanges. People are co-creators of interactions with other people, and perceive themselves as acting in the real world. Neisser writes that a close match between the intentions and the outcome of a behavior establishes a strong sense of agency and of effectiveness. A person's sense of self can be understood as the behavioral expressions that he or she thinks are possible in a given situation (Bergner & Holmes, 2000). In affect phobia the self is understood as part of the affective dynamics. In the conflict triangle "self" is written in the middle. If a person can experience and express his or her affects in socially adaptive ways, the person will experience a strong sense of self. If, however, a person feels that he or she cannot tolerate or bear to experience or express affects, the sense of self tends to be weaker. Often one will hear patients with a weaker sense of self express things like "I don't deserve to ask for anything," "I have never felt proud of myself," or "I focus on what other people want; I don't know what I want for myself."

People with a stronger sense of self might need shorter treatments. Therapists tend to be able to start with an affect exposure, which is described below, early in treatment. Often these patients have acquired an affect phobia later in life, and treatment focuses on a specific event or on the influence of a particular person (like a demeaning boss). For example, a soldier who was trained to be stoic at age 18 may only need to focus on one specific trauma of military training to resolve symptoms. However, if a patient was repeatedly hit or ridiculed by his father for crying when he was a child, treatment may be more complex because the affect phobia is more ingrained. The patient might have a harder time with recognizing or experiencing the affects and may become confused by his or her affective experiences. The sense of such a patient is that if he or she experiences the avoided affect he or she would catastrophically disintegrate. Patients with a weaker sense of self might need interventions to help them strengthen this sense of self. These interventions include exposing the patient for feelings of closeness and self-compassion (which are placed at the bottom corner of the conflict triangle along with other activating affects), with the therapist adopting an empathic and accepting stance. In this way the therapist is providing an emotionally corrective experience with regard to the patient's sense of self. Interventions aimed at the sense of self are interspersed between exposures to warded-off affects to help the patient regulate his or her affective reactions to these distressing emotions.

Introduction to Therapy

APT uses the theoretical framework we discussed by helping the person experience and express previously warded-off adaptive, activating affect. The therapist aims at preventing the patient from resorting to defensive behavior, focuses on the activating affect, and helps regulate the inhibitory affect. Throughout this process attention is given to understanding the foundation of the phobia and the function the maladaptive pattern serves. In order to achieve these goals, therapists must be acutely aware of the affects experienced by the patient when talking about important events in the patient's life. The therapist pays close attention to the facial expressions and bodily movements of the patient, the pitch and tone of the patient's verbal expression, and how well these responses reflect the content of the verbal report of the patient, and whether or not important details are left out of the verbal report.

A primary characteristic of APT sessions is the elicitation of the adaptive activating affect, which serves as an exposure. Through inhibitory affects and defenses, the patient is unable or unwilling to express an adaptive activating affect. The therapist works to encourage the patient to experience and express the affect in the therapy session, and the therapist emphasizes that the patient can do this without being punished, humiliated, or criticized, as was likely the case for the patient in other circumstances in his or her life. Instead, the therapist will praise the patient for having the courage to express these difficult emotions. This process serves as an exposure, as the patient engages in the avoided behavior (i.e., expressing a particular emotion) in a safe context. Repeated exposures to the adaptive activating affect teaches the patient that the associations between the activating affects and inhibiting affect and defenses can be changed. The affect exposures typically are repeated several times, with the therapist pointing out the progress the patient is making in experiencing more of the activating affect, less of the inhibitory affect, and less frequent or more mature use of defenses. The exposures are repeated until the patient freely can experience the affects in the session. The exposure process can involve affects that are present when the patient is thinking of situations in his or her life by helping the patient re-experience situations using imagery exposures or by working with affects that are present between the patient and therapist. In order to help the patient experience the affects fully and freely, it is often necessary to help the patient experience affects and express them in ways that would not be possible or socially adaptive outside of the therapy room. After this is accomplished, efforts are made to make sure the patient understands the difference between the therapeutic work in a psychotherapy session and the adaptive expression of affect outside of the therapy room.

Take, for example, a woman coming to therapy after her son committed suicide, presenting with clear symptoms of depression and anxiety. She had a stiff and unmoving body when talking about the day when her son committed suicide. There were some signs that her eyes were tearing up as she talked about the events that day, but her voice was flat and she talked quickly and in a "matter of fact" kind of way, with little emotional content. She jumped from when her husband came running in to the house screaming that their son was lying dead in the garage to the day she was standing at the son's grave a week later, after the coffin had been lowered down into the grave. There was clearly avoidance of sadness and grief, and perhaps anger, in her description of the events. The therapist was able to aid the patient by empathically helping her experience the affects she had for these events. The therapist helped her to slow down her pace of talking, allowing her not to rush through the experiences, but to pay attention to what was happening to her as she told the story. The therapist then talked about how affects carry important information and why it is important to pay attention to grief and specifically about how grief worked in the body (i.e., psychoeducation about affect). As the patient was telling the story, the therapist emphatically pointed out when the patient was rushing her words, and when she was avoiding painful material, such as her seeing the dead body in the garage, helping her regulate the intense emotional pain she was experiencing, continuously and empathically orienting her toward the warded-off grief.

When the patient was ready, the therapist proposed an imagery exposure, having the patient imagine being alone with her son while he was lying in the coffin, and being present in the church before the funeral. The patient was able to express, with much emotionality in her voice, face, and body, her feelings of grief, love, and loss to her son, before she was able to say good-bye to him. The therapy then went on to focus on the meaning of loss and her identity as a mother. She expressed that as a child she felt she was unwanted by her parents. Her emotional reactions were never validated, but were often punished. She felt like she could not express who she was, and the first time she felt joy and a sense of worth in her life was when she could be a mother.

The remainder of this chapter presents research in support of the treatment orientation and interventions used in APT, before moving on to a more detailed description of how APT is conducted.

Evidence in Support of APT

APT utilizes techniques from several approaches to psychotherapy, including cognitive, Gestalt, and learning approaches, but the fundamental framework is psychodynamic. The interventions used in APT therefore have research support from several traditions. APT is typically regarded as a short-term psychodynamic psychotherapy. Shedler (2010) summarized the evidence for the general effect of psychodynamic therapy, whereas Leichsenring, Klein, and Salzer (2014), Leichsenring, Rabung, and Leibing (2004), and Abbass, Hancock, Henderson, and Kisely (2006) found evidence for the efficacy of short-term dynamic therapy for common psychiatric disorders. For personality disorders, Abbass, Sheldon, Gyra, and Kalpin (2008), Winston et al. (1994), McCullough et al. (1991), and Svartberg, Stiles, and Seltzer (2004) have found evidence supporting the efficacy of short-term dynamic approaches. Research on DSM-IV Axis I disorders and short-term dynamic approaches have found evidence for the effectiveness of these treatments for depression (Bressi, Porcellana, Marinaccio, Nocito, & Magri, 2010; Driessen et al., 2010; Leichsenring, 2001), generalized anxiety disorder (Leichsenring et al., 2009; Salzer, Winkelbach, Leweke, Leibing, & Leichsenring, 2011), anxiety disorders in general (Bressi et al., 2010), and somatic disorders (Abbass, Kisely, & Kroenke, 2009).

APT has in particular been studied in personality disorders with encouraging results. Using a first-generation APT, Winston et al. (1991) studied 32 patients with anxious–avoidant, histrionic, or mixed personality disorders randomly assigned to brief adaptational therapy (BAT) or to APT and then compared the results with a wait-list control. The two active treatment groups showed significant improvement on outcome and were significantly different from the wait-list control at termination of therapy. APT had larger effect sizes than BAT but the difference did not reach significance. In Winston et al. (1994) the previous study was expanded, with a larger sample size ($n = 81$), and the findings were largely replicated. In addition, the study also reported that improvement in target complaints were maintained at follow-up (mean time to follow-up 1.5 years, $n = 38$). Svartberg et al. (2004) studied 50 patients with anxious and avoidant personality disorders, many of whom also reported comorbidity with Axis I disorders. The patients were randomly assigned to either cognitive therapy (CT) or the current model of APT. At termination, the patients showed significant improvements on symptoms, interpersonal relations, and personality functioning, and results were similar at 2-year follow-up although there were no significant differences between the two treatments. At 2-year follow-up 54% of APT patient had recovered symptomatically, whereas 40% of the CT patients had done the same (Svartberg et al., 2004).

As already mentioned, APT has three treatment objectives: defense restructuring, affect restructuring, and self and other restructuring, all with their respective foundation in research and theory. Diener, Hilsenroth, and Weinberger (2007) found a relationship between therapist facilitation of affect and outcome for psychodynamic psychotherapy. Several studies of dynamic therapy have explored this relationship in more detail. Coady (1991), Hilsenroth, Ackerman, Blagys, Baity, and Mooney (2003) and Jones, Parke, and Pulos (1992) found that patients who had a therapist who focused or oriented the patient toward affect had better outcomes than patients who had therapists who did not focus on affect. McCullough et al. (1991) found that interventions that were followed by an affective response in the patient were associated with a positive outcome, and particular therapist interventions (viz., confrontation, clarification, and support) were important for the patient's affect experiencing (Town, Hardy, McCullough, & Stride, 2011). In fact, Ulvenes et al. (2012) found that avoiding affect was not associated with good outcomes, even if avoiding affect was associated with a good bond, and the bond often is found to be predictive of good outcomes. This finding has been interpreted to imply that within APT focusing on problematic affect is so important that it must be done even if it interferes with the formation of the therapeutic bond because the focus on affect leads to better outcomes, despite the attenuation of the bond. Sometimes it appears that patients know they have to do difficult work even though they would prefer to avoid it (see also Wampold & Kim, 1989).

There is evidence from theoretical orientations that are integrated into the APT model that support various therapeutic actions. Process–outcome research points toward the importance of both deepening and engaging in exploration of emotions (Greenberg, 1984; Greenberg, 1979; Mackay, 1995) and of engaging in imaginal confrontations (Greenberg & Malcolm, 2002; McMain, Goldman, & Greenberg, 1996) for producing good outcomes. However, there is also evidence that purely emotional activation (i.e., catharsis) may not be helpful (Bohart, 1977, 1980), and that an integrated experience of affect, self-narrative, and reflection is superior to only emotional arousal (Elliott, Greenberg, & Lietaer, 2004; Greenberg, Auszra, & Herrmann, 2007; Mergenthaler, 1996; Purton, 2004; Stalikas & Fitzpatrick, 1995; Warwar & Greenberg, 2000), which indicates the importance of working on all three therapeutic objectives in APT: helping the patient experience and express the conflicted affect, understand and reflect on the development and function of the defenses (or maladaptive behavioral patterns), and see the significance of this work related to the patient's experience of him- or herself and other people.

Practical Introduction to Therapy

To illustrate the process of APT, a transcript based on an American Psychological Association (2012) PsychTHERAPY video recording from a therapy session with Leigh McCullough, the developer of APT, is included below, with descriptions of nonverbal behavior and explanation of the therapist's intentions. The session is a good illustration of how working with the triangle of conflict is accomplished. There is, however, much happening in the session, including work on the triangle of the person and on the patient's sense of self and sense of others. Due to space limitations, only a transcript of the beginning of the session is presented to give a sense of how a session can unfold. The material relates specifically to how affect can be worked with in therapy and exemplifies the moment-to-moment tracking of affect as well as the therapist's effort to help expose the patient to activating affects in session.

The patient is a male in his late 30s. He has a son from an earlier relationship, but does not have much contact with him or his earlier partner. He is planning to get married, and this new relationship is triggering his sadness over being separated from his son. The patient is showing signs of anxiety.

THERAPIST: What would you like to focus on?
PATIENT: Ah, my son.

The patient is stuttering, trying hard to find words. His body is leaning over to one side, one arm clutching the other. It looks like he is trying to control an activation of his body. He is avoiding eye contact, and his facial expression is similar to one experiencing physical pain. He takes a long break before starting to talk. The therapist infers that the patient is trying hard to manage something inside of himself. As can be seen here, the APT therapist is focused on the nonverbal behavior and its inconsistency with the patient's verbal report.

THERAPIST: Is this hard for you to even talk about?
PATIENT: (*Laughs.*) Yes.

The therapist is trying to bring attention to the patient's activating affect by orienting him toward the difficulty he is experiencing when talking about what is problematic to him. The patient is displaying a defensive reaction. He has learned how to avoid the activating affect, and in an instant he is laughing while at the same time confirming that it is difficult to talk about his son. Clearly, it is hard for him to talk about what is troubling him.

THERAPIST: You are putting on a big smile.

The therapist is empathically validating the defense, but at the same time mirroring what the therapist hypothesizes to be the avoided activating feeling, a sadness.

THERAPIST: (*gesturing toward her chest*) What's the feeling that's coming up?

PATIENT: (*smiling*) It's rough.

While smiling, the patient confirms that it is difficult for him to be in contact with his problematic emotions.

THERAPIST: If you didn't smile, what would you be feeling?

The therapist is empathically probing for the avoided feeling. The therapist observes that the patient is able to take away the smile for less than a second and that he is thinking about or experiencing something, but the defenses are activated again, and a strong burst of laughter is present.

PATIENT: (*laughing*) Right, right.

The therapist notices that the patient is clutching his arm tighter, looking like he is striving to control himself, but the rest of his body is moving about like he is laughing cheerfully. Paying attention to his eyes and mouth, the therapist is able to infer that sadness is present.

THERAPIST: That smile helps shove it down, doesn't it?

The therapist is again orienting the patient toward the underlying feeling and commenting on the defense.

PATIENT: Hmmm, hmmm. (*His eyes and mouth suggests sadness.*)

THERAPIST: What has been the hardest?

PATIENT: (*Looks calmer, but not in touch with his feelings.*) With him? You know, we're close you know, we're close. (*Looks a lot calmer, but the smile disappears.*)

THERAPIST: You are close?

PATIENT: (*Nods.*)
THERAPIST: And you haven't been able to see him?

    The therapist is trying to build momentum for the sadness to come to the surface.

PATIENT: No, no (*shaking his head, looking down, with feelings of sadness more present*), not regularly. (*He is avoiding eye contact and his voice is not much affected by sadness, but he is swallowing.*)

    The therapist interpreted swallowing as a sign of anxiety or inhibition, as often swallowing is due to a dry mouth.

THERAPIST: Let me just point out, you had a big wave of sadness just now.

    The therapist has noticed signs of sadness and points out the underlying but not experienced feeling.

PATIENT: (*Looks interested but with a smile on his face.*)
THERAPIST: And you pushed it down. Can you feel yourself doing that?

    The therapist is helping the patient see that this is something the patient is doing actively himself, not an automatic process outside of his control. That is, the therapist is making the unconscious conscious, in a sense.

PATIENT: Sure, sure. It is interesting. Wow. (*laughing, and is looking with affection at the therapist*)
THERAPIST: You hadn't realized. People do these things automatically. What would it have been like to let that show here with me?

    The therapist is simultaneously acknowledging and normalizing the defenses. She is also using the person triangle by bringing herself, the therapist, into the dynamic of the affects, thus using the transference relationship therapeutically.

PATIENT: I have no idea (*still smiling affectionately*). I don't know (*speaking in a soothing voice*).
THERAPIST: Would it have been hard to do that?

    The therapist is exploring the inhibitory reactions.

PATIENT: (*Looks interested and thoughtful.*) Yeah, I think so, I think that would have been hard.

THERAPIST: Let us look at that because that is what we are here for right now. To look at things that are difficult. You know you have to stuff them down all through the day. It would be a shame to do that here.

PATIENT: It is weird, it is like, it's like it's all concentrated now (*pointing to chest, laughing*) it is so freaky (*hand covering his face while laughing*). Whatever the feeling is, whatever the thing is, you know. Now it is a little less, you know, I guess it's because I'm a little more animated. When I started talking a little more it gets less. You know I get to use my hands, and I get to be animated, and I get to forget about it. That's a little strange.

The patient is noticing how his behavior with the therapist is helping him manage and control his affects.

THERAPIST: But you are paying attention to it. That is good, let us pay attention to it, watch it go up and down.

After less than 2 minutes into the therapy session a few things are becoming clear on the triangle of conflict. Initially what was most apparent was the patient's defenses. The affective conflict was so uncomfortable and so ingrained that it was hard to see both the activating feeling and the inhibition associated with it, although the therapist was quite aware that the patient was suppressing the activating feeling of grief, as exhibited by smiling while talking about difficulties with his son. As the therapist continuously helped the patient examine the activating feeling, the patient was able to both identify that he is avoiding some affect, and how he was doing it. He is also able to understand that it is a feeling of pain and of roughness that prevents him from experiencing sadness. Mapping this exchange onto the triangle of conflict, we would have sadness or grief at the bottom corner, pain and maybe other inhibitory affects on the right corner, and defensive reactions like laughing, avoiding eye contact, becoming animated, and the like on the left corner.

THERAPIST: Is there any sadness left right now?

The therapist again is orienting the patient toward the sadness.

THERAPIST: Where do you feel it in your body?
PATIENT: Right here. (*pointing toward his heart*)
THERAPIST: What is there? (*looking empathically at patient*)

The therapist is actively using herself as part of the person triangle. She is communicating that the experience of the sadness is understood by the therapist (empathy) and that this feeling is accepted by the therapist (reinforcement).

PATIENT: What is here? Oh, that is my heart.
THERAPIST: You feel your sadness in your heart.

The therapist is anchoring the affect in the body, and orienting the patient again toward his feelings of sadness. In APT, it is recognized that affects have a bodily felt component, although the patient uses defenses so that it is not "experienced." Thus, the APT therapist will frequently focus on the somatic sensation of affect, and help the patient pay attention to and notice when affects create sensations in the body.

PATIENT: But it is more at the top of my stomach, yeah the same area.
THERAPIST: Is there pain there?

The therapist is trying to identify any inhibitory affects, again using somatic sensations.

PATIENT: Pain?
THERAPIST: Or is it sad?
PATIENT: Not like hurt pain but, probably like, I mean, if I, I would say, the feeling that I had, and since I'm rambling now it is not there. But the feeling that I had was probably thick.
THERAPIST: Thick?
PATIENT: Yeah, strange.
THERAPIST: And it really showed on you, you welled up. And you have a way of, as you say, you are rambling now, you have a lighthearted way of moving, it seems to pull you away from it.

The therapist is commenting on the patient's defenses, but in an empathic manner.

PATIENT: Yes, yes.
THERAPIST: That is something you developed no doubt to stay afloat and stay buoyant.

The therapist is acknowledging the defenses or maladaptive patterns, which were developed sometime in the patient's life. The therapist is also acknowledging that these defenses have helped the patient in his life at some point. It is central in APT, as well as other dynamic therapies, to recognize that defenses are adaptive in some instances or in some developmental periods, but that they are related to the patient's difficulties in the current situation, a theme that is pursued in the next few interchanges.

PATIENT: Yes.

THERAPIST: Are you typically very buoyant, like this?

PATIENT: Yes.

THERAPIST: That is a tremendous strength in life. It gets you through rough times, doesn't it?

The therapist is again validating the defenses, pointing to them as resources the patient has used to good advantage in many instances, but which are causing the patient difficulty in the present circumstance. The therapeutic strategy is therefore to not have the patient defend against the activating feelings, but to block the function of defenses in the session and try to bring the patient into contact with the avoided feeling.

It should be recognized that the goal of APT is not simply to have the patient experience the affect (e.g., grief/sadness in the present situation), but to utilize the affect to respond adaptively. The patient will be making some decisions about how to structure his relationship with his son, given his impending marriage. Decisions will be more adaptive for the patient when he is able to experience and express his grief. The patient will then be basing his decision on a fuller range of his affects that inform the patient what he is feeling about the situation. Because of the motivational function of affects, having access to a fuller range of affects will help the patient be motivated to choose more adaptive behaviors with his relationship to his son. The function of grief can be understood as motivation to help the person reflect and reorganize his life and future after a loss. Experiencing adaptive grief will enable other affects and behavioral tendencies to surface and help the patient navigate his circumstances and relationships. Having desensitized the associations between the adaptive, activating affect and the inhibition and defenses, the patient is also better prepared to handle situations in his future wherein experiencing grief will help him not become anxious or depressed.

In the present case, avoiding feelings of grief and sadness may lead the patient to accept the situation with his son; he would then tolerate not seeing him and being involved in his life. On the other hand, experiencing grief and sadness may motivate the patient to assertively ask his ex-partner for increased visitation rights and to demand that the ex-partner function better as a parent. The patient may determine that if the ex-partner is not adequately parenting the child, he may seek custody. None of these actions is likely without experiencing the loss of his son, as his inhibition has led to inaction and passivity.

PATIENT: I think so.

THERAPIST: But here we need to try to set that aside if we can, and help you touch into this pool of pain you are sitting on. Right, that's right there. About your son.

PATIENT: (*Sadness wells up, visible on the frown his mouth is making and the tightening of his eyebrows.*)

After having affirmed the adaptive aspect of the defense, the therapist is directing the patient back again to the activating affect that is being avoided. The therapist is helping the patient identify the feelings that are present and how his pattern of behaving is moving him away from his felt sensations of affect. The therapist has recognized the maladaptive pattern, empathizing with the patient and pointing out how the defense has served a purpose and was developed to help him in various aspects in his life, but that it might not help him in the current situation.

The therapist goes on to explore what inhibitions are present that prevent the experience of affects.

THERAPIST: As I say that, does it come up again?

PATIENT: No, but I am thinking about trying to let it, thinking about, OK, let me put my hands down and open up a little bit, because I'm kind of like closed.

THERAPIST: Right, right, good to notice that. The other thing that I think would help is just to be, let's just be, for a moment about, what it would be like to let down and open up and show that sadness. Are you able to do that in your life?

The therapist is exploring what inhibitory affects might be present that prevent him from experiencing his activating affects. This is also an attempt to expose the patient to affect. The therapist is checking if the patient is able to let go of his inhibitions and experience the avoided affect freely.

PATIENT: You know, people are eh, people have expectations (*smiling*) you know, they have expectations and hmm (*a slight expression of contempt is visible*).

The patient is using another defense here involving what others will think of him. The patient is feeling some expectations put on him from the outside. He believes that he is expected to behave in certain ways, and that these expectations are in conflict with his affective responses. We can infer that violating these expectations will lead to feelings of either shame or guilt and to the discomfort associated with feeling these inhibitory responses are obstructing the experience of sadness.

THERAPIST: What kind of expectations?

PATIENT: That, hmm (*looking down, tightening of lips, eyebrows clenched together, almost closed eyes, a facial expression mixing concentration and pain, and now looking up again*), I'm not sure, it just feels like it is inappropriate.

THERAPIST: I see, well certainly men in our culture are taught that boys don't cry. Right?

PATIENT: Right.

THERAPIST: But when you say people have expectations, that you are not to have feelings, that you are not to lean, is that it?

The therapist is testing out assumptions connected to the pain that is inhibiting his expression of affect, challenging the defense.

PATIENT: Yeah, well I don't know. I think I'm . . . It is hard not to concentrate on the camera now.

THERAPIST: That is all right, you don't have to apologize. Let's take a minute and think about that. This is being videotaped, what does that bring up?

When possible, the APT therapist works on the feelings present in the therapy room. These often occur when talking about troublesome issues, but here the therapeutic context is brought up by the patient, perhaps as a defense, so the therapist works with these feelings, as they are related to the central triangle of conflict.

PATIENT: Guard. There's 10 million people (*burst of laughter*).

THERAPIST: Ten million people, that is a hard thing. It takes a lot of courage for you to be here, doesn't it?

The therapist is accepting the inhibitory affect, while at the same time reinforcing a strong sense of self, another key component of APT. Here, the therapist hypothesizes that a low sense-of-self is also inhibiting feelings of sadness and therefore attending to the sense-of-self will increase the likelihood that the patient will express the warded-off affect.

THERAPIST: So let's take 1 minute and see what do you think me and the 10 million other people might be thinking?

PATIENT: Ahh, you know (*slight pained expression on his face*).

THERAPIST: Of you, if you were to let down.

The therapist is again testing assumptions related to the inhibitory feeling.

PATIENT: I don't know, you know, if I think about it for a minute, probably, I'm not sure, I don't think, I'm not sure, you know.

THERAPIST: Well, just let the thoughts come, there is some projection you are doing. You know that term? You project something out thinking there is going to be some way that you are going to be viewed. It makes you put up your guard.

The therapist has identified some thoughts and also some projections that refer to the patient's sense of others. These thoughts and projections interfere with the patient's experience of affects, and the therapist will continue to work on them and reduce their impact on the activating affect.

THERAPIST: So there is something that you are projecting out, I am going to ask you one more time. Let's just see if you can put some words on it. Let's imagine someone watching this session right now.

PATIENT: Pity.

THERAPIST: That they would pity you. And how would that make you feel?

PATIENT: I don't need pity.

THERAPIST: You don't need pity. There is a guard right there. It is a shame response. You'd be ashamed if someone pitied you. If they saw you so sad. As sad as you are in your heart.

The therapist is first pointing out the inhibitory affect, before accentuating that he is not showing the sadness in his heart, as a way of emphasizing the cost of his defenses.

PATIENT: Yeah.

THERAPIST: Well, let me put it this way, if there was a man sitting here (*pointing toward an adjacent area, opposite of patient*), telling the same story, and he was open and he could really show his sorrow, how would you feel toward him?

PATIENT: I would accept the guy, you know, I would.

THERAPIST: Is it hard for you to think to feel that others might feel that toward you?

The therapist is pointing out that he is not letting himself have the same understanding or compassion toward himself that he would for another. He has different standards for himself than for other people. The therapist is trying to regulate the inhibitory response.

PATIENT: (*slight pained expression*) I'm not sure. Perhaps you know.

THERAPIST: Perhaps they could feel accepting toward you.

PATIENT: Sure.

THERAPIST: That is hard for you to feel deeply. Is that what you are telling me?

PATIENT: It is hard to wrap my mind around why, . . . why are you guarded, you know, it's not the easiest thing to fit in.

The therapist has identified a feeling of pity and shame that is associated with displaying affect. The inhibitory affect is preventing the expression of affect in the session and in the patient's life in general. There is also an understanding that this is something the patient is putting on himself; he was able to feel acceptance toward someone else telling the same story and opening up. After working with reducing the inhibitory and defensive reactions, the therapist now moves back to try and help the patient experience the sadness associated with his son.

THERAPIST: You were starting to talk about your son and how awful it has been for you.

The therapist is redirecting the patient back toward experiencing the avoided activating feeling.

PATIENT: It's been hard. (*He is calmer and more attuned with the therapist, but a sad grimace appears on his face briefly.*)

THERAPIST: Just that flush of pain right there, you want to tell me about the worst part?

The therapist is again focusing in on the worst part to arouse the avoided activating feeling. This is a good example of the therapist utilizing the facial expression of emotion to infer an internal state.

PATIENT: You know, him, he's just seven (*hesitating a bit, rubs his face, looks down, inhibition rising*). He's smart.

THERAPIST: He's just a little guy.

PATIENT: Yeah, he's a little guy, he's behind in school (*continues to rub his eyes*). He's behind, he's behind (*tears seems to be appearing*) the curve, every time . . .

THERAPIST: Yeah, yeah.

The therapist is empathically supporting the patient's initial expressions of the activating feeling, encouraging him to continue experiencing the sadness.

PATIENT: I get to see him for a year, and then he is gone for a year.
THERAPIST: You didn't get to see him for a year.

The therapist is restating the patients' response to help him experience the significance of what he is talking about

PATIENT: No, and ah.
THERAPIST: What must that have done to you?

The therapist is again focusing in on the patient's emotionally felt experience of his separation from his son.

PATIENT: It was terrible, you know you think about, not every day, I don't think about him every day, but I think about him often.
THERAPIST: And what would you be feeling in your heart?

The therapist is orienting the patient toward his affective reaction rooted in his heart, where he identified the somatic experience of his affective response.

PATIENT: Mad, sad, mad, you know.
THERAPIST: Mad, sad, and all those.
PATIENT: Sure, you know it's rough, some days some nights I wait long.
THERAPIST: You'll have a long painful worry, what do you worry the most about?

The therapist is restating the patient's response to encourage sadness. Notice how the patient also brought up that he was feeling angry. While anger certainly can be an adaptive response to his experience with his expartner, the response is now interfering with experiencing sadness and actually has a defensive function, as we discussed earlier. Notice that the therapist did not say that the anger is maladaptive. There is a refocus of attention, and the anger might be brought back up at a later time in therapy. The therapist is therefore trying to redirect the patient to experiencing the sadness. This illustrates two important points. First, it is important for the therapist to follow his or her conceptualization of the client, based on the conflict triangle; here the therapist has conceptualized sadness/grief as the central suppressed activating affect and that anger is being used defensively. Second, such conceptualizations should, however, be considered hypotheses, and the continuing work will determine the role of anger for this patient. The therapist will want to keep in mind the uncertainty about the role of anger and to test his or her hypothesis that sadness and grief are central, but for now, the therapist follows the working conceptualization of this client.

PATIENT: (*sorrow starting to appear; he is rubbing his eyes again*) That he is not getting what he needs. His mother [inaudible] she is smart, you know, but, for instance (*looks sad, swallows, tears rolling down his cheeks*) first time when he came to live with me for a stay . . .

THERAPIST: He lived with you for 5 months.

PATIENT: Yeah, but then his mother came and snatched him up. I didn't see him for a year before that, and then she kind of just dropped him off—"I'm moving to Arizona"—you know, I saw him for a couple of weeks before that. And when I got him, he couldn't wipe himself properly, he couldn't tie his shoes . . .

THERAPIST: Let me just slow you down a little bit. One way you stay away from the feeling is talking fast. Let's just take a deep breath and stay with it, 'cause that must have broken your heart.

The therapist observes that there is a mismatch between the displayed emotion and the story the patient is telling. The therapist is trying to help him experience the grief by allowing it to have space to come to the surface. Reducing the pace of his talking allows him to pay attention to bodily activations associated with his story.

THERAPIST: When you got him back he'd been gone for a year, and he couldn't wipe himself . . .

The therapist is restarting the history from the beginning to help him experience the affect in his story.

PATIENT: Right, not properly.

THERAPIST: So he really seemed to be neglected.

The therapist is trying to redirect the patient toward the hardest parts of his story, what holds most potential for the patient to experience the avoided sadness.

PATIENT: He sat in front of the TV you know (*getting more in touch with sadness*). He was watching movies he shouldn't watch.

The therapist is continuing to orient the patient toward sadness, the avoided activating affect. The excerpt of the session has showed how initially just talking about the avoided affect led the patient to defensive laughter, but that the patient was made aware of this and the function it served. After the strong association between the activating affect (sadness) and the defenses (laughter) had been pointed out and worked with, the therapist's effort turns to helping the patient experience the sadness that had been inhibited. A sense of pity and shame was activated when getting close to sadness, and this greatly reduced the patient's experience of the activating affect. As shame is related to the belief of someone observing and judging the person, the therapist focused on testing out and changing the assumptions the patient had about shame. Another strong force in changing shame is the therapist's reaction when the patient was expressing whatever affects or behavior with which the shame is associated. After working with helping the patient to experience more adaptive levels of shame and having a more realistic view of other people, the therapist oriented the patient back to experiencing the sadness connected to the separation from his son. Although this summary displays the parts as fairly separated objectives that is worked with in a chronological way, the process is often very dynamic, with the therapist switching back and forth from working on the different corners of the triangle of conflict, but with the same aim in sight: helping the patient resolve the affect phobia. The triangle of conflict for this patient had sadness or grief at the bottom corner, shame as the primary inhibitory affect, and laughter as a prominent defense. However, in the remainder of the session it became clear that another activating affect with a lesser phobia attached to it was anger. The therapist chose to work with sadness first for two reasons: the phobia seemed to be stronger for grief, and anger was aroused when the patient was getting in touch with the sadness. This could indicate that aggression served a defensive function to help the patient avoid experiencing the sadness, in addition to a healthy activating self-asserting affect connected to the ex-partner's behavior with his son.

It is evident in the session that the patient was beginning to experience previously avoided affects, recognize and understand his maladaptive patterns in light of the triangle of the person, and reorganize his view of himself and of others in important areas. Continuation of the therapy would have proceeded along the lines of this session, with efforts made to tie this work into his current relationships with his son and his new family.

Future Directions

APT is at its core a transdiagnostic approach. That is not to say that every patient is treated equally, but that every patient has his or her unique formulation of the triangle of conflict and the triangle of person. The therapist must investigate and test out his or her hypothesis and develop an understanding for the patient's affect phobias. APT is best delivered by a skilled therapist who is not afraid of strong feelings, feelings that some might find uncomfortable to experience even in the setting of a therapeutic relationship. The therapeutic work is aimed directly at the patient and his or her affect phobias as they arise experientially in session. Because the affect phobias are often developed in close attachment situations, this raises possibilities of transporting affects from other relationships into the therapeutic relationship (i.e., transference and countertransference reactions). These reactions can be challenging for the patient, as well as for the therapist, even if one is aware of the function of the affect. With some experience and guidance the approach is manageable to most therapists, however.

Principles from APT are transferrable to other therapy orientations. In particular understanding the relationship between defenses, activating and inhibiting affects, their function and how they interfere with each other to regulate, diminish, or block each other can be central to understanding the patient's reactions in therapy and in the patient's life. Further, interventions from APT can be integrated with other therapy orientations to help arouse affects, regulate affects, and handle maladaptive defenses, both from the triangle of conflict directly, but also from the triangle of person indirectly.

In CBT, the focus is often on regulating emotions that are explicitly problematic by attenuating their expression. For example, the CBT therapist might work toward managing one's anger or using relaxation and cognitive reappraisals to reduce fear. Clearly, there are instances when the CBT therapist wants to activate the patient, which would be the case for depression, but this is usually done through behavioral (e.g., behavioral activation) or cognitive strategies (e.g., Beckian cognitive therapy). APT provides a complementary strategy that focuses directly on the expression of activating affects that are being avoided. Incorporation of APT techniques provides the CBT therapist with a range of options for intervention that would include behavior, cognition, and affect.

Further Resources

- For a manual detailing the treatment objectives and suggestions for interventions, see McCullough et al. (2004).
- For a more in-depth description of the foundation for APT, see McCullough Vaillant (1997).
- APT has an online teaching tool for learning how to identify central objectives in the patient during therapy. See *www.ATOStrainer.com*, and McCullough, Bahtia, Ulvenes, Berggraf, and Osborn (2011).
- A video recording of an affect phobia therapy session has been published through the American Psychological Association (affect-focused dynamic psychotherapy; see *www.apa.org/pubs/videos/4310728.aspx*).

References

Abbass, A., Hancock, J., Henderson, J., & Kisely, S. (2006). Short-term psychodynamic psychotherapies for common mental disorders. *Cochrane Database of Systematic Reviews, 4*.

Abbass, A., Kisely, S., & Kroenke, K. (2009). Short-term psychodynamic psychotherapy for somatic disorders. *Psychotherapy and Psychosomatics, 78*(5), 265–274.

Abbass, A., Sheldon, A., Gyra, J., & Kalpin, A. (2008). Intensive short-term dynamic psychotherapy for DSM-IV personality disorders: A randomized controlled trial. *Journal of Nervous and Mental Disease, 196*(3), 211–216.

American Psychological Association (Producer). (2012). *Working with attachment behavior in affect-focused dynamic therapy* [streaming video]. Retrieved from PsycTHERAPY database.

Bergner, R., & Holmes, J. (2000). Self-concepts and self-concept change: A status dynamic approach. *Psychotherapy, 37*, 36–44.

Bohart, A. C. (1977). Role playing and interpersonal-conflict reduction. *Journal of Counseling Psychology, 24*(1), 15–24.

Bohart, A. C. (1980). Toward a cognitive theory of catharsis. *Psychotherapy: Theory, Research and Practice, 17*(2), 192–201.

Bressi, C., Porcellana, M., Marinaccio, P. M., Nocito, E. P., & Magri, L. (2010). Short-term psychodynamic psychotherapy versus treatment as usual for depressive and anxiety disorders: a randomized clinical trial of efficacy. *Journal of Nervous and Mental Disease, 198*(9), 647–652.

Coady, N. F. (1991). The association between complex types of therapist interventions and outcomes in psychodynamic psychotherapy. *Research on Social Work Practice, 1*(3), 257–277.

Cramer, P. (1998). Coping and defense mechanisms: What's the difference? *Journal of Personality, 66*(6), 919–946.

Diener, M., Hilsenroth, M. J., & Weinberger, J. (2007). Therapist affect focus and patient outcomes in psychodynamic psychotherapy: A meta-analysis. *American Journal of Psychiatry, 164*(6), 936–941.

Driessen, E., Cuijpers, P., de Maat, S., Abbass, A. A., de Jonghe, F., & Dekker, J. J. (2010). The efficacy of short-term psychodynamic psychotherapy for depression: A meta-analysis. *Clinical Psychology Review, 30*(1), 25–36.

Elliott, R., Greenberg, L. S., & Lietaer, G. (2004). Research on experiential psychotherapies. *Bergin and Garfield's handbook of psychotherapy and behavior change, 5*, 139–193.

Fischer, A. H., & Manstead, A. S. R. (2008). Social functions of emotion. *Handbook of Emotions, 3*, 456–468.

Fridja, N. (1986). *The emotion: Studies in emotion and social interaction*. Cambridge, UK: Cambridge University Press.

Greenberg, L. S., Auszra, L., & Herrmann, I. (2007). The relationship among emotional productivity, emotional arousal and outcome in experiential therapy of depression. *Psychotherapy Research, 17*(4), 482–493.

Greenberg, L. S. (1979). Resolving splits: Use of the two chair technique. *Psychotherapy: Theory, Research and Practice, 16*(3), 316–324.

Greenberg, L. S. (1984). A task analysis of intrapersonal conflict resolution. In N. L. Rice & L. S. Gredenberg (Eds.), *Patterns of change: Intensive analysis of psychotherapy process* (pp. 67–123). New York: Guilford Press.

Greenberg, L. S., & Malcolm, W. (2002). Resolving unfinished business: Relating process to outcome. *Journal of Consulting and Clinical Psychology, 70*(2), 406–416.

Gross, J. J. (1998). The emerging field of emotion regulation: An integrative review. *Review of General Psychology, 2*(3), 271–299.
Gross, J. J. (1999). Emotion regulation: Past, present, future. *Cognition and Emotion, 13*(5), 551–573.
Gross, J. J., & Muñoz, R. F. (1995). Emotion regulation and mental health. *Clinical Psychology: Science and Practice, 2*(2), 151–164.
Hilsenroth, M. J., Ackerman, S. J., Blagys, M. D., Baity, M. R., & Mooney, M. A. (2003). Short-term psychodynamic psychotherapy for depression: An examination of statistical, clinically significant, and technique-specific change. *Journal of Nervous and Mental Disease, 191*(6), 349–357.
James, W. (1890/2011). *The principles of psychology* (Vol. 1). Boston: Digireads.com. (Original work published 1890)
Jones, E., Parke, L., & Pulos, S. (1992). How therapy is conducted in the private consulting room: A multidimensional description of brief psychodynamic treatments. *Psychotherapy Research, 2*(1), 16–30.
Leichsenring, F. (2001). Comparative effects of short-term psychodynamic psychotherapy and cognitive-behavioral therapy in depression: A meta-analytic approach. *Clinical Psychology Review, 21*, 401–419.
Leichsenring, F., Klein, S., & Salzer, S. (in press). The efficacy of psychodynamic psychotherapy in specific mental disorders—A 2013 update of empirical evidence. *Contemporary Psychoanalysis*.
Leichsenring, F., Rabung, S., & Leibing, E. (2004). The efficacy of short-term psychodynamic psychotherapy in specific psychiatric disorders: A meta-analysis. *Archives of General Psychiatry, 61*(12), 1208–1216.
Leichsenring, F., Salzer, S., Jaeger, U., Kächele, H., Kreische, R., Leweke, F., et al. (2009). Short-term psychodynamic psychotherapy and cognitive-behavioral therapy in generalized anxiety disorder: A randomized, controlled trial. *American Journal of Psychiatry, 166*(8), 875–881.
Leonard, E. M., Miles, L. E., & Van der Kar, C. S. (1944). *The child at home and school*. Woodstock, GA: American Book Co.
Mackay, B. N. (1995). *The Gestalt two-chair technique: How it relates to theory*. Vancouver: University of British Columbia.
Malan, D. H. (1979). *Individual psychotherapy and the science of psychodynamics*: London: Butterworths.
McCullough, L., Bhatia, M., Ulvenes, P., Berggraf, L., & Osborn, K. (2011). Learning how to rate video-recorded therapy sessions: A practical guide for trainees and advanced clinicians. *Psychotherapy, 48*(2), 127–137.
McCullough, L., Kuhn, N., Andrews, S., Kaplan, A., Wolf, J., & Lanza Hurley, C. (2004). *Treating affect phobia: A manual for short-term dynamic psychotherapy*. New York: Guilford Press.
McCullough, L., Winston, A., Farber, B. A., Porter, F., Pollack, J., Vingiano, W., et al. (1991). The relationship of patient–therapist interaction to outcome in brief psychotherapy. *Psychotherapy: Theory, Research, Practice, Training, 28*(4), 525–533.
McCullough Vaillant, L. (1997). *Changing character: Short-term anxiety regulating psychotherapy for restructuring defences, affects and attachment*. New York: Basic Books.
McMain, S., Goldman, R., & Greenberg, L. (1996). Resolving unfinished business: A program of study. In W. Dryden (Ed.), *Research in counselling and psychotherapy: Practical applications* (pp. 211–232). Thousand Oaks, CA: Sage
Menninger, K. A., & Holzman, P. S. (1958). *Theory of psychoanalytic technique* (Vol. 12). New York: Basic Books.
Mergenthaler, E. (1996). Emotion-abstraction patterns in verbatim protocols: A new

way of describing psychotherapeutic processes. *Journal of Consulting and Clinical Psychology, 64*(6), 1306–1315.

Neisser, U., & Jopling, D. A. (1997). *The conceptual self in context: Culture, experience, self-understanding.* New York: Cambridge University Press.

Post, R. M. (2003). Introduction: Emotion and psychopathology. In R. J. Davidson, K. R. Scherer, & H. H. Goldsmith (Eds.), *Handbook of affective sciences* (pp. 899–903). New York: Oxford University Press.

Purton, C. (2004). *Person-centered therapy: The focusing-oriented approach.* Basingstoke, UK: Palgrave Macmillan.

Salzer, S., Winkelbach, C., Leweke, F., Leibing, E., & Leichsenring, F. (2011). Long-term effects of short-term psychodynamic psychotherapy and cognitive-behavioural therapy in generalized anxiety disorder: 12-month follow-up. *Canadian Journal of Psychiatry/Revue Canadienne de Psychiatrie, 56*(8), 503–508.

Schore, A. N. (2003). *Affect dysregulation and disorders of the self.* New York: Norton.

Shedler, J. (2010). The efficacy of psychodynamic psychotherapy. *American Psychologist, 65*(2), 98–109.

Southam Gerow, M. A., & Kendall, P. C. (2002). Emotion regulation and understanding: Implications for child psychopathology and therapy. *Clinical Psychology Review, 22*(2), 189–222.

Stalikas, A., & Fitzpatrick, M. (1995). Client good moments: An intensive analysis of a single session. *Canadian Journal of Counselling, 29*(2), 160–175.

Svartberg, M., Stiles, T. C., & Seltzer, M. H. (2004). Randomized, controlled trial of the effectiveness of short-term dynamic psychotherapy and cognitive therapy for Cluster C personality disorders. *American Journal of Psychiatry, 161,* 810–817.

Tomkins, S. (1995). The quest for primary motives: Biography and autobiography of an idea. In E. V. Demos (Ed.), *Exploring affect: The selected writings of Silvan Tomkins* (pp. 27–63). Cambridge, UK: Cambridge University Press.

Town, J. M., Hardy, G. E., McCullough, L., & Stride, C. (2011). Patient affect experiencing following therapist interventions in short-term dynamic psychotherapy. *Psychotherapy Research, 22*(2), 208–219.

Ulvenes, P. G., Berggraf, L., Hoffart, A., Stiles, T. C., Svartberg, M., McCullough, L., et al. (2012). Different processes for different therapies: Therapist actions, therapeutic bond, and outcome. *Psychotherapy, 49*(3), 291–302.

Wampold, B. E., & Kim, K. (1989). Sequential analysis applied to counseling process and outcome: A case study revisited. *Journal of Counseling Psychology, 36,* 357–364.

Warwar, S., & Greenberg, L. S. (2000). Advances in theories of change and counseling. In S. D. Brown & R. W. Lent (Eds.), *Handbook of counseling psychology* (3rd ed., pp. 571–600). Hoboken, NJ: Wiley.

Winston, A., Laikin, M., Pollack, J., Wallner Samstag, L., McCullough, L., & Muran, J. C. (1994). Short-term psychotherapy of personality disorders. *American Journal of Psychiatry, 151*(2), 190–194.

Winston, A., Pollack, J., McCullough, L., Flegenheimer, W., Kestenbaum, R., & Trujillo, M. (1991). Brief psychotherapy of personality disorders. *Journal of Nervous and Mental Disease, 179*(4), 188–193.

Part III

Using Imagery to Connect with Emotions and Transform Maladaptive Schemas and Beliefs

CHAPTER 8

Imagery Rescripting for Personality Disorders
Healing Early Maladaptive Schemas

Arnoud Arntz

The view that personality disorders (PDs) are unchangeable was prominent until two decades ago and lead to therapeutic pessimism. This view has radically changed in recent years, and a variety of treatment approaches with empirical support are now available. However, traditional cognitive-behavioral therapy (CBT), which has been highly successful in the treatment of syndromal disorders, has shown only limited effects in the treatment of PDs (e.g., Davidson et al., 2006), perhaps with the exception of Cluster C PDs (e.g., Emmelkamp et al., 2006). Patients with PDs might be quite resistant to the kind of rational approach that is so prominent in most CBT, and experiential methods might be needed to bring about the deeper changes that lead to healthier views of the self and others. Most therapists know the type of patients that respond to challenging their negative views by verbal methods or by experiments by stating, "I understand what you are saying, but it just doesn't feel like that to me."

The problem of patients not responding to rational techniques can be understood from schema theory. According to this paradigm, people form knowledge structures about the world (including themselves) that govern information processing, including the regulation of attention, information selection, and giving meaning to information. An important aspect of the schema construct as it was developed in basic cognitive psychology is that a schema is not necessarily (fully) open to conscious inspection and that its content is not necessarily restricted to verbal information. The distinction is important in the context of PDs, as very early (preverbal) experiences are thought to play a role in personality development. An important example is attachment, which is a process active from birth on and is nonverbal—mainly communicated (at least initially) through bodily contact. Early attachment experiences contribute strongly to the development of schemas—which in turn influence how the individual later in life regulates stress and relates to other people, for example, whether the individual trusts others or not. PDs are generally thought to develop as the result of an interplay between constitutional and environmental factors, and there are indeed indications for strong environmental influences (Joyce et al., 2003; Kendler et al., 2008). Many people with PDs have experienced severe maltreatment during childhood (Bernstein, Stein, & Handelsman, 1998; Bierer et al., 2003; Cohen et al., 2013; Lobbestael, Arntz, & Bernstein, 2010; Hernandez, Arntz, Gaviria, Labad, & Gutiérrez-Zotes, 2012), and there are longitudinal studies supporting a causal link (Horwitz, Widom, McLaughlin, & White, 2001; Johnson, Cohen, Brown, Smailes, & Bernstein, 1999; Johnson, Cohen, Chen, Kasen, & Brook, 2006; Johnson et al., 2001; Johnson, Smailes, Cohen, Brown, & Bernstein, 2000). Thus, there are at least two reasons to use imagery rescripting (ImRs) in the treatment of PDs. First, the nonverbal ("feeling") aspects of dysfunctional views call for techniques that can address the nonverbal content of underlying schemas directly. Second, the influences of early childhood experiences on the formation of dysfunctional schemas call for techniques that address these early experiences. ImRs is a powerful technique to achieve these goals.

Rationale for ImRs

Before going into the details of ImRs, it is good to discuss why the use of imagery—as opposed to verbal cognition or real experience—is helpful. First, imagery evokes more emotions than just talking about issues (Holmes, Arntz, & Smucker, 2007), and basic experiments testing the effects of experimentally manipulated interpretation biases on stress responsivity demonstrated that the experimental manipulation of interpretations is strongly enhanced by having participants imagine the situation (Holmes, Mathews, Dalgleish, & MacKintosh, 2006). Second, in many respects, the brain does not differentiate between real and imagined experiences; thus imagined experiences have highly similar brain responses to real experiences, and imagining skills is the second best option after real practice (Holmes & Mathews, 2010). Third, imagined stimuli can act as conditioned and unconditioned stimuli, similar to real stimuli (Dadds, Bovbjerg, Redd, & Cutmore, 1997). Thus, imagery is a powerful mental activity, in emotional and behavioral impact superior to verbal reasoning, approaching the effects of a real experience.

The basic idea of ImRs in the treatment of PDs is to activate memories of childhood events that contributed to the formation of dysfunctional schemas, reexperience the event, and imagine a different ending that better matches the needs of the child. Through this process a change of the meaning of the original event is created, which leads to a change in the schema. Although the current theory is that the change of meaning of the memory representation of the original event is central, another (or additional) possibility is that the expression of needs and feelings, which were inhibited at the time, usually because of survival reasons, is a healing factor (e.g., Arntz, 2012). That said, reprocessing of experiences from childhood is the central aim, and several aspects of ImRs are probably important in explaining why it is such a powerful technique (Arntz, 2011):

1. *Reattribution.* Patients start to attribute what has happened to other causes than they did when they were a child. For instance, the lack of attention the patient received in childhood when in need of emotional reassurance is no longer attributed to the inherent worthlessness of the patient, but to psychological problems that the parents had in dealing with emotions and attaching to any child.

2. *Emotional processing.* Difficult experiences from childhood are usually not emotionally processed in patients with PD. Lack of safety or even straightforward threats these patients got when expressing emotions and trying to get emotional support prevented this. For instance, one of the author's patients, as a child, was locked in her room when she became emotional, and was not released until she stopped crying. The rejection and abandonment when in need of safe attachment caused abandonment panic in the child, making the parent even madder. As an adult, the patient still felt very uncomfortable with emotions. Most patients with PDs are afraid or ashamed of their emotions. ImRs helps them to feel more comfortable with emotions and to process them. This changes the basic dysfunctional views of patients about emotions. ImRs also teaches them how to deal with emotions so that their emotion regulation improves.

3. *Receiving care.* As we have seen, many patients with PD were emotionally neglected during childhood, if not abused. In ImRs they experience, although in fantasy, somebody taking care of them as a child, often for the first time in their life. Allowing and experiencing that somebody sincerely cares about you is an important and necessary aspect of healthy development, and underlies the capacity to form healthy relationships later in life, and good parenting of one's own children.

4. *Changing meaning on the child level.* The use of corrective information at the adult level (e.g., rational verbal reasoning) might have only

limited impact on knowledge that was stored in memory during childhood, when other levels of information processing were prominent. It is helpful to adjust the corrective information to levels on which children process information. This can be accomplished by activating the childhood memory and providing corrective experiences and other types of information to the child in the image, in a way one would do to a real child. The therapist can adjust the content and the reasoning style to the child level, but can also adapt the channel thru which the information is given. For example, for children, bodily contact with a safe figure is the primary channel through which safety and soothing is conveyed. In ImRs, the patient can imagine being soothed as a child by a trustworthy person.

5. *Transforming the rule to the exception.* Children view their environment as a prototypical representation of the world in general. For instance, if their caregivers react with threats to their needs, they start to believe that everybody will do this and that nobody can be trusted. With ImRs, patients start to learn that their environment was the exception. The same holds for moral issues: moral rules and values that were misunderstood to be universal can also be changed with ImRs.

Empirical Evidence

ImRs has not been tested extensively as an isolated technique for PDs, as it is typically used in conjunction with other cognitive, behavioral, and experiential methods when applied to patients with PD. However, ImRs is thought to be a particularly powerful method in part due to evidence that the use of imagery can have more impact than verbal methods in fostering cognitive and emotional change (Holmes et al., 2007; Holmes & Mathews, 2010). ImRs has been tested as an isolated technique as a treatment of traumas in a variety of syndromal disorders (Arntz, 2012). ImRs seems especially effective for maladaptive but ego-syntonic views of the self and others, which have their roots in earlier negative experiences, a central issue in addressing PDs (for a review, see Arntz, 2012).

One treatment study focusing specifically on patients with PD ($N = 21$) compared experiential techniques directed at processing childhood memories to more common CBT techniques focusing on present problems, using a crossover design (Weertman & Arntz, 2007). ImRs was the most often used experiential technique. The two sets of techniques were equally effective in the short term. Interestingly, some cases profited more from the experiential techniques, others from the more common CBT techniques. The crossover design, wherein participants received both treatment techniques, cannot answer what the long-term effects of ImRs are in the treatment of PD. Nevertheless, this study is important because it proved that experiential techniques focusing on childhood memories are as effective as more common CBT techniques for patients with PD, and might help cases that don't respond well to common CBT.

A laboratory experiment in patients with borderline personality disorder (BPD) demonstrated that imagery work was superior to distraction and a neutral condition in increasing positive emotions after watching a stressful movie, and as effective in reducing negative emotions as distraction (Jacob et al., 2011). Note, however, that the study did not assess therapeutic change by imagery *rescripting*; the focus was on the use of imagery as an emotion regulation strategy. Though using imagery with the primary goal of improving emotion regulation is not the topic of the present chapter, the study demonstrated that imagery can have powerful positive effects in patients with BPD. ImRs as described in this chapter is an important ingredient of schema therapy (ST) for PDs (Arntz & van Genderen, 2009; Arntz & Jacob, 2012; Farrell & Shaw, 2012; Young, Klosko, & Weishaar, 2003). ST as a treatment for BPD has been tested in several trials and found to be more effective and cost-effective, while having fewer dropouts, than transference-focused psychotherapy and usual treatment (Giesen-Bloo et al., 2006; van Asselt et al., 2008; Farrell, Shaw, & Webber, 2009; for reviews, see Jacob & Arntz, 2013; Sempérteguia, Karremana, Arntz, & Becker, 2013). Nadort et al. (2009) demonstrated that ST for BPD can be successfully implemented in regular mental health care. ST for six other PDs (avoidant, dependent, obsessive–compulsive, paranoid, histrionic, narcissistic) was found to be more effective in recovery from PD diagnosis and comorbid depressive disorder; and in general and social functioning than usual psychological treatment and another new specialized psychotherapy for PDs, clarification-oriented psychotherapy. Again, ST had fewer dropouts, superior cost-effectiveness, and more completed treatments in the study's time window (Bamelis, Evers, Spinhoven, & Arntz, 2014a; Bamelis, Arntz, Wetzelaer, Verdoorn, & Evers, 2014b). An important finding in the Bamelis et al. (2014a) study is that a significant effect resulted from the type of ST therapists' training: those who were trained in a highly structured format, involving role plays (thus, experiential learning) had superior effects compared to those who were trained mainly by lecturing.

A randomized controlled trial comparing ST for forensic patients with PDs to usual treatment is under way (Bernstein et al., 2012), and preliminary results suggest strong effects of ST even in patients with high psychopathic traits.

Future studies should investigate how much ImRs adds to standard CBT for PDs, especially in the long term. Additionally, future studies are needed to validate the proposed mechanisms of change in ImRs for PDs. Clinical observations and patient reports indicate that ImRs is a powerful technique addressing aspects of patient problems not easily addressed by standard CBT techniques, contributing to a deep change in PD pathology

(Napel-Schutz et al., 2011). It is important that this impression is tested in an empirical study.

Application with PDs

Four applications will be discussed: first, imagery of a safe place; second, the use of diagnostic imagery; third, ImRs of childhood memories; and fourth, the use of ImRs in addressing current and future problems.

Imagery of a Safe Place

Imagery of a safe place is an option, not a necessity. However, for patients who easily experience high anxiety, it is a helpful method to help them find safety. One can start introducing imagery work by teaching the patient to imagine a safe place, so that the patient gets used to imagery. With a powerful image of a safe place, patients can return to that safe place at any time if the other imagery exercises evoke too high levels of negative emotions. They can also use the image any time they are in need of safety. Ask the patient to close his or her eyes or, if he or she finds this too uncomfortable, to pick a point on the floor and stare at it. Then ask the patient to imagine a safe place. This can be a real place that the patient has been to, or it can be a fantasy. If the patient cannot create a safe place in imagery, the therapist can suggest a place in nature; a pleasant memory of being with a friend or a pet; or imagining a big balloon around him or her that protects the patient from everything; or the like. A minority of patients cannot imagine a safe place because the world is too dangerous. For these patients it is important that the therapist develops a very strong, safe therapeutic relationship. In such cases it is essential that the therapist actively protects the patient during ImRs, so that safety is brought in by the therapist. If the patient cannot imagine a safe place, the therapist reassures the patient and proceeds with ImRs.

Diagnostic Imagery and Imagery Rescripting of Memories from Childhood

From an empirical perspective, it is not clear yet what is the best approach to introduce ImRs in the treatment of PDs. A recent qualitative study into patients with PDs' opinions about ImRs suggests that some patients preferred more preparation and explanation of the technique than their therapists did. However, patients who were in treatment for a longer time had a different view, as by practicing ImRs they understood it better, were less afraid of it, and acknowledged its effectiveness (Napels-Schutz, Abma, Bamelis, & Arntz, 2011). One could argue that lengthy explanations could lead to high levels of anticipatory fear and avoidance or refusal—some therapists therefore prefer to not make a big deal of the technique and to start with it after a short introduction as a completely normal part of therapy. If the patient feels rather overwhelmed, care is then taken after the exercise that the emotions are validated, that the technique is fully explained, and that emotional support is given.

In ImRs, an image of a childhood memory is "rescripted" by having an adult person enter the scene and intervene, thus changing the script. In the early stages of treatment of patients with PD it is advised that the therapist enters the image and rescripts. There are at least two reasons for this. First, these patients usually don't have a strong enough healthy part to intervene themselves. They might easily feel overwhelmed or threatened; or agree with the views of the persons who maltreated the child, lacking healthy views on the situation and on what the child needs; or don't know what to say or how to behave. Second, most patients with PD did not get adequate protection and care as a child, and they should learn, on the child level, to receive and accept this, as this is essential for healthy development. When devising the protocol, it was thought that the basic approach should be that patients themselves enter the image to intervene (Arntz & Weertman, 1999). Our experience with patients with PD has indicated that this is not a good approach, and that initially the therapist should intervene. For patients with PD, the following approach is suggested (Arntz, 2011).

1. Start with a problem from the last week (or a strong feeling emerging during the session).

2. Ask the patient to close his or her eyes and get an image of the recent problem. Let the patient describe in here-and-now terms, from his or her own perspective, what happens and what he or she experiences. Ask for emotions and needs.

3. Instruct the patient to stick with the feeling but to let the image go, and to see whether an image from childhood appears. The patient should not try to find an image in a rational way—ask him or her to let it come spontaneously.

4. Ask the patient how old he or she is, where he or she is, with whom, and what happens. Let the patient talk in the present tense, from the perspective of the child. Gently correct if the patient uses another perspective, or doesn't use the present tense. After factual details are clear, ask for emotions, then thoughts, and then needs. It is always good to ask for needs. But the patient might not yet be able to express any need, or only something rather unarticulated (avoidance, denial, and overcompensation are defining characteristics of PDs). If severe abuse is (nearly) happening, don't wait but intervene. If it is not completely clear what is happening and what the emotional problem is, let the image continue. The basic questions are:

"What do you see [hear, smell, etc.]? What is happening?"
"What do you feel?"
"What do you think?"
"What do you need?"

After each intervention in the script, these questions can be asked again.

In the early phases of treatment the exercise can stop here and the experiences can be used to complete the case formulation. This is called "diagnostic imagery." Using the procedure up to this point can be helpful in gaining an understanding of what kinds of difficult early experiences the patient went through to shape who he or she has become. Importantly, diagnostic imagery also helps the therapist to get a sense of what kind of needs (e.g., for safety, reassurance, empathy, encouragement, praise, love) have gone chronically unmet for the patient. In the case of diagnostic imagery, the exercise would end here, and the therapist and patient would discuss and explore the experience and what it revealed. If the patient has already had one imagery session that has gone up to this point that was used for case formulation and diagnostic purposes, the therapist will continue on to the rescripting phase.

5. Here the "rescripting" begins. Tell the patient that you will now enter the scene. Don't ask permission—chances are high that you won't get it! Act on your own healthy views. It might help to visualize the situation yourself, so that you see the little child who is in a nasty situation. Act as if you are responsible for the child. Do what you feel you need to do. The patient might protest (e.g., the patient prefers to avoid or to comply, because he or she is too afraid and might want you to do the same), but you have to trust that what you do is healthy. When you intervene, describe to the patient what you are doing and what you are saying. If there is abuse or the threat of abuse, stop or prevent it. Ask the patient what happens next in the image, how he or she feels now, and what he or she needs. Rescript further until the threat is under control. Every time you ask the patient what happens in the image, what he or she feels, and what he or she needs (as a little child). Then take care of the little child. Create safety (which might involve taking the child out of the house, and bringing it to another family, or to your own family). Comfort the child, or find a trustworthy person who can do that (e.g., the mother of the child's friend, or an aunt). For comforting a sad or stressed child, bodily contact is the most important channel. So if the patient expresses the need for bodily contact, let the patient imagine that he or she is comforted with bodily contact, as one would do with any child (but don't force it). Correct misinterpretations that the child makes, explain what is wrong with the parent's behavior, why you intervened, and

so on. Finally, ask the child whether he or she wants to do something pleasant, like playing.

6. When it is OK for the patient, ask him or her to slowly open his or her eyes and to return to the therapy room. Discuss the exercise, but expect that most of the effects have already started on an experiential level—thus the discussion afterward is not the essence of the method. It is designed more to check how the exercise was received and whether changes in the rescripting are indicated. Ask the patient to listen to the recording you made and to try to do the whole exercise at home (but don't be disappointed if the patient avoids doing that; this is to be expected with patients with PD—accept it as being too difficult at the moment, but continue to suggest that the patient tries it at home).

7. If the patient is not satisfied, don't worry. Just try another way of rescripting. It is a fantasy, so we can easily rewind the movie and rescript in another way. Invite the patient to develop variations of the scripts and to try them out.

A typical start of a session would be to ask the patient how he or she has been doing since the last session. The patient's response informs the therapist about the state the patient presently is in, and also informs the therapist about emotional events that took place after the last session. The therapist can use a recent important emotional experience as starting point to find and address a childhood memory. Alternatively, the therapist can use the present emotional state of the patient to find a childhood image. Both of these options use an "affect bridge" to get to a relevant childhood image—using recent or current affect to link to a related affective state as a child. The following is excerpted from Arntz (2011):

THERAPIST: Was there anything in particular that was bothering you during or after last session? Can you try to tell me?

PATIENT: Well, I started to realize that I have always felt very lonely. Not only now, but already as a child. A feeling I rather not want to feel.

THERAPIST: OK, I understand this is a difficult feeling that you would rather avoid and that you remember already from your childhood. I would like to do an exercise with you, in which we return, in fantasy, to your childhood and assist little Ben in his loneliness. I'll ask you to close your eyes, and get an image of yourself when you were a child and had this dreadful feeling of loneliness. I'll then enter the image to support little Ben. In a way, we will rescript the image and give it a new, better outcome. Or, if that is not possible, we will organize emotional support for little Ben to help him to deal with the difficulties he experienced. It may sound strange, but although we cannot change the reality of what happened in patients' childhoods, with this technique we can help them process the emotions that are related to these childhood experiences, which lie at the root of their problems, and we can help them to give new and more adaptive meanings to these early experiences. The whole exercise will take about 30 minutes. Do you have any questions?

PATIENT: Not really. Seems quite strange, but let's give it a try.

THERAPIST: If that is OK with you, can you then close your eyes and focus on the loneliness you have been feeling?

Therapists can also ask patients to directly get an image of a memory of an adverse event in their childhood. For example, the therapist might know of maltreatment or important childhood experiences, like the loss of a parent, and these can be directly addressed. Last, the therapist can ask the patient to close his or her eyes and find a safe image. If the patient has a safe image, the therapist can instruct the patient to let the image go, and to see whether an image from childhood appears. Usually a childhood image with opposite meaning is triggered, which can be addressed in ImRs. Note that it is possible to use three or more images in succession; for example, start with an image of a difficult situation last week, then have the safe place imagined, then a childhood image, and after rescripting return to the safe place, before opening the eyes.

The most frequently used method to get to a childhood image suitable for ImRs is the use of an affect bridge between the image of a recent difficult situation and childhood images. Here is a complete example of an ImRS exercise starting with a recent difficult feeling (from Arntz, 2011).

THERAPIST: Can you close your eyes and get an image of this experience last week when you felt so guilty?

PATIENT: Yes, I have it.

THERAPIST: Can you tell where you are?

PATIENT: I am at the office.

THERAPIST: What is happening?

PATIENT: I already worked an hour's overtime. Everybody has left, now my boss also leaves. I was not able to complete all the tasks.

THERAPIST: What do you feel?

PATIENT: I feel guilty, I feel that I failed. And I am panicking. I'm afraid that I will be fired.

THERAPIST: What would you need?

PATIENT: Certainty. Less work to do. Reassurance that I will not be fired.

THERAPIST: OK. Could you now keep the feeling but let the image go and see whether a memory from your childhood pops up?

PATIENT: Mhm. (*after some time*) Yes, I have an image.

THERAPIST: Can you tell where you are?

PATIENT: I am in the kitchen.

THERAPIST: How old are you?

PATIENT: 9 or 10, I guess.

THERAPIST: What is happening?

PATIENT: My mother just left. She was disappointed in me and now she went to bed. I know she will lie in bed the coming days and will not talk to me.

THERAPIST: How come?

PATIENT: I had a low grade in school and now I have to do extra homework and cannot help on the farm.

THERAPIST: What do you feel?

PATIENT: Guilt. Failure. And panic. I caused my mother to get depressed again. I am afraid she will not recover.

THERAPIST: What would you need?

PATIENT: To not have this burden on me.

THERAPIST: OK. Now imagine that I am with you. I am with you in the room. Can you see me?

PATIENT: Yes.

THERAPIST: We walk to your mother's bedroom and this is what I say to your mother: "Madam, I understand that you are disappointed that Peter had a low grade in school and you worry about how all the work on the farm has to be done now that Peter has to do extra homework. But your reaction is excessive. By lying in bed, feeling depressed, and not talking to Peter you punish him for something he did not do on purpose. And you punish him excessively. He feels extremely guilty and anxious about your condition. You should not charge a child with responsibility for your excessive reaction. What Peter needs is understanding and reassurance that it is not a problem that he had a low grade and that with some extra homework everything will be fine. So can you get out of your bed and take care of him? He really needs you." What is happening? How is your mother reacting?

PATIENT: She says that she is not able to get out of her bed because she is feeling too depressed.

THERAPIST: "But Peter is really upset now. He is very frightened. He is still a child and he needs you to take care of him." How is your mother reacting?

PATIENT: She says that she feels too bad to do something.

THERAPIST: Then I say to her: "Madam, if you are too depressed to come out of your bed, that is bad enough, but don't blame Peter for it. I think you are emotionally not healthy and that you need professional help. I'll arrange that you will get treatment for your depression." Come, Peter, we leave the room and return to the kitchen. We are now in the kitchen. How are you feeling?

PATIENT: A little bit relieved because you said so clearly that it wasn't my fault.

THERAPIST: Yes, it is not your fault. You must understand that every child has now and then a problem with learning and that every child needs a parent that reassures him and tells him that that is not a problem. You know, I really think your mother has an emotional problem. You are not to blame for her despair and depression. Somehow, she cannot handle a minor disappointment. I understand she gives you the feeling that it is your fault that she feels like that, but it isn't your fault. She has an emotional problem and somebody has to take care of her, and I'll arrange that. So that means that you don't have to worry about that anymore. How do you feel now?

PATIENT: Relieved, but still not at ease. I am so afraid of my mother's despair and her suicide threats . . . I don't want to stay here . . .

THERAPIST: So what is it what you need?

PATIENT: I need a home where I can live without all these worries.

THERAPIST: Is there someone you can imagine you would like to live with?

PATIENT: My aunt.

THERAPIST: OK, then imagine that I take you to your aunt. We leave the house and I bring you to your aunt. Can you see that?

PATIENT: Yes.

THERAPIST: OK. And I say to your aunt: "Madam, Peter and I have come to ask you whether Peter can live with you. His mother is so depressed and stressed, and with even a minor disappointment she lies for days in bed and doesn't talk anymore to Peter. He is feeling so guilty and so panicky that it is not sensible that he stays with her, at least not until her emotional problems are treated. Peter needs a safe home, and he needs somebody who takes care of him and reassures him and doesn't make him feel guilty when he has a minor problem at school. Could he live with you?" What is your aunt saying?

PATIENT: She says that is OK.

THERAPIST: How do you feel now?

PATIENT: Better now.

THERAPIST: Is there anything else you need?
PATIENT: I feel sad. I need to be soothed.
THERAPIST: Can you aunt comfort you? What could she do?
PATIENT: I want her to hold me.
THERAPIST: OK, ask her to hold you.
PATIENT: Aunt, can you hold me, I feel so sad.
THERAPIST: OK, and imagine that your aunt holds you—feel how she holds you.
PATIENT: (*Starts to cry—emotional release.*)
THERAPIST: That is OK (*after a while, when the patient calms down*) How do you feel now?
PATIENT: Quiet.
THERAPIST: Is there anything else you need?
PATIENT: I want to play. I want to play with my nephew.
THERAPIST: That's OK. Can you imagine playing with your nephew now?
PATIENT: Mhm.
THERAPIST: (*after some time*) How are you feeling now?
PATIENT: Fine.
THERAPIST: Is there anything else you need?
PATIENT: No, I am fine.
THERAPIST: OK, then you can slowly open your eyes and return to this room.

From this example it is clear that stopping the threatening event is only half of the story. Care was taken that needs that became apparent when the threat was taken away were addressed. Furthermore, the father was completely missing. Therefore, ImRs addressing the father's role was done in a later session.

In some cases the therapist must be very determined and strong to win from the abuser. The therapist should not allow the abuse to continue.

THERAPIST: I say to your father "Stop hitting Steve. Parents are not allowed to beat up their children."
PATIENT: Watch out, my father is very strong.
THERAPIST: Don't worry, I may be small, but I'm also very strong. I have a degree in karate and in judo. If you father tries to attack him, I'll put him in a hold. What happens now?
PATIENT: My father is very angry at you. But he doesn't dare to hit me as long as you're here.

THERAPIST: "Mr. X, you better not try to attack me as I have a degree in karate and in judo. So you better listen to me. Fathers are not allowed to beat up their children. It is not good that you do that, it is illegal, and Steve does not deserve it. Steve needs a good father who loves him and cares about him, not a father who beats him up when he is drunk and irritated. You have an alcohol problem, and instead of being a mean drunk and making Steve the victim of your problems, you should do something about your drinking problems."

PATIENT: Now my father is swearing at you and says that I'm no good . . .

THERAPIST: "Stop that immediately and leave us alone. Go away. You are drunk and I cannot allow that you talk this bullshit. Go away. I'll talk with you when you are sober."

PATIENT: He wants to hit you.

THERAPIST: I throw him out of balance, grab his arm, and hold it behind his back. I bring him to the door and put him out, and close the door. He cannot enter the house anymore. He's gone!

PATIENT: Yeah now he can't hit you.

THERAPIST: And he can't hit you either. I won't allow him to come back as long as he drinks too much and beats you up.

Therapists should be prepared to deal with abusers who were, at least in the eyes of the child, extremely powerful and sometimes unconquerable. Thus, they might tell the patient that they are specialists in fighting sports, or that they will bring in four very strong policemen, or that they have a secret weapon that temporarily paralyzes the abuser, or the like.

As just mentioned, the therapist should not forget to take care of the child after the abuse has stopped. But first safety should be created. It the child is afraid that the abuser will take revenge, it might help to give the child a secret apparatus that warns the therapist if there is danger so that the therapist can return immediately to intervene again. Other options include taking the child out of the abusive situation and finding a safe home for the child; enforcing treatment on the abuser; or putting the abuser in jail. There is a debate over the degree to which it is therapeutic to let patients imagine revenge or to have abusers killed. Some argue that it is healthy to fantasize about taking revenge, as it makes one's revenge fantasies less frightening, and acting aggressive revengeful impulses out in fantasy might actually lead to better anger control (see Arntz, Tiesema, & Kindt, 2007, for empirical evidence that ImRs was associated with increased anger control, and reduced anger; and Seebauer, Froß, Dubaschny, Schönberger, & Jacob, 2014, for empirical evidence that there is no short-term risk of acting out revenge in ImRs). Others doubt whether this is safe with patients with PD who have aggressive acting-out problems. I once had a patient who killed her extremely abusive father in fantasy, after which she was dissatisfied, so the image was rewound and the father was put in jail, which satisfied the patient more. The following week she set, for the first time, healthy limits to the abusive behavior of her partner, without any physical threat (she told him she would call the police—similar to what was done initially in the ImRs exercise when her abusive father had to be stopped). This approach suggests that one can allow patients to imagine revenge fantasies, and that patients can develop healthy ways of handling their anger in real life. Another question is how far the therapist would go in exercising the revenge wished by the patient in the rescripting. The advice is to respect your own limits and not do anything you feel uncomfortable with in the imagery rescripting.

Following creating safety and satisfying possible feelings of justice and revenge, the therapist should take care of the further needs of the patient. Usually there is the need to be comforted, and the therapist can ask the patient who could do that or comfort the child him- or herself. A common next need is the need for recreation, joy, or playfulness. Thus, the child likes to relax, to play, and to have fun. The example continuous as follows:

THERAPIST: How are you doing, Steve?

PATIENT: I'm still scared because he might come back in and hit me. And now he's even madder because you threw him out.

THERAPIST: Then I think it's a good idea if he's locked up somewhere so that he cannot return. Where shall I have him locked up? In jail?

PATIENT: Yes, put him in jail.

THERAPIST: OK, I'll have him locked up in jail. I explain to the police that he is drunk and beat you up, and that he is going to do this again and again if he is not forced to stop. As he is a real danger for you, they put him in jail. Can you picture that? (*The patient nods.*) How do you feel now?

PATIENT: Calmer but I feel sad.

THERAPIST: You're sad. What do you need?

PATIENT: I don't know. I feel so alone now! (*crying*)

THERAPIST: Shall I come and sit next to you? Would you like a tissue? Let me put my arm around you. It's OK, he's gone now and I am with you. It is OK to be sad. (*The patient sighs and slowly begins to stop crying.*) How do you feel now?

PATIENT: Much better.

THERAPIST: Is there something else you want to say?

PATIENT: Yeah, I'm scared that my father will come back and really let me have it because I said you should lock him up.

THERAPIST: So you're scared of being left here alone?

PATIENT: Yes...

THERAPIST: Is there anybody who you could live with? Anybody who is nice to you and who would like to take care of you?

PATIENT: Perhaps the family of my friend Bob... his parents are always nice to me.

THERAPIST: Shall I take you to Bob's family? You'll be safe there and you can call me if you need to. Can you picture that I bring you to Bob's? (*The patient nods yes.*) I take you to his house.... So, here we are. Let's ring the bell. Who is opening the door?

PATIENT: Bob's mother. (*Nods and smiles.*)

THERAPIST: Hello, madam, I've brought Steve to you; he is not safe at home because his father is often drunk and beats him up. His father is in jail now anyhow and cannot take care of him. Steve would like to stay with you, if that is possible. He knows you are always fond of him.

THERAPIST: (*to the patient*) What does Bob's mother say?

PATIENT: She says it is fine and has me sit on the sofa and makes me a hot chocolate.

THERAPIST: How do you feel now? Is there anything you need?

PATIENT: I would like to play with Bob.

THERAPIST: OK, I'll visit you now and then, and you can always call me if you need me. What do you think of that?

PATIENT: That's nice.

THERAPIST: OK, then go to play with Bob! Can you picture that?

PATIENT: Yes!

THERAPIST: If you need anything else, tell me—if not, enjoy your play with Bob!

PATIENT: No, this is good. I'm glad that I can stay with Bob and that you'll visit me.

There are some general guidelines for ImRs for treating the childhood roots of PD problems:

1. The younger the child in the image is, the better the technique works. This is partly because earlier experiences lie closer to the root of the problems, and partly because it is more convincing for the patient that he or she not be guilty of the problems when the patient was very young. Some patients strongly avoid memories of when they were young because they are afraid of the strong emotions that they evoke. In such cases it might take

some time (and psychoeducation) before they are able to address memories of earlier childhood.

2. It is not essential whether the memory is correct or not for ImRs to be effective. If the patient doubts the reality of the memory, but the memory is disturbing and seems clinically important, ImRs can still be used. Note that ImRs is a powerful part of an evidence-based and very effective treatment for nightmares and that many nightmares are fantasy (the patient rescripts the nightmare by giving it a more satisfying end; see Arntz, 2012). Therapists should explain this to patients. The same holds for the rescripting: it is not real, and can be completely unrealistic. Nevertheless, it can be very effective. In a certain sense, the brain does not differentiate between real and imagined experiences, even though the patient is aware of the fact that the new script is imagined—that is why the technique is so effective. Thus, therapists can explain this and reassure the patient. Of course, one doesn't want to create false memories. Thus, the fact that the patient gets an image is not in itself a proof of its correctness, and therapist and patient can agree that it is not clear whether the memory represents something that happened in reality, while still processing it with ImRs.

3. Third, when there was extreme trauma, it is not necessary, and even contra-indicated to relive the whole trauma. Therapists should enter the scene when the trauma is going to happen (so emotional expectation is high), but before the trauma proper takes place, prevent the abuse from taking place and create safety. It might be helpful to explain this to the patient and reassure him or her. This will help patients to engage, especially those who are too afraid to reexperience the whole trauma or who dissociate during reexperiencing. Unlike prolonged imaginal exposure, the technique is not based on confrontation with all details of the trauma, but on actively changing the meaning of the trauma and its interpersonal context. Note, however, that the expectation that the trauma is going to happen (in the imagery) is necessary—it is the unexpected change in what happens after this expectation is fully triggered that is an essential factor in the meaning change of the emotional memory representation (Arntz, 2012).

4. The therapist should know that imagery rescripting can bring about a period of mourning—when the patient realizes that his or her basic needs were not met in childhood and will never be met by the parents, either because it is too late (the patient no longer is a child), and/or because the parents are still incapable or unwilling to meet the patient's needs. Thus, rather than magically repairing what did not go well during childhood, the technique brings about a shift in meaning, which confronts the patient with the reality of his or her childhood. Explain this to the patient and reassure him or her; and don't forget to bring in comfort in the image when the little child is sad.

5. As noted, in general we allow patients to have revenge acted out in the rescripting if they feel a need for it. However, the therapist should feel free to refuse to execute it if he or she feels it as a moral transgression (e.g., the therapist killing a perpetrator). With patients with a history of poor control of impulsive aggression, the therapist might negotiate with the patient that an aggressive revenge will only be imagined under the condition that it is not acted out in reality and that the patient contacts the therapist if he or she feels that it gets difficult to control aggressive impulses. However, so far we have never observed increases in aggression. On the contrary, we have observed improvements in control over aggressive outbursts.

Later Treatment Phases: Patient Rescripts

Later in treatment, the therapist invites the patient to enter the scene as an adult to rescript. Basic questions to the patient as an adult are:

"What do you see? What is happening?"
"What do you feel?"
"What do you think about the situation?"
"Is there anything you would like to do?" ("Is there anything that should be done?")

First, the patient experiences the adverse event from the child's perspective. When the moment for an intervention has come, the therapist asks the patient to step into the scene as an adult. As the patient is usually not yet strong enough, the therapist initially assists the patient. So the instruction could be (from Arntz, 2011):

THERAPIST: OK, I would like you to enter the image as an adult, and I'll join you. Can you imagine that we are both standing in the same room as little Rose is?
PATIENT: Yes, I can see that.
THERAPIST: Good. What do you see? [etc.]
Therapist and patient then discuss in the image what has to be done and intervene together.
PATIENT: I feel that Rose's brother should stop abusing her.
THERAPIST: OK, and how could we stop him?
PATIENT: Perhaps we can tell him to stop.
THERAPIST: Good idea. Imagine that we tell him to stop.
PATIENT: Stop this! You are not allowed to abuse Rose.
THERAPIST: Excellent. What happens now in the image?
PATIENT: He is getting really angry. I'm afraid.

THERAPIST: Is there anything you want to do?

PATIENT: I want that he stops threatening me but I don't know how.

THERAPIST: Don't be afraid, I am with you. Let us discuss what we can do to stop him from threatening you.

PATIENT: I have no idea.

THERAPIST: Well, we could take him up and throw him out of the house. Or tell him that if he doesn't stop threatening, we will alarm our four policemen who will put him in jail. Or we could bind him up and tape his mouth so that he cannot speak anymore.

PATIENT: that is a good idea! Yes, let's do that.

One or more of these methods of stopping the maltreatment is then imagined in the rescripting.

After the maltreatment has stopped, the therapist asks the patient (as an adult) to look at the little child—as patients sometimes forget to take care of the child.

THERAPIST: Now look at little Rose. What do you see?

PATIENT: She looks sad.

THERAPIST: What do you think?

PATIENT: I think she needs to be comforted.

THERAPIST: What would you like to do?

PATIENT: Hold her and comfort her.

THERAPIST: OK, do that!

The cycle is repeated until the patient (as an adult) feels satisfied. An important next step is to let the patient experience the whole intervention by the adult patient and the therapist again, but now from the perspective of the little child.

THERAPIST: OK, now I would like you to experience the whole rescripting again, but now from the perspective of little Rose. Can you please rewind the image and be little Rose again, and imagine that the abuse threatens to happen again?

PATIENT: OK, yes, I have the image again.

THERAPIST: What happens [etc.]? (*after the whole image is vivid again and emotions are triggered*) Now adult Rose and I are entering the room. Can you see us?

PATIENT: Yes.

THERAPIST: What happens? What are they doing?

PATIENT: They tell my brother to stop abusing me. He gets angry at them, but they bind him on a chair and tape his mouth.
THERAPIST: What do you feel (if unclear: as little Rose)?
PATIENT: Relief. But still angry.
THERAPIST: What do you need?
PATIENT: That he is punished.
THERAPIST: What kind of punishment do you have in mind?
PATIENT: He should clean the toilets for the coming five years.
THERAPIST: OK, ask adult Rose and me to punish him with this.

Thus, from the child's perspective new needs may come up, and the therapist asks the patient to ask her adult self to fulfill them.

With this perspective reversal, the child might experience other needs than the patient realized as an adult (e.g., to be comforted, or to live elsewhere). That is one of the main reasons for this reversal of perspectives. The other main reason is that we found that using ImRs without feeding the new experiences into the child level was not as effective. The adult intervening is one thing, the child experiencing the intervention is probably more important (Arntz & Weertman, 1999).

Frequency of Application of ImRs

Although one good ImRs session sometimes brings about impressive changes, it should be used repeatedly in its application to PDs. Usually there are many childhood experiences that are related to the patients' problems that should be addressed. In the case of PDs, adverse childhood experiences were not isolated phenomena. On the other hand, there is no need to target every experience. Usually, many of the adverse events were repeatedly experienced (otherwise, they would probably not have contributed to the origination of a PD), and it suffices to address some prototypical examples. Usually we trust that the events that come up spontaneously in the process are good ones to address, but sometimes it is obvious that some important experiences are not addressed when the therapists only relies on letting the patient come up with an image. Examples include traumatic events that the patient avoids addressing, or the role of more passive or absent parents in the child's problems. In such cases, the therapist should propose to address these events directly with ImRs.

Imagery Rescripting of Present and Future Situations

ImRs can also be used to address current and anticipated problems. This is usually in the later phases of therapy, when patients have already undergone a considerable change, but still need to make changes on a behavioral level in their present life (e.g., Young et al., 2003; Arntz, 2014; Arntz & van Genderen, 2009). Insight is one thing, but actually changing one's behavior is another. ImRs can be used to help the patient to bring about actual behavioral change. Here the therapist asks the patient to imagine a recent or an anticipated difficult situation. The patient describes what happened—or what he or she expects to happen. Usually the way the patient felt and acted is dominated by old patterns—that is why the situation is still problematic (or is feared). Next, the therapist asks the patient to rewind and to act, in the image, in a new, more functional way. It helps to ask the patient what he or she needs and would like to say or do, and to stimulate the patient to try it out—if the patient doesn't like it after trying out, he or she can try out something else. In the beginning, the therapist might support and coach the patient in the image. Thus, the patient imagines that the therapist is also present to support him or her and the patient and the therapist discuss in the image what options there are to address the problem. For many patients, ImRs with difficult situations in their present or future life is very empowering.

Difficulties with the Application of ImRs

The major difficulties that can be encountered with the application of ImRs and how they can be addressed are summarized below. More details can be found in Arntz and Weertman (1999) and Arntz and van Genderen (2009).

1. *The patient does not dare to close his or her eyes.* The therapist should try to find out what the reason is. Some patients are very distrustful and are afraid that the therapist will laugh at them when they close their eyes. If the reason is clear, therapist and patient can work on a solution. For distrustful patients, therapists can reassure them that the therapist will also close his or her eyes and that the patient may check that occasionally. Another option is to place the chairs with their backs to each other, so that the therapist cannot look at the patient's face. In other cases, the therapist initially allows the patient to keep his or her eyes open in order to get used to the technique. Later the therapist stimulates to try to close the eyes (as ImRs will have more impact with eyes closed).

2. *The patient does not get a memory of a young child.* Again, the reasons for this phenomenon have to be clarified before any solution can be tried. McNally (2003) discusses factors that interfere with memory retrieval. Patients might, for instance, avoid remembering, and the reasons for the avoidance should be explored. Some patients think, for instance, that they should start immediately with the most severe traumas and that they will be fully exposed to them in imagery. In such

cases, the therapist should explain that it is better to start with less severe memories.

3. *The patient dissociates.* This is one of the most complicated issues, as dissociation might block information processing (Kleindienst et al., 2011; Olsen & Beck, 2012), so the patient does not profit from treatment. As soon as dissociative symptoms appear, the therapist should bring the patient back to reality; for example, by opening his or her eyes, walking around with the patient, and so on. Dissociation suggests high fear levels; thus, perhaps less frightening memories should be tried out first. It is important that the therapist brings safety into the image as soon as possible. The use of imagery of a safe place is also indicated with these patients. Last, patients should learn to detect early signs of the dissociative shift and prevent it from happening—often patients are capable of controlling this more than they (and their therapists) might initially think.

4. *The patient feels disloyal to his or her parent(s).* Feelings of being disloyal to the parent(s) might lead to resistance to rescripting. Therapists can explain that if they address the parent in the image, they are not addressing the complete parent, but only his or her behavior at that moment. They can also explain that there are two kinds of loyalty: positive and negative. Positive loyalty is feeling loyal to other people or to a group because you get positive things from them; for example, for children, care, love, and protection. Negative loyalty is feeling loyal to other people because you are afraid that if you are disloyal, you will be punished. This is not the kind of loyalty that should be used toward children (it is more what the Mafia uses). If negative loyalty is prominent in the patient's actual present life, the therapist should help the patient to get away from the threats of the family. If that is not possible, the therapeutic possibilities are probably limited. In general this explanation helps patients to get a different view of their resistance. It also helps to make clear that parents often maltreated their children because of their own psychological problems (see the ImRs example discussed, and where this is weaved into the rescripting). Last, therapists can explain that it is ultimately up to patients to decide what they want to do in reality with their parents or family in general. Some patients can talk the issues over with their parents and come to a mutual understanding, others find a way to deal with them, and still others break with them.

When and How to Use ImRs in CBT of PDs

ImRs is a standard technique of ST, but not of other forms of CBT for PDs, although it has been described in Beck et al. (2004) and Layden, Newman, Freeman, and Morse (1993) as an optional technique. ImRs can be easily integrated in regular CBT, and it is a good idea to add it to the more verbal and rational CT work and to use it before the focus of treatment is on behavioral change. There are some specific indications for using ImRs in the context of a CBT treatment. First, it is useful when patients have trouble emotionally integrating new beliefs. The classic example that of a patient who agrees that his idea that he is inferior is not rational and that he should feel differently, but who doesn't succeed in profiting from that insight on a "gut level." In such cases, it might be good to go back to early experiences where he got this feeling of being inferior and to use ImRs to change the meaning if those experiences. Second, there might be traumas or other adversities that the patient wants to process or that the therapists feels that processing would be helpful. ImRs offers an excellent processing method, as it places early adversities in the interpersonal context that is so important for personality development. Moreover, it does not require lengthy confrontation with all the trauma details, as the focus is on the (interpersonal) meaning and not on the perceptual details. Third, ImRs of childhood memories is most indicated in the earlier and mid-treatment phases, as the later phases of treatment should focus more on the present and future, and necessary behavioral change. Of course, ImRs work of focusing on present and future situations can be used in the later phases, especially if the patients reports strong emotional barriers to a change in behavior. On the other hand, ImRs of severe traumas is contraindicated very early in treatment when the therapeutic relationship is not so strong yet, and patients have to get used to discussing problems and emotions anyway. A possible exception is the patient who comes to treatment for trauma processing; in such a case, ImRs can start after a short preparatory phase.

An ImRs exercise takes about 20 minutes, but because it is difficult to predict when the exercise is finished, therapists are advised to start it within the first 20 minutes (if your session is about 50 minutes). We generally found that if therapists don't start to use any experiential technique within this time frame, the session ends in a talking session—and is by hindsight often "lost." It is thus advised to include in every other session an experiential exercise and start this within 10–20 minutes, to prevent both therapist and patient from remaining stuck in a talking (instead of experiencing) mode. The talking can be done after the exercise and is often more productive after such an exercise.

It is a good idea to change techniques within and for different sessions— thus use thinking, feeling, and behavior as channels to bring about integrated change. ImRs can be prepared with cognitive techniques; for example, the session before the ImRs work can be devoted to rationally challenging beliefs about the self or others, whereas the ImRs uses these new insights to correct the old beliefs and bring in new functional beliefs in the memory of events that are associated with these beliefs. It should be noted, however, that we don't know yet whether or not ImRs has better effects when the patient is cognitively prepared (see Arntz, 2012), and too much planning might lead to losing contact with his or her emotions of the moment—as between the sessions other issues might have been triggered that are more open for therapeutic work.

There is no specific indication when ImRs work can be considered completed, although a good sign is when patients are capable of taking the lead as an adult in the rescripting and report that ImRs improves their functioning. ImRs is a powerful technique that can be used repeatedly, but when patients do well and the focus of treatment is more on continuation of change, its use is usually reduced. Quite another issue is when the patient seems to profit more from other types of experiential work, like chair work and historical role plays. Some people seem to profit more from imagery work, and others from role plays, and the therapist is encouraged to follow the format preferred by the patient, realizing that a lot of "rescripting" can also be done with other methods.

Future Directions

One of the attractive aspects of using ImRs in the treatment of PDs is the possibility of processing memories of childhood experiences that lie at the root of personality problems. It is an appealing idea that processing such memories leads to very fundamental changes in core schemas and coping strategies. But as far as the present author knows, there is no empirical evidence that treatments that incorporate techniques like ImRs to process such early memories have superior effects compared to treatments that don't. Although we know that such techniques are effective, and that some patients seem to profit more from them while others seem to profit more from techniques focusing on present problems (Weertman & Arntz, 2007), we don't know whether adding techniques like ImRs to usual CBT techniques improves the long-term outcome—although the good effects of ST suggest so. Dismantling studies are needed here to investigate this issue. The rapid dissemination of ST will also contribute to dissemination of ImRs as a technique in the treatment of PDs. It is to be expected that CBT therapists will increasingly use ImRs when treating patients with PDs, since there don't seem to be specific problems with integrating ImRs into common CBT. A relatively new development is group ST—and the application of ImRs in groups clearly requires adaptations to the group format (e.g., see Farrell & Shaw, 2012). How this can best be done has not been completely crystalized– but it is to be expected that in the coming decade standardized ways to use ImRs in groups of patients with PD will be developed and empirically tested. More research is also needed into the basic mechanisms underlying ImRs, especially how and under what conditions the mechanism differs from exposure procedures (see also Arntz, Chapter 9, this volume). Last, one of the most common barriers to applying ImRs with difficult patients like those with PDs is that therapists hesitate to use it and often would rather stick with talking than to do this kind of emotive work. Helping therapists to not fall into this pitfall is an important issue for training, supervision, and quality control systems.

Further Resources

- For DVD examples of ImRs, see Bernstein and van den Wijngaart (2010) and Nadort (2005).
- For books discussing ImRs, and other experiential techniques in the treatment of PDs, see Arntz and van Genderen (2009), Arntz and Jacob (2012), and Farrell and Shaw (2012).
- For information about schema therapy, go to *www.isst-online.com*.

Author Note

This chapter is partially based on Arntz (2011) and Arntz and van Genderen (2009).

References

Arntz, A. (2011). Imagery rescripting for personality disorders. *Cognitive and Behavioral Practice, 18,* 466–481.
Arntz, A. (2012). Imagery rescripting as a therapeutic technique: Review of clinical trials, basic studies, and research agenda. *Journal of Experimental Psychopathology, 3,*189–208.
Arntz, A. (2014). Borderline personality disorder. In A. T, Beck, D. D. Davis, A. Freeman, & Associates (Eds.), *Cognitive therapy of personality disorders* (3rd ed.). New York: Guilford Press.
Arntz, A. & Jacob, G. (2012). *Schema therapy in practice*. Chichester, UK: Wiley.
Arntz, A., & van Genderen, H. (2009). *Schema therapy for borderline personality disorder*. Chichester, UK: Wiley.
Arntz, A., Tiesema, M., & Kindt, M. (2007). Treatment of PTSD: A comparison of imaginal exposure with and without imagery rescripting. *Journal of Behavior Therapy and Experimental Psychiatry, 38,* 345–370.
Arntz, A., & Weertman, A. (1999). Treatment of childhood memories: Theory and practice. *Behaviour Research and Therapy, 37,* 715–740.
Bamelis, L. L. M., Evers, S. M. A. A., Spinhoven, P., & Arntz, A. (2014a). Results of a multicentered randomised controlled trial on the clinical effectiveness of schema therapy for personality disorders. *American Journal of Psychiatry, 171,* 20–25.
Bamelis, L. L. M., Arntz, A., Wetzelaer, P., Verdoorn, R. & Evers, S. M. A. A. (2014b). Economic evaluation of schema therapy for personality disorders. Submitted for publication.
Beck, A. T., Freeman, A., Davis, D. D., & Associates. (2004). *Cognitive therapy of personality disorders* (2nd ed.). New York: Guilford Press.
Bernstein, D. P., Nijman, H. L. I., Karos, K., Keulen-de Vos, M., Vogel, V., & Lucker, T. P. (2012). Schema therapy for forensic patients with personality disorders: Design

and preliminary findings of a multicenter randomized clinical trial in the Netherlands. *International Journal of Forensic Mental Health, 11,* 312–324.

Bernstein, D. P., Stein, J. A., & Handelsman, L. (1998). Predicting personality pathology among adult patients with substance use disorders: Effects of childhood maltreatment. *Addictive Behavior, 23,* 855–868.

Bernstein, D. P., & van der Wijngaart, R. (2010). *Schema therapy: Working with modes* [DVD]. Available at *www.schematherapy.nl*.

Bierer, L. M., Yehuda, R., Schmeidler, J., Mitropoulou, V., New, A. S., Silverman, J. M., et al. (2003). Abuse and neglect in childhood: Relationship to personality disorder diagnoses. *CNS Spectrums, 8,* 737–754.

Cohen, L. J., Foster, M., Nesci, C., Tanis, T., Halmi, W., & Galynker, I. (2013). How do different types of childhood maltreatment relate to adult personality pathology? *Journal of Nervous and Mental Disease, 201,* 234–243.

Dadds, M. R., Bovbjerg, D. H., Redd, W. H., & Cutmore, T. R. (1997). Imagery in human classical conditioning. *Psychological Bulletin, 122,* 89–103.

Davidson, K., Norrie, J., Tyrer, P., Gumley, A., Tata, P., Murray, H., et al. (2006). The effectiveness of cognitive behavior therapy for borderline personality disorder: Results from the Borderline Personality Disorder Study of Cognitive Therapy (BOSCOT) trial. *Journal of Personality Disorders, 20,* 450–465.

Emmelkamp, P. M. G., Benner, A., Kuipers, A., Feiertag, G., Koster, H. C., & van Apeldoorn, F. J. (2006). Comparison of brief dynamic and cognitive-behavioural therapies in avoidant personality disorder. *British Journal of Psychiatry, 89,* 60–64.

Farrell, J. M., & Shaw, I. A. (2012). *Group schema therapy for borderline personality disorder: A step-by-step treatment manual with patient workbook.* New York: Wiley.

Farrell, J. M., Shaw, I. A., & Webber, M. A. (2009). A schema-focused approach to group psychotherapy for outpatients with borderline personality disorder: A randomized controlled trial. *Journal of Behavior Therapy and Experimental Psychiatry, 40,* 317–328.

Giesen-Bloo, J., van Dyck, R., Spinhoven, P., van Tilburg, W., Dirksen, C., van Asselt, T., et al. (2006). Outpatient psychotherapy for borderline personality disorder: A randomized controlled trial of schema-focused therapy versus transference focused psychotherapy. *Archives of General Psychiatry, 63,* 649–658.

Hernandez, A., Arntz, A., Gaviria, A. M., Labad, A. & Gutiérrez-Zotes, J. A. (2012). Relationships between childhood maltreatment, parenting style and borderline personality disorder criteria. *Journal of Personality Disorders, 26,* 727–736.

Holmes, E. A., Arntz, A., & Smucker, M. R. (2007). Imagery rescripting in cognitive behaviour therapy: Images, treatment techniques and outcomes. *Journal of Behavior Therapy and Experimental Psychiatry, 38,* 297–305.

Holmes, E. A., & Mathews, A. (2010). Mental imagery in emotion and emotional disorders. *Clinical Psychology Review, 30,* 349–362.

Holmes, E. A., Mathews, A., Dalgleish, T., & Mackintosh, B. (2006). Positive interpretation training: Effects of mental imagery training versus verbal training on positive mood. *Behavior Therapy, 37,* 237–247.

Horwitz, A. V., Widom, C. S., McLaughlin, J., & White, H. R. (2001). The impact of childhood abuse and neglect on adult mental health: A prospective study. *Journal of Health and Social Behavior, 42,* 184–201.

Jacob, G. A., & Arntz, A. (2013). Schema therapy for personality disorders—A review. *International Journal of Cognitive Psychotherapy, 6,* 170–184.

Jacob, G., Arendt, J., Kolley, L., Scheel, C. N., Bader, K., Lieb, K., et al. (2011). Comparison of different strategies to decrease negative affect and increase positive affect in women with borderline personality disorder. *Behaviour Research and Therapy, 49,* 68–73.

Johnson, J. G., Cohen, P., Brown, J., Smailes, E. M., & Bernstein, D. P. (1999). Childhood maltreatment increases risk for personality disorders during early adulthood. *Archives of General Psychiatry, 56,* 600–606.

Johnson, J. G., Cohen, P., Chen, H., Kasen, S., & Brook, J. S. (2006). Parenting behaviors associated with risk for offspring personality disorder during adulthood. *Archives of General Psychiatry, 63,* 579–587.

Johnson, J. G., Cohen, P., Smailes, E. M., Skodol, A. E., Brown, J., & Oldham, J. M. (2001). Childhood verbal abuse and risk for personality disorders during adolescence and early adulthood. *Comprehensive Psychiatry. 42,* 16–23.

Johnson, J. G., Smailes, E. M., Cohen, P., Brown, J., & Bernstein, D. P. (2000) Associations between four types of childhood neglect and personality disorder symptoms during adolescence and early adulthood: Findings of a community-based longitudinal study. *Journal of Personality Disorders, 14,* 171–187.

Joyce, P. R., McKenzie, J. M., Luty, S. E., Mulder, R. T., Carter, J. D., Sullivan, P. F., et al. (2003). Temperament, childhood environment and psychopathology as risk factors for avoidant and borderline personality disorders. *Australian and New Zealand Journal of Psychiatry, 37,* 756–764.

Kendler, K. S., Aggen, S. H., Czajkowski, N, Roysamb, E., Tambs, K., Torgersen, S., et al. (2008). The structure of genetic and environmental risk factors for DSM-IV personality disorders: A multivariate twin study. *Archives of General Psychiatry, 65,* 1438–1446.

Kleindienst, N., Limberger, M. F., Ebner-Priemer, U. W., Keibel-Mauchnik, J., Dyer, A., Berger, M., et al. (2011). Dissociation predicts poor response to dialectial behavioral therapy in female patients with borderline personality disorder. *Journal of Personality Disorders, 25,* 432–447.

Layden, M. A., Newman, C. F., Freeman, A., & Morse, S. B. (1993). *Cognitive therapy of borderline personality disorder.* Boston: Allyn & Bacon.

Lobbestael, J., & Arntz, A. (2010). Emotional, cognitive and physiological correlates of abuse-related stress in borderline and antisocial personality disorder. *Behaviour Research and Therapy, 48,* 116–124.

Lobbestael, J., Arntz, A., & Bernstein, D. P. (2010). Disentangling the relationship between different types of childhood maltreatment and personality disorders. *Journal of Personality Disorders, 24*(3), 285–295.

McNally, R. J. (2003). *Remembering trauma.* Cambridge, MA: Harvard University Press.

Nadort, M. (2005). *Schema therapy for borderline personality disorder* [DVD]. Available at *www.schematherapie.nl.*

Nadort, M., Arntz, A., Smit, J. H., Giesen-Bloo, J., Eikelenboom, M., Spinhoven, P., et al. (2009). Implementation of outpatient schema therapy for borderline personality disorder with versus without crisis support by the therapist outside office hours: A randomized trial. *Behaviour Research and Therapy, 47,* 961–973.

Napel-Schutz, M. C., ten, Abma, T. A., Bamelis, L., & Arntz, A. (2011). Personality disorder patients' perspectives on the introduction of imagery within schema therapy: A qualitative study of patients' experiences. *Cognitive and Behavioral Practice, 18,* 482–490.

Olsen, S. A., & Beck, J. G. (2012). The effects of dissociation on information processing for analogue trauma and neutral stimuli: A laboratory study. *Journal of Anxiety Disorders, 26,* 225–232.

Seebauer, L., Froß, S., Dubaschny, L., Schönberger, M., & Jacob, G. A. (2014). Is it dangerous to fantasize revenge in imagery exercises?: An experimental study. *Journal of Behavior Therapy and Experimental Psychiatry, 45*, 20–25.

Sempérteguia, G. A., Karremana, A., Arntz, A., & Bekker, M. H. J. (2013). Schema therapy for borderline personality disorder: A comprehensive review of its empirical foundations, effectiveness and implementation possibilities. *Clinical Psychological Review, 33*, 426–447.

van Asselt, A. D. I., Dirksen, C. D., Arntz, A., Giesen-Bloo, J. H., van Dyck, R., Spinhoven, P., et al. (2008). Outpatient psychotherapy for borderline personality disorder: Cost-effectiveness of schema-focused therapy versus transference-focused psychotherapy. *British Journal of Psychiatry, 192*(6), 450–457.

Weertman, A., & Arntz, A. (2007). Effectiveness of treatment of childhood memories in cognitive therapy for personality disorders: A controlled study contrasting methods focusing on the present and methods focusing on childhood memories. *Behaviour Research and Therapy, 45*, 2133–2143.

Young, J. E., Klosko, J. S., & Weishaar, M. E. (2003). *Schema therapy: A practitioner's guide*. New York: Guilford Press.

CHAPTER 9

Imagery Rescripting for Posttraumatic Stress Disorder

Arnoud Arntz

Although imagery rescripting (ImRs) as a treatment for posttraumatic stress disorder (PTSD) has attracted less attention from researchers than imaginal exposure and eye movement desensitization and reprocessing (EMDR), it is a powerful treatment with high acceptability that can be used for simple as well as complex PTSD. In fact, variations of ImRs have been used in various forms of psychotherapy for more than a century (Edwards, 2007). However, it is only recently that ImRs has been accepted in mainstream cognitive-behavioral therapy (CBT), which is clear from the fact that scientific studies about its effectiveness and underlying processes have been increasing in number and quality (Arntz, 2012). This chapter discusses how ImRs can be used to treat PTSD, starting with the theoretical rationale, then a brief review of the empirical evidence for its effectiveness, and finally with further delineation of its clinical application.

Rationale for ImRs

The basic idea of ImRs in the treatment of PTSD is to activate the trauma memory and imagine a different ending that better matches the needs of the patient. The therapeutic effects are not based on a simple replacement of the original memory by a new memory, as research shows that the facts of the original trauma memory are not forgotten or overwritten by rescripting (Arntz, 2012). The mechanism seems to be a change in the meaning of the trauma memory, brought about by experiencing in fantasy what one needed in the situation and getting these lingering, unmet needs met in fantasy. In learning theory terms this is called "US revaluation"—the change in meaning of the original unconditioned stimulus (US), the traumatic experience.

This is a different mechanism than extinction, on which exposure treatment is based (Arntz, 2012). With extinction, people learn that in a certain context the conditioned stimulus (CS), that is, a trauma reminder, no longer predicts the occurrence of the US, that is, the trauma. However, the original CS–US association remains stored in memory, and a change to another context than that in which extinction (i.e., exposure treatment) took place can trigger the original memory trace again, so that the CS again leads to the expectation of the US. Thus, exposure treatment does not change the meaning of the trauma memory itself, but leads to the formation of an alternative memory trace. Confronted with a trauma reminder, there is a competition between the original and the new memory traces, and it depends on variables, like the context, which trace "wins" the competition, that is, whether the person feels safe or expects a reoccurrence of the trauma.

With US revaluation, new information is fed into the memory representation of the US, the trauma itself. If this information is helpful, it will reduce the dysfunctional meaning of the trauma memory. Independent of context, a trauma reminder will trigger the changed memory representation of the trauma (the US) and, if the meaning change was successful, this memory will no longer lead to dysfunctional responses, like anxious expectation that the trauma will take place again. The effects of treatment using this mechanism are not context-dependent, as is the case with extinction.

The kind of needs that patients want to be met during ImRs can range widely, from being more powerful to ward off a natural disaster or the attack by a perpetrator, to having the assistance of others, up to changing the aftermaths of a traumatic event, such as giving an appropriate funeral to the deceased. Although the current theory is that the change of meaning of the trauma memory is central, another (or additional) possibility is that the expression of needs, feelings, and actions, which were inhibited at the time, usually because of survival reasons, is a healing factor (e.g., Arntz, 2012). ImRs has been applied for a wide range of PTSD, with traumas ranging from single accidents during adulthood to complex repeated traumas with severe consequences for interpersonal trust in childhood.

Empirical Evidence

Smucker and coworkers developed an ImRs protocol for incest-related PTSD (Smucker & Niederee, 1995), but the results of the trial testing were never published. An open trial tested whether ImRs is a helpful treatment when imaginal exposure for accident-related PTSD fails (Grunert, Weis, Smucker & Christianson, 2007). Twenty-three patients with PTSD resulting from industrial accidents participated, all of whom were nonresponders to standard imaginal exposure. Eighteen of the 23 patients showed a full recovery from PTSD after ImRs. It should be noted that the study was uncontrolled: ImRs was not compared to an alternative second treatment. The authors suggest that when fear is not the predominant emotion related to the trauma, but emotions like anger, shame, or guilt dominate, prolonged imaginal exposure is not very helpful and ImRs is a better treatment. When fear is predominant, exposure would be the optimal treatment. However, more research is needed to test this proposition, as some findings suggest that exposure is also effective for nonfear emotions, and other studies suggest that ImRs is also effective when fear is predominant.

The effects of adding ImRs to prolonged imaginal exposure (IE) for PTSD were studied in an RCT by comparing the combined IE–ImRs treatment to IE alone and both to wait list (Arntz, Tiesema, & Kindt, 2007). The mixed trauma sample of 71 chronic PTSD patients had mosly suffered multiple traumas and were highly dysfunctional and chronic. The waitlist condition showed no evidence of any improvement. Active treatment, however, was superior to wait list, showing reductions in symptoms with medium-to-large effects. The study further demonstrated that the addition of ImRs to IE led to a significant reduction of treatment dropouts, and better effects on anger, anger control, shame and guilt, compared to IE alone.

Therapists tended to prefer ImRs instead of IE, as they felt less helpless listening to the trauma relivings and experienced less distress with ImRs. In an open trial Kindt, Buck, Arntz, and Soeter (2007) assessed the effects of ImRs combined with imaginal exposure in 25 chronic PTSD patients with a varying trauma background (the majority had experienced multiple physical or sexual assaults). The study primarily focused on a hypothesized underlying mechanism in treatment of PTSD, which is the activation of perceptual trauma memories, and which should be followed by their transformation from perceptual to conceptual encoding. Large effects on PTSD complaints of ImRs were found, as well as evidence for the mechanism. A third study tested 10 sessions of ImRs as treatment for war-related PTSD in refugees in a multiple-baseline case series design. There were large effects on PTSD and depression, as well as a strong reduction in the use of psychoactive medication (Arntz, Sofi, & van Breukelen, 2013)—despite the complexities of this group, including poor social integration and the use of interpreters in many treatments. Fourth, Steil developed and tested a very effective ImRs protocol for survivors of childhood sexual abuse who suffer from a continuous feeling of being contaminated (Steil, Jung, & Stangier, 2011; Jung & Steil, 2013). Not only did the contamination feelings decrease dramatically, but also the PTSD symptoms were reduced, with high effect sizes.

Further evidence stems from research into Ehlers and Clark's CT for PTSD, which has ImRs as an integrated part (Ehlers & Clark, 2000; Ehlers, Clark, Hackmann, McManus, & Fennell, 2005). On the average 3 out of

12 sessions involve imagery work (Ehlers et al., 2005). As an example of their use of ImRs, Ehlers et al. (2005) describe the case of a woman who suffered from feeling unattractive as a result of her rapist telling her she was ugly:

> For example, a woman who had been raped identified a moment when her assailant said she was ugly and turned her over, as the worst 'hot spot.' Ever since the rape she had felt unattractive and, more recently, had been engaging in frequent casual sex in an apparent attempt to convince herself that she was attractive. Socratic questioning was used to identify an alternative appraisal, which was that the rapist had identified her because she is attractive and his comment was because he is unable to become aroused without abusing and humiliating women. During a subsequent imaginal reliving, she introduced the new appraisal into the 'hot spot' by standing up in the image and saying it to the rapist at the moment that he verbally abused her. (p. 415)

Very strong effects of the Ehlers and Clark package have been reported (Ehlers et al., 2003, 2005; Duffy, Gillespie, & Clark, 2007). An important difference to some other ImRs applications is that the rescripting is carefully prepared before imagined, to correct dysfunctional appraisals of the traumatic event. The rescripting is then implemented in a rather directive way, with the therapist instructing the patient to imagine the prepared new script. In other approaches, patients try out rescripting on the basis of needs they experience while imagining the trauma; and in still other approaches the therapists develop the script. Apart from how the script is developed, the basic principles are the same (Clark, 2011; Duffy, personal communication) and it is an empirical issue for future research what method to develop and imagine the new script is optimal.

ImRs is also an effective treatment of PTSD-associated chronic nightmares. In short, patients rescript the nightmare into a more benign ending and rehearse that daily (Davis & Wright, 2005; Krakow & Zadra, 2006). Strong effects have been found in well-controlled trials (e.g., Krakow et al., 2001; Davis & Wright, 2007). For an overview of studies into ImRs for nightmares, see Long and Quevillon (2009).

In summary, studies of ImRs for PTSD show positive results, especially regarding dysfunctional interpretations and emotional problems like anger and shame. Future studies should test ImRs alone by comparing it to other effective treatments.

Application with PTSD

Simple Trauma

With simple trauma, there is no need to decide on what trauma should be focused on first, and the therapist can start with gathering the usual information about the trauma: what happened, when took it place, what were the preceding factors, and what were the effects. It is helpful to get an idea what the current imagery symptoms are (intrusions, nightmares); what sensory modalities are involved; what they mean to the patient; and how the patient tries to deal with them. Such reliving symptoms might form a helpful focus for ImRs, as they are often central to the dysfunctional meaning the patient gave to the trauma (and/or to the trauma symptoms), and often represent signals of the feared catastrophe (like death; Ehlers et al., 2002; Hackmann, 2011). The meaning of the traumatic event for the patient should also be explored, as well as emotions and action tendencies that were activated but could not be expressed. Sometimes these emotions and the related action tendencies start to develop after the trauma proper, but they are nonetheless informative about what patients' unfulfilled needs are.

In the next session the therapist can either start ImRs directly, or do a cognitive preparation. With the latter approach, the central dysfunctional meanings associated with the trauma should be clarified and a functional alternative should be formulated that can be used to base the ImRs on. An example was already given when discussing the Ehlers and Clark protocol (pp. 205–206). Depending on the time this takes, ImRs can be tried out during the very same session or in the next session.

With the first approach, the therapist starts with an explanation of the ImRs procedure. Important parts of the explanation are:

1. Imagery is a more powerful way than talking to change traumatic memories and the associated meaning and emotions. The therapist might want to refer to the scientific tests by Emily Holmes (e.g., training of positive interpretations; Holmes, Mathews, Dalgleish, & Mackintosh, 2006), the successful and proven use of imagery to rehearse (musicians, sportsmen), and the neuroscience findings that the brain responds almost equally to imagined as to real events (e.g., Holmes & Mathews, 2010).

2. During a traumatic event it is natural that all kinds of needs, emotions, and action tendencies are triggered, but they usually cannot be fully actualized—as this is impossible (e.g., one is immobilized) or too dangerous (e.g., attacking a perpetrator might lead to the perpetrator killing you). It is healthy and corrective to imagine emotions to be expressed, actions to be carried out, and needs to be met. The effects are much stronger if we imagine this process as if it was really done in the context of the actual trauma, not just talked about (see 1).

3. The effect of ImRs is not that the original memory of the facts is replaced by a new memory (in fact, a "false memory"). Research shows that the memory of the facts of the traumatic event is not damaged by ImRs (Hagenaars & Arntz, 2012; Spinhoven, Bamelis, Haringsma, Marc Molendijk, & Arntz, 2012). Rather, a cognitive and emotional processing of the event is brought about by ImRs, which leads to reduction of the

vividness of the memory, a change in its meaning, a reduction of fear of the memory, and reduced intrusions and nightmares. Thus though many qualities of the memory become less intense, the memory of the facts is not damaged.

4. The patient can imagine all kinds of changes in the script that meet his or her needs. It is not important whether these changes are realistic, as long as they are experienced during ImRs as having a powerful impact and satisfying the patient's needs. Thus patients might fantasize that troops fly into the scene to kill the terrorists and rescue them; that Superman helps them; that they give a proper funeral to the deceased; that they torture the torturers; that they visit the deceased in heaven and get his or her permission to stop mourning; and so on. Creativity and suggestions by the therapist help!

5. If the patient is not (completely) satisfied with the rescripting, there is no problem, as additions to the script, or completely different scripts can be tried out. Additionally, during rescripting, the "film" can be rewound and a different rescripting can be tried out.

6. It is helpful if the patient rehearses the ImRs several times during the week, for example, by practicing while listening to a recording of the ImRs during the session.

When the general explanation is given and questions by the patient have been addressed, the therapist then invites the patient to sit comfortably, close his or her eyes, and start imagining and describing the sequence of events that led to the trauma. Questions like "Where are you?", "What do you see, hear, smell?", and "What is happening?" help the patient emerge in imagery. While initially the focus is on perceptions, the next questions focus on emotions ("What do you feel?"), and (after the emotions) on cognitions ("What are you thinking? What do you think of the situation?"). If it is clear that distress is getting high, the therapist asks what the patient needs ("What do you need?"). When the patient's needs are clear, the patient is invited to change the script so that his or her needs are better met by imagining the new script as vividly as possible. Usually patients imagine that they behave differently themselves, or that other people are there to help them. Thus, the perspective remains the point of view of the patient. Many changes in the script can be made, for example, preventing the trauma from taking place, changing the aftermath of the trauma, or bringing in reality in the image at the most horrible moment (e.g., realizing that one's partner will arrive in time to rescue you from choking). The therapist helps the patient to imagine the rescripting as vividly as possible by asking the same questions as before, first focusing on perceptions ("What do you see?", "What is happening?", etc.), then on emotions, then on cognitions, and then on possible further needs ("Is there anything else you need?"). If more needs are expressed, additional rescripting is used, and the cycle is repeated, until the patient states that everything is fine. Here are some examples of what patients imagined during rescripting:

- A victim of a violent robbery imagined scaring away the assailant by his superior skills in martial arts.
- Ehlers et al. (2005) give an example of a woman who identified the worst moment of her memory of the rape when the assailant said she was ugly and turned her over. She imagined telling the rapist that he lied, that he had identified her because she was attractive, and that he needed to abuse and humiliate women to become aroused (p. 415).
- One of the participants of the Arntz et al. (2013) trial imagined that his family got a decent funeral, following the rituals of his religion—whereas in fact his family was brutally slaughtered and the remains were left in the open air by the terrorists.

For therapists who were trained in imaginal exposure as treatment of PTSD, it is important to know that ImRs does *not* require full exposure to all details of the trauma. Whereas in imaginal exposure treatment this would be seen as avoidance, in ImRs the rescripting can start just before the trauma proper happens. ImRs can also address only parts of the trauma memory, whether they are preceding the trauma proper, part of it, or part of its aftermath. The patient usually indicates which part of the memory is most troublesome and where he or she would have liked for something different to have happened, or where he or she would, if possible, had liked to have acted differently. The rescripting can then focus on this part. However, therapists should be aware that patients might avoid addressing parts of the memory that play a role in maintaining the problems, and this possibility should be discussed with the patient. Moreover, we don't encourage rescripting to start before a clear expectation of the trauma is built up, and associated emotions are triggered. ImRs might be particularly effective as a method to change the meaning of the trauma memory because the rescripting brings an unexpected change into an expected sequence (see Arntz, 2012, for a detailed discussion of this possible fundamental mechanism), but to capitalize on this mechanism, a clear expectation on both a cognitive and an emotional level should be activated.

Multiple Traumas

With multiple traumas it might be necessary to make a list of the traumas that should be addressed and to decide what trauma to address first. The list can be flexible, in the sense that items may be added or removed, and the order can be changed, according to the patient's wishes. There is no need for a hierarchical order, and the therapist can leave the choice of which trauma to start with to the patient. However, if fear of specific memories is very high, or the patient tends to respond with dissociative responses, it is helpful to start with a memory of a less distressing trauma. The therapist therefore checks with the patient whether he or she is not asking too much from him- or herself when choosing to start with a very difficult memory. Some patients don't mention any less severe traumas, so some extra exploration might be helpful. To reduce the fear of trauma processing with ImRs, even a memory of a distressing event that strictly speaking does not qualify for PTSD could be taken.

A usual therapeutic process is to work with one trauma memory every session, and to take each session a new trauma. However, it is wise to adapt to the processing speed of the patient—some patients need more sessions with one memory, others may be able to address two or three memories in one session. Often, once the patient has become used to the technique and has found effective rescripting strategies, several traumas can be addressed in one session (e.g., see Arntz et al., 2013).

The ImRs work in the session can be recorded and patient can rehearse the rescripting at home while listening to the recording. Often he or she initially reports problems with imagining as vividly as in the session, but over time they usually get better at this.

Complex PTSD

With complex PTSD there has usually been extended childhood abuse in a context of lack of safety, and this issue has considerably damaged interpersonal trust and self-views. Like in the treatment of severe personality disorders (see Arntz, Chapter 8, this volume), it is then indicated that the therapist initially leads the rescripting, preventing the abuse, creating safety, correcting the abusers, and taking care of the child after this has been done. Extended examples are provided in Chapter 8. One of the reasons to do this is that these patients often are too frightened during the imagery to be able to fantasize any rescripting. Another reason is that for this kind of early abuse it might be an extra healing factor for the patient to experience a healthy adult patient protecting the child and taking care of him or her (see Arntz, Chapter 8, this volume). During treatment, the patient can gradually take the lead in the rescripting—initially coached and assisted by the therapist, to be able to rescript him- or herself at the end of treatment (Arntz & Weertman, 1999). A typical way to do this is to ask the patient to step into the image as an adult, look at the (threatening) abuse of the child, realize the emotions and needs this evokes, and intervene. Of course the adult can get help from others (including the therapist) in the rescripting.

Difficulties with the Application of ImRs

1. *The patient does not dare to close his or her eyes.* The therapist should try to find out what the reason is. Often it is the fear of being overwhelmed by memories. If so, the therapist can reassure the patient that the rescripting can start before the actual trauma happens, to prevent being overwhelmed. A script can be worked out. The therapist can also initially allow the patient to keep his or her eyes open in order to get used to the technique. Later the therapist asks the patient to try to close his or her eyes.

2. *The patient dissociates.* As soon as dissociative symptoms appear, the therapist should bring the patient back to reality; for example, by opening his or her eyes, walking around with the patient, and the like. Signs that should warn the therapist include the patient stops responding to the therapist, or responds in a robot-like fashion; the patient starts to hum; the patient reports an inability to focus on the image; the patient states that he or she is going to faint; and so on. Dissociation suggests high fear levels; thus, perhaps less frightening memories should be tried out first. It is important that the therapist brings safety into the image as soon as possible. Remember, ImRs does not require full exposure to all the horrible details of the trauma, and patients should be reassured about this method. Last, patients should learn to detect early signs of the dissociative shift and prevent it from happening—often patients can control this more than they initially think.

3. *The patient wants to take revenge in imagery.* Some patients express a need to take revenge toward perpetrators or people who maltreated them, for example, after the trauma (e.g., the police or a medical doctor humiliating the victim of sexual or physical abuse). Therapists might feel reluctance to consent to act this out in ImRs, as they might wonder whether this activity would increase the risks of actual aggression. Luckily, there are some empirical data about this problem. In the Arntz et al. (2007) RCT, imagining revenge during ImRs was allowed. The results showed that adding ImRs to imaginal exposure had positive effects on anger and on anger control, compared to imaginal exposure alone. Thus this trial suggests that with the average PTSD patient there is even a reduction of risk of actual aggressive acting out with ImRs. One reason for this reduced risk is that taking revenge in fantasy satisfies the revenge needs more than trying to suppress it; it also normalizes it and makes it more acceptable and less frightening—possibly reducing the risk of loss of control in difficult circumstances. Laboratory work at Freiburg University has so far also indicated that there is no indication of adverse effects by using revenge in ImRs (Seebauer, Froß, Dubaschny, Schönberger, & Jacob, 2014). However, one might argue that with specific populations (e.g., forensic patients with a known history of losing control over aggression, or patients who

lose control over aggressive impulses when intoxicated by alcohol or drugs) there might be problems. Lacking empirical data, therapists might want to reach agreement about reducing risk factors with such patients before allowing them to act out revenge during ImRs. For example, therapists can agree with patients that use of (excessive) alcohol should be stopped (in any case better for PTSD treatment!) and check to ensure that patients do not ruminate with plans for actual aggression. A healthy response to a successful ImRs session involving imagined revenge is a reduction in revenge impulses and fantasies; when the opposite takes place, it should be considered a warning signal, and the clinician should conduct a risk assessment.

4. *The patient goes into a mourning process.* Sometimes the rescripting, though satisfying needs as experienced during imagery, nevertheless triggers a mourning process. There might have been losses associated with the trauma, or the contrast between what the patient needed (as realized during ImRs) and what actually happened leads to a mourning process. In essence, this is a natural and healthy process, and the therapist should explain this process to the patient, validate his or her sadness, and support the patient. If the mourning process gets stuck, factors that prevent resolution should be explored. Often they can also be addressed in ImRs, like visiting the deceased in heaven and asking him or her permission to stop mourning.

See Arntz (Chapter 8, this volume) for how to deal with problems with more complex traumas.

When and How to Use ImRs for PTSD

ImRs can be given as a full treatment for PTSD and will then usually take between five and 20 sessions. It can also be combined with other CBT techniques, like rational challenging dysfunctional interpretations and exposure *in vivo*; and is a standard part of Ehlers and Clark's cognitive therapy for PTDS. An ImRs exercise takes about 20 minutes, but as it is difficult to predict when it is finished, therapists are advised to start it within the first 20 minutes (if your session is about 60 minutes); and two or three ImRs exercises can be done in one session. Sessions can be taped and the patient can rehearse the ImRs while listening to the recording as homework.

Usually patients with PTSD indicate when symptoms are reduced enough to lead a satisfactorily life, and therapy can then be stopped.

Future Directions

Given the increasing interest in ImRs as a treatment for PTSD, new developments are to be expected. Among them are the development and empirical validation of specific rescripting techniques to deal with complex trauma-related phenomena, as we have seen with nightmares (Krakow & Zadra, 2006) and feelings of disgust resulting from sexual abuse (Steil et al., 2011). The question of how to address revenge feelings with ImRs has only very recently lead to empirical studies (Seebauer et al., 2014), but the most important questions—whether it is helpful or not to fantasize revenge against perpetrators in ImRs and whether or not it is dangerous in specific populations, have still to be addressed. The finding in social psychology that revenge needs are satisfied if the other person shows an understanding of the reason for the revenge, but doesn't depend so much on the degree of suffering of the offender, might be important to develop effective ways to deal with revenge issues in treatment (Gollwitzer & Denzler, 2009). Another important clinical issue is deciding when it is indicated that therapists guide the rescipting and when it is better that patients do it. Early applications of ImRs in the context of CBT relied on the patient leading the rescripting, but work with patients with more severe early maltreatment histories showed that patients are often incapable of doing so—which necessitated variants in which the therapist takes the lead. Interestingly, there are indications that even patients with much less severe forms of psychopathology positively experience the therapist taking care of the rescripting—perhaps because this meets a basic need in them (Voncken, personal communication). This clearly calls for empirical investigations. Research is also necessary to further clarify what are the exact mechanisms that underlie ImRs. The possibility that ImRs can change the meaning of the trauma memory itself—in contrast to the mechanism in imaginal exposure (the formation of an alternative memory trace that has to compete with the orginal memory trace)—is fascinating but needs more basic experimental work (e.g., Dibbets, Poort, & Arntz, 2012). This work should also clarify what are the necessary conditions for such a memory change, which can help to improve applications in clinical practice. ImRs has been integrated into standard CBT—for example, with CT (cognitive challenging to develop a script which is then imagined; Ehler's CT-protocol for PTSD, and with imaginal exposure (e.g., Arntz et al., 2007); but it is unclear whether such integration leads to better results than when ImRs is applied as a standalone technique—again an important issue for the research agenda.

Further Resources
- For an excellent treatise of ImRs for PTSD, see Hackman (2011).
- For ImRs of nightmares, see Krakow and Zadra (2006).
- See Hackmann, Bennett-Levy, and Holmes (2011) for a book on imagery and ImRs.
- See Arntz and Weertman (1999) for an extensive text on treatment of childhood memories of maltreatment.

References

Arntz, A. (2012). Imagery rescripting as a therapeutic technique: Review of clinical trials, basic studies, and research agenda. *Journal of Experimental Psychopathology,3*,189–208.

Arntz, A., Sofi, D., & van Breukelen, G. (2013). Imagery rescripting as treatment for complicated PTSD in refugees: A multiple baseline case series study. *Behaviour Research and Therapy, 51*, 274–283.

Arntz, A., Tiesema, M., & Kindt, M. (2007). Treatment of PTSD: A comparison of imaginal exposure with and without imagery rescripting. *Journal of Behavior Therapy and Experimental Psychiatry, 38*, 345–370.

Arntz, A., & Weertman, A. (1999). Treatment of childhood memories: Theory and practice. *Behaviour Research and Therapy, 37*, 715–740.

Clark, D. M. (2011, August 31). *Developing and disseminating effective psychological treatments: Science, practice, and economics.* Keynote presented at the 41st annual EABCT Congress, Reykjavik, Iceland.

Davis, J. L., & Wright, D. C. (2005). Case series utilizing exposure, relaxation and rescripting treatment: Impact on nightmares, sleep quality, and psychological distress. *Behavioral Sleep Medicine, 3*, 151–157.

Davis, J. L., & Wright, D. C. (2007). Randomized clinical trial for treatment of chronic nightmares in trauma-exposed adults. *Journal of Traumatic Stress, 20*, 123–133.

Dibbets, P., Poort, H., & Arntz, A. (2012). Adding imagery rescripting during extinction leads to less ABA renewal. *Journal of Behavior Therapy and Experimental Psychiatry, 43*(1), 614–624.

Duffy, M., Gillespie, K., & Clark, D. M. (2007). Post-traumatic stress disorder in the context of terrorism and other civil conflict in Northern Ireland: Randomized controlled trial. *British Medical Journal, 334*, 1147–1150.

Edwards, D. (2007). Restructuring implicational meaning through memory based imagery: Some historical notes. *Journal of Behavior Therapy and Experimental Psychiatry, 38*, 306–316.

Ehlers, A., & Clark, D. M. (2000). A cognitive model of posttraumatic stress disorder. *Behaviour Research and Therapy, 38*, 319–345.

Ehlers, A., Clark, D. M., Hackmann, A., McManus, F., & Fennell, M. (2005). Cognitive therapy for posttraumatic stress disorder: Development and evaluation. *Behaviour Research and Therapy, 43*, 413–431.

Ehlers, A., Clark, D. M., Hackmann, A., McManus, F., Fennell, M., Herbert, C., et al. (2003). A randomized controlled trial of cognitive therapy, a self-help booklet, and repeated assessments as early interventions for posttraumatic stress disorder. *Archives of General Psychiatry, 60*, 1024–1032.

Ehlers, A., Hackmann, A., Steil, R., Clohessy, S., Wenninger, K., & Winter, H. (2002). The nature of intrusive memories after trauma: The warning signal hypothesis. *Behaviour Research and Therapy, 40*, 995–1002.

Gollwitzer, M., & Denzler, M. (2009). What makes revenge sweet: Seeing the offender suffer or delivering a message? *Journal of Experimental Social Psychology, 45*, 840–844.

Grunert, B. K., Weis, J. M., Smucker, M. R., & Christianson, H. F. (2007). Imagery rescripting and reprocessing therapy after failed prolonged exposure for post-traumatic stress disorder following industrial injury. *Journal of Behavior Therapy and Experimental Psychiatry, 38*, 317–328.

Hackmann, A. (2011). Imagery rescripting in posttraumatic stress disorder. *Cognitive and Behavioral Practice, 18*, 424–432.

Hackmann, A., Bennett-Levy, J., & Holmes, E. (2011). *Oxford guide to imagery in cognitive therapy*. Oxford, UK: Oxford University Press.

Hagenaars, M. A., & Arntz, A. (2012). Reduced intrusion development after post-trauma imagery rescripting: An experimental study. *Journal of Behavior Therapy and Experimental Psychiatry, 44*, 808–814.

Holmes, E. A., & Mathews, A. (2010). Mental imagery in emotion and emotional disorders. *Clinical Psychology Review, 30*, 349–362.

Holmes, E. A., Mathews, A., Dalgleish, T., & Mackintosh, B. (2006). Positive interpretation training: Effects of mental imagery training versus verbal training on positive mood. *Behavior Therapy, 37*, 237–247.

Jung, K., & Steil, R. (2013). A randomized controlled trial on cognitive restructuring and imagery modification to reduce the feeling of being contaminated in adult survivors of childhood sexual abuse suffering from posttraumatic stress disorder. *Psychotherapy and Psychosomatics, 82*, 213–220.

Kindt, M., Buck, N., Arntz, A., & Soeter, M. (2007). Perceptual and conceptual processing as predictors of treatment outcome in PTSD. *Journal of Behavior Therapy and Experimental Psychiatry, 38*, 491–506.

Krakow, B., Hollifield, M., Johnston, L., Koss, M., Schrader, R., Warner, T. D., et al. (2001). Imagery rehearsal therapy for chronic nightmares in sexual assault survivors with posttraumatic stress disorder: A randomized controlled trial. *Journal of the American Medical Association, 286*, 537–545.

Krakow, B., & Zadra, A. (2006). Clinical management of chronic nightmares: Imagery rehearsal therapy. *Behavioural Sleep Medicine, 4*, 45–70.

Long, M. E., & Quevillon, R. (2009). Imagery rescripting in the treatment of posttraumatic stress disorder. *Journal of Cognitive Psychotherapy, 23*, 67–76.

Seebauer, L., Froß, S., Dubaschny, L., Schönberger, M., Jacob, G. A. (2014). Is it dangerous to fantasize revenge in imagery exercises?: An experimental study. *Journal of Behavior Therapy and Experimental Psychiatry, 45*, 20–25.

Smucker, M. R., & Niederee, J. (1995). Treating incest-related PTSD and pathogenic schemas through imaginal exposure and rescripting. *Cognitive and Behavioral Practice, 2*, 63–93.

Spinhoven, P., Bamelis, L., Haringsma, R., Marc Molendijk, M., & Arntz, A. (2012). Consistency of reporting sexual and physical abuse during psychological treatment of personality disorder: An explorative study. *Journal of Behavior Therapy and Experimental Psychiatry, 43*, S43–S50.

Steil, R., Jung, K., & Stangier, U. (2011). Efficacy of a two-session program of cognitive restructuring and imagery modification to reduce the feeling of being contaminated in adult survivors of childhood sexual abuse: A pilot study. *Journal of Behavior Therapy and Experimental Psychiatry, 42*, 325–329.

CHAPTER 10

Experiential Exercises and Imagery Rescripting in Social Anxiety Disorder

New Perspectives on Changing Beliefs

Jennifer Wild
David M. Clark

Many successful and well-known people throughout history have reported symptoms of social anxiety. Sir Winston Churchill reported a fear of stuttering before speaking in public. For a period in his life, Sir Laurence Olivier suffered extreme anxiety before acting in front of live audiences, and Barbra Streisand has described feeling terrified of performing in public. Social anxiety is one of the most common (Pilling et al., 2013) and persistent of the anxiety disorders in the absence of treatment (Bruce et al., 2005). People with social anxiety fear they will make a poor impression on other people and so avoid social and performance situations, such as participating in meetings, going to parties, telephoning in public, and public speaking. They typically underperform at school and work, establish fewer social relationships, and unsurprisingly, often suffer from depression and alcohol and substance dependence as a result.

A network meta-analysis recently performed by the National Institute for Health and Care Excellence (NICE) concluded that individual cognitive-behavioral therapy (CBT) based on the Clark and Wells (1995) cognitive therapy (CT) model or Rapee and Heimberg's (1997) model is the most cost-effective treatment for social anxiety disorder (NICE, 2013). As a consequence, individual CT/CBT is recommended as the first-line treatment in

NICE clinical guidelines. CT for social anxiety based on Clark and Wells (1995) is a 14-session treatment that targets key factors hypothesized to maintain the disorder, such as patients' self-focused attention, their use of safety behaviors, and their persistent negative beliefs about themselves and their social world. Linked to their negative self-beliefs, patients with social anxiety often experience negative self-images or impressions of how they fear they will come across to other people. In their negative self-images, they tend to see their worst fears being realized. A patient with a fear of his mind going blank when chatting to colleagues, for example, may have images in which his face predominates and he sees himself frozen with his mouth open, people pointing and laughing at him. Wild and Clark (2011) report that the negative self-images appear to maintain social fears in a number of ways. First, patients believe their negative self-images are a true reflection of how they come across to other people. They therefore think they come across much worse than they actually do, which reinforces rather than disconfirms their beliefs about performing inadequately. Second, the negative imagery motivates patients to use safety-seeking behaviors, which can interfere with their social performance (Alden & Taylor, 2004; Clark & Wells, 1995; Hirsch, Meynen, & Clark, 2004; Rapee & Heimberg, 1997) and cause them to feel negative emotions, notably anxiety (Hirsch, Clark, Mathews, & Williams, 2003). Third, the negative imagery blocks positive interpretation bias (Hirsch, Mathews, Clark, Williams, & Morrison, 2003), which means that when faced with an ambiguous social cue, such as a smile from a conversational partner, patients with social anxiety are unlikely to make a positive interpretation about the smile and so miss opportunities to benefit from the very feedback that could help them to reevaluate their beliefs and reduce their anxiety. Fourth, negative imagery facilitates selective retrieval of negative memories (Stopa & Jenkins, 2007) and may lead patients to overestimate the likelihood of negative outcomes in future social situations because of the accessibility of their past negative memories (Wild & Clark, 2011).

In this chapter, we present an overview of CT for social anxiety disorder, with a focus on the experiential exercises aimed at transforming negative imagery linked to persistent negative beliefs.

Overview of CT for Social Anxiety Disorder

Cognitive therapy for social anxiety based on the Clark and Wells (1995) model of social anxiety aims to reverse the maintaining processes specified in the model (Clark, 2001). The model highlights three key maintaining processes: negative self-processing, self-focused attention, and safety-seeking behaviors. Negative self-processing refers to negative patterns of thinking that are influenced by particular assumptions patients have developed on the basis of early experience and include (1) excessively high standards for social performance (e.g., "I must always appear witty and intelligent," "I should not have pauses in my conversations"), (2) beliefs concerning the consequences of performing in a certain way (e.g., "If I blush or sweat appears on my forehead, people will think that I am odd or incompetent"), and (3) beliefs about the self (e.g., "I'm odd or different," "I'm unlikeable," "I'm boring") (Clark, 2001). These beliefs may be coupled with negative imagery in which patients also see themselves as looking odd or as coming across as boring, for example, or as failing to meet their high standards for social performance and of people responding to them in a negative, humiliating way when they are in social situations.

When patients with social anxiety disorder believe they are in danger of negative evaluation by others, they shift their attention away from the environment to a detailed monitoring and observation of themselves. This process refers to self-focused attention and is another maintaining process that CT for social anxiety aims to reverse. Once self-focused, patients then use the internal information made accessible by self-monitoring to infer how they appear to other people and what other people are thinking of them (Clark, 2001).

The third key maintaining process refers to safety-seeking behaviors. It is common for patients with social anxiety to engage in a number of safety behaviors with the aim of preventing their feared catastrophe from happening and of ensuring they come across well (Clark, 2001). However, the safety behaviors can create some of the symptoms that patients with social anxiety fear. For example, rehearsing what to say to prevent one's mind from going blank makes it difficult to keep track of a conversation and can make patients appear less interested in other people than they really are. Some safety behaviors draw more attention rather than less attention from other people. For example, a patient who has a fear of blushing and covers her face with her hands to hide a blush is more likely to draw more attention than less attention from other people.

Figure 10.1 depicts an example of a collaboratively completed cognitive model of social anxiety with a patient, Fran, a 23-year-old woman who had a fear of blushing and of coming across as unlikeable to other people. The model demonstrates how the three processes described above maintained Fran's social anxiety. The arrows within the model demonstrate the vicious circles that kept her anxiety going.

When in a feared social situation, such as chatting to colleagues over coffee at work, Fran's negative patterns of thinking (negative self-processing) were activated. Some of her thoughts, beliefs about herself, and assumptions that formed her negative self-processing included: "If I blush, my colleagues will think I am odd." "I have to be interesting." "I must appear witty." "If I run out of things to say, they will think I am dull." "I am inadequate." "I should fill any pauses or gaps in the conversation or they will feel awkward and think I am unlikeable." Believing that she was in danger of negative

Figure 10.1

Situation: Chatting to colleagues over coffee at work

Thoughts: If I blush, they will think I am odd. I have to be interesting. I must appear witty. If I run out of things to say, they will think I am dull. I am inadequate. I should fill any pauses or gaps in the conversation or they will feel awkward and think I am unlikeable.

Focus on Self: Self-focused attention. Negative image of looking like a clown with red cheeks.

Safety Behaviors: Covering face with hair to hide a blush. Rehearsing what to say in advance. Censoring myself. Monitoring my performance.

Anxiety: Flushed in the face. Tense. Sweaty palms.

Early Events: Humiliated at school when friends encircled me and pointed at my clown-like face.

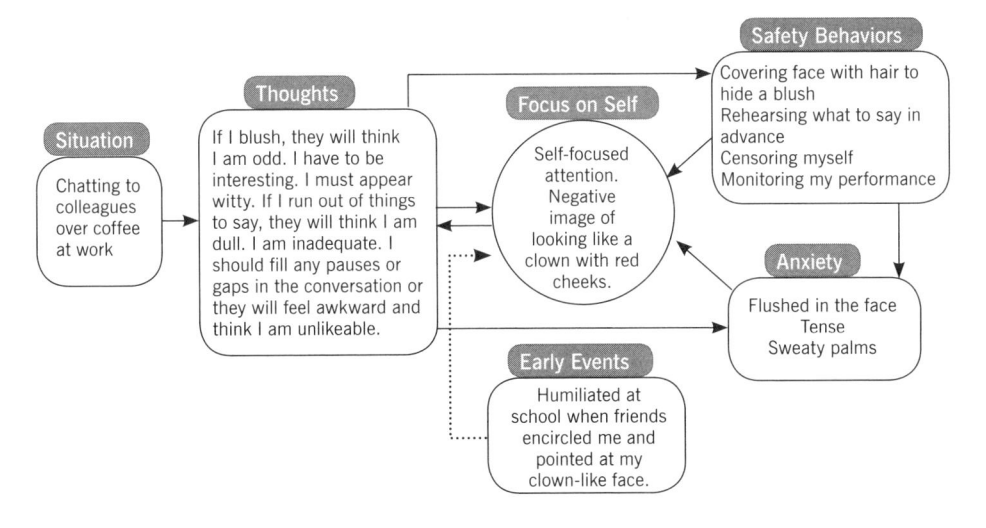

FIGURE 10.1. A cognitive conceptualization of Fran's social anxiety. Based on Clark and Wells (1995).

evaluation by others, Fran shifted her attention away from the environment to a detailed monitoring of herself. Her self-monitoring tuned her attention to internal signs of anxiety and she noticed that she felt flushed in the face, tense, and the palms of her hands were sweaty. Having noticed signs of anxiety reinforced her self-focused attention. When self-focused, her beliefs about herself and fears of how the conversation would progress felt more true to her. To ensure that she came across well and to prevent other people from noticing her fears, Fran engaged in safety behaviors, such as covering her face with her hair to hide a blush, rehearsing what to say so that she did not run out of things to say, censoring what she said so that she did not say anything stupid, and monitoring her performance. Engaging in these safety behaviors kept Fran's attention self-focused, reinforcing a vicious cycle linking her self-focused attention, beliefs, safety behaviors, and anxiety symptoms. When Fran's attention was self-focused, her negative patterns of thinking felt as though they carried more weight, and she was more likely to notice her anxiety symptoms and to engage in safety behaviors, which kept her attention focused on herself. When she was self-focused, she was more likely to generate a negative self-impression or image of how she was coming across, which was based on how anxious she was feeling. In her negative image, she saw herself with bright red cheeks, which stood out on a white face like a clown, with people snickering and laughing at her. Her negative imagery facilitated retrieval of negative memories, in particular, a memory of an early event in which her friends encircled her at school, pointing and laughing at her clown-like, flushed face.

CT for social anxiety based on the Clark and Wells (1995) model incorporates a number of experiential techniques to target maintaining processes, and many of these target negative beliefs and linked imagery. For many patients, their negative self-images appear to be linked in meaning and content to past socially traumatic events, such as being bullied or humiliated at school or criticized by a parent or teacher (Hackmann, Clark, & McManus, 2000). Therefore, in CT for social anxiety, two sets of interventions aim to update negative beliefs and frequently linked negative imagery. These are present- and past-focused interventions. Present-focused interventions include video feedback, attention training, behavioral experiments, surveys, and decatastrophizing experiments. Past-focused interventions, which directly consider the content and meaning of past socially traumatic events, are stimulus discrimination and imagery rescripting. The interventions will be discussed with reference to how they transform negative imagery, beliefs, and emotions.

Empirical Evidence

Several randomized controlled trials (e.g., Clark et al., 2003; Clark et al., 2006; Stangier, Heidenreich, Peitz, Lauterbach, & Clark, 2003; Stangier, Schramm, Heidenreich, Bergen, & Clark, 2011; Mortberg, Clark, Sundin, & Wisted, 2007; Leichsenring et al. 2013) demonstrate the effectiveness of Clark's (1999) CT for social anxiety disorder. In the first trial of their treatment, Clark et al. (2003) randomly assigned 60 patients with social anxiety disorder to one of three treatments: cognitive therapy, fluoxetine plus self-exposure, or placebo plus self-exposure. CT was superior to both fluoxetine and pill placebo. In their next trial, Clark et al. (2006) compared CT for social anxiety disorder with an established behavioral treatment: exposure and applied relaxation. Sixty-two patients with social anxiety disorder were randomly assigned to receive cognitive therapy, exposure, and applied relaxation or to a wait-list period of 14 weeks. Seventy-six per cent of patients who received cognitive therapy recovered compared to only 38% who received exposure and applied relaxation.

Two studies (Stangier et al., 2003; Mortberg et al., 2007) have compared individual CT with group CBT interventions. Stangier et al. (2003) assigned 71 patients to CT, to group CBT, or to a wait-list control. CT was superior to group CBT, with 84% of patients showing reliable and clinically significant change compared to 44% in group CBT. Both treatments were superior to the wait-list control. Mortberg et al. (2007) assigned 100 patients to individual CT, an intensive group CT, or medication-based treatment as usual (TAU). Individual CT was superior to both alternatives with 56% of patients achieving reliable and clinically significant change compared to 20% for group-intensive CT and 24% for TAU. Stangier et al. (2011) compared CT with interpersonal psychotherapy (IPT). One hundred and seventeen patients were assigned to CT, IPT, or a wait-list control.

CT was superior to IPT, and both treatments were better than no treatment (wait). Sixty-six percent of patients who received CT were classified as responders compared to 42% in IPT and 7% in the wait-list group. Finally, Liechsenring et al. (2013) compared a modified version of CT with psychodynamic psychotherapy (PDT) and wait list. Four hundred and ninety-five patients were randomized. The main modifications were to extend the treatment over 9 months rather than the usual 3 to 4 months (in order to match psychodynamic psychotherapy) and a reduction in the use of behavioral experiments. Both of these modifications are a source of concern (see Clark, 2013). As we discuss in this chapter, behavioral experiments are a key component of CT. In addition, Herbert et al. (2004) showed that extending a standard CBT program for social anxiety disorder over a longer period than usual reduced its effectiveness. Despite these modifications, Liechsenring et al. (2013) found that CT was superior to PDT, with both being superior to no treatment. Remission rates were lower than in previous studies (36% for CT vs. 20% for PDT).

These trials demonstrate that Clark's CT for social anxiety disorder is an effective treatment consistently leading to reliable and clinically significant change. Preliminary evidence demonstrates that treatment change in social anxiety is preceded by a change in maintaining beliefs that individuals may hold about the probability of the occurrence of negative social events and their costs (i.e., Hofmann, 2004; Hoffart, Borge, Sexton, & Clark, 2009), inspiring investigation into what leads to a change in beliefs in the treatment of social anxiety. A number of studies (e.g., McManus et al., 2009; Wild, Hackmann, & Clark, 2007; Wild, Hackmann, & Clark, 2008; Mortberg, Hoffart, Boecking, & Clark, 2013; Hedman et al., 2013) suggest that experiential exercises that engage attention and emotion contribute to the clinical improvement seen with CT for social anxiety disorder. For example, Wild et al. (2007) demonstrated that imagery rescripting of socially traumatic memories led to significant change in maintaining beliefs. McManus et al. (2009) investigated the effects of manipulating safety behaviors and self-focused attention in an experiential intervention that is conducted in Session 2 of Clark's (1999) CT for social anxiety disorder, demonstrating that the intervention led to significant improvements in negative self-impressions. The authors also investigated the effects of video feedback, a core experiential intervention, which is first conducted in Session 3 of Clark's (1999) protocol, demonstrating that video feedback of the self-focus and safety behaviors experiment consistently led patients to make less negative ratings of their social performance after viewing the video than before viewing the video and contributed to a significant proportion of the overall improvement achieved in treatment. Thirty-two out of the 34 (94%) patients in the study rated their social performance more positively after having viewed themselves on video. Video feedback appears to be highly successful in demonstrating to patients that their impressions and beliefs of how they come across are excessively negative.

Updating Negative Beliefs and Linked Imagery in CT for Social Anxiety

Experiential Present-Focused Techniques

In this section, we discuss five experiential present-focused techniques: video feedback, therapist-directed attention training, behavioral experiments, decatastrophizing experiments, and surveys.

Video Feedback

Video feedback is used in CT for social anxiety to demonstrate for patients the discrepancy between how they look and how they feel, and to update their negative self-imagery with a more realistic image. The therapist will record on video many behavioral experiments, beginning with the safety behavior and attention experiment, which takes place in Session 2. In this experiment, the patient most often has a conversation with a stranger (a colleague of the therapist) under two conditions: one in which he or she adopts his or her usual safety behaviors and maintains self-focused attention and one in which he or she aims to adopt few, if any, safety behaviors and try to externalize his or her attention. Patients are encouraged to adopt self-focused evaluative attention, where they focus their attention on themselves and evaluate how they are coming across in the first condition, and in the second condition to adopt externally focused nonevaluative attention, where they aim to fully absorb their attention on the conversation and their conversational partner without evaluating how they are coming across. The purpose of recording this experiment is fivefold: (1) to help demonstrate to patients the discrepancy between how they feel they come across to other people and how they objectively come across on video, which helps to update their negative self-beliefs; (2) to demonstrate that even when they are adopting safety behaviors, maintaining self-focused attention, and feeling anxious, they still come across much better than how they feel they do; (3) to demonstrate the difference between self-focused evaluative and externally focused nonevaluative attention and the effects on anxiety; (4) to demonstrate that predictions based on feelings about their performance and how other people will respond are inaccurate; and (5) to provide a more realistic image about how they come across. Other behavioral experiments are also video-recorded, where possible, to continue to demonstrate to patients that they come across much better than how they feel they do, which serves to update their negative self-beliefs and self-images or impressions of themselves.

To enhance the benefits of video feedback, we have found that it is useful to spend some time preparing the patient prior to viewing the video. Cognitive preparation for video feedback includes three steps: (1) predicting in detail the contents of the video, (2) forming an image of the performance, and (3) watching the video as an objective observer (Harvey, Clark, Ehlers, & Rapee, 2000). Before watching the recording, the therapist encourages patients to think in detail about what they predict they will see when they watch themselves on video. The therapist encourages patients to describe their image of how they think they will appear on video and to predict and rate the social fears they expect to see. Finally, the therapist encourages patients to watch the recording as if they are an objective observer. The therapist may suggest watching the recording as if they are watching a stranger on television. Afterward the therapist will ask the patients to describe what they saw on the video and to rerate their initial predictions. The therapist will ask the patient to summarize what they have learned and to summarize the differences between their negative imagery and the actual image of how they came across on video after they watched their recording.

Video feedback is a powerful corrective tool that helps to update negative self-imagery and self-beliefs and replace them with more realistic outcomes. While patients understandably feel apprehensive and often anxious about seeing themselves on a video recording, many report feeling surprised at how much better they came across than they had thought they would. Occasionally, video feedback leads to emotions of sadness when patients simultaneously realize that they have been judging themselves harshly for many years, having mistakenly equated feeling anxious with looking anxious.

Therapist-Directed Attention Training

The central component of the Clark and Wells (1995) model of social anxiety hinges on attentional focus: the more patients are able to externally focus their attention, the less true their negative self-beliefs appear and the less likely they are then motivated to engage in safety behaviors. Therapist-directed attention training gives patients the experience of externally focusing their attention outside of social situations before attempting to focus their attention externally in social situations. The aim is to help patients to gain confidence in externally focusing their attention, and also to gain familiarity with this experience. Therapist-directed attention training in CT for social anxiety (Clark, 1999) begins in Session 4 with a homework task in which the patient is asked to practice listening to different sounds on a CD, tuning into individual instruments and then to the whole of the track. Patients are then urged to practice for 2–3 minutes walking outside, paying attention only to what they can hear, see, and smell, not on what they are feeling or what they are thinking. The idea is that patients focus their attention on what is happening in the present in their environment rather than on their social fears and somatic experience of anxiety, thereby increasing the opportunity to notice benign or even positive feedback from other people when they are in a social situation. Attention training indirectly helps to update negative self-beliefs and imagery because patients are more likely to experience how they come across to other people according to objective evidence rather than through the lens of their negative self-beliefs or their own well-rehearsed distorted imagery. The therapist monitors a patient's attentional focus every week through his or her self-report of how externally focused he or she has been in social situations. If patients appear to have struggled with externally focusing their attention in the previous week, then the therapist may conduct guided in-session attention training. This is likely to occur after Session 4 and before Session 8.

In therapist-guided attention training, the therapist asks the patient to first focus on themselves while simultaneously completing a task, such as identifying three sounds in the office. The therapist then has the patient focus externally and complete the same task. The patient is asked to consider what feels more threatening: focusing on themselves and identifying three sounds or focusing externally and identifying three sounds? The same process is repeated for colors, shadows, and a passage that the therapist reads, in which the patient is asked to switch between self- and externally focused attention at the sound of random knocks that sound while the therapist reads.

Behavioral Experiments

Behavioral experiments are a key component of CT for social anxiety disorder. Behavioral experiments help patients test their thoughts about how they fear they appear to other people while dropping safety behaviors and focusing their attention externally. Since models of learning (i.e., Cahill, Gorski, & Le, 2003) suggest that there must be sufficient anxiety to facilitate learning, behavioral experiments are ideal ways to facilitating new learning to update negative self-beliefs and linked images because the patient is encouraged to test his beliefs in social situations in which he feels anxious, such as making a telephone call in public, giving a presentation, or talking to a stranger. The therapist helps the patient to identify what he is worried will happen in the situation and then put it to the test. The patient may also be encouraged to think of an image of how he thinks he will appear and to operationalize his image and fears. For example, if a patient thinks that he will blush like a red beetroot while speaking up in a meeting, causing people to then laugh and point, the therapist first helps the patient to specify how much he believes he will blush out of 100%, what color that may look like on a pink to red paint chart, and crucially, how he envisages other people reacting. The patient is encouraged to complete the experiment while dropping his usual safety behaviors, which may mean purposely avoiding covering his face with his hands or refraining from commenting that the room feels hot. The patient is encouraged to focus externally on what is happening rather than on how he is feeling since this will help him to attend to how people really respond to him. The patient will then speak up in a meeting, one of his feared situations, focusing externally on how other people are responding to him.

After the experiment, the patient is required to note what actually happened and to think more broadly about what he has learned in terms of how he comes across to other people in social situations. These experiments help patients to gather this evidence, which helps some patients to update their negative imagery and self-beliefs because they discover that they come across much more favorably than they have previously believed and more favorably than the content of their negative self-images has suggested.

Decatastrophizing Experiments

Decatastrophizing experiments encourage patients to fake their worst fears to discover whether or not other people notice and whether or not they respond more favorably than predicted. Patients are encouraged to fake their worst fear and if they have a negative image of what that looks like, then to make themselves look as though they appear in their negative image. Examples of decatastrophizing experiments would be to cover one's face with blusher and then speak up in a meeting, to cover one's shirt and face with water to make it look as though one is sweating and then give a presentation, to intentionally pause while chatting to a colleague at work, to purposely make one's hands shake while paying a cashier at a supermarket, or to purposely say something boring or stupid while talking to other people.

These challenging experiments help patients to update their beliefs about catastrophes happening and how people respond to them if their fears occur. Patients typically learn that few people notice their fears and even if they do, they are uninterested in judging them harshly or responding negatively, giving patients valuable information to correct their negative self-beliefs and linked images of how other people may respond to them. Coupled with video feedback of behavioral experiments, patients learn that even when they have made themselves look as though they fear in their image, their fears look much less catastrophic than previously thought, helping them to update their negative imagery.

Surveys

In CT for social anxiety, the therapist may construct a survey with patients, which the therapist will give to other people, usually colleagues of the therapist, to gather information about how commonly other people also experience similar social fears and how other people respond when they do notice a social fear being exhibited by another individual. The therapist does not include the patient's name, thereby keeping his or her identity anonymous. Surveys help to normalize patients' social fears, some of which will be linked to negative self-images. For example, a patient may have a fear of her mind going blank and may picture other people pointing and laughing as a response. A survey to address a client's fear of his mind going blank may include questions such as "Has your mind ever gone blank in a meeting? If so, what did you do? How did other people respond to you? If you noticed a colleague's mind going blank, what would you think of them? How would you respond to them?" The therapist would then give the survey to colleagues and collect responses for the following session. Surveys help patients to discover that other people also experience some of their social concerns and that they typically respond more favorably than the patient may have predicted. This helps patients to update their negative imagery and linked beliefs about being odd or different, for example, for having social fears and symptoms of anxiety.

Experiential Past-Focused Techniques

While randomized controlled trials of CT for social anxiety (e.g., Clark et al., 2006) suggest that many patients respond to the present-focused techniques alone, Clark et al. (2006) report that for a subset of patients these techniques were insufficient to fully update patients' recurrent negative imagery and negative beliefs. Since patients' negative self-images are often linked to past socially unpleasant events, such as being bullied at school or criticized by a parent or teacher, specific techniques may be required to target these memories and linked images and beliefs directly. There are two interventions the therapist may use to help patients more clearly consider how they come across in the present and to help them make a distinction between what happened in the past (their memory), what they fear will happen in the present (their image), and what actually happens (now, their present reality). These are stimulus discrimination and imagery rescripting.

Stimulus Discrimination

To help patients consider the present more clearly without the negative influence of their past unpleasant memories, the therapist will encourage the patient to look at the differences between *then* (their socially unpleasant memory) and *now* (how people respond to them today). In CT for social anxiety disorder, this is called stimulus discrimination: discriminating between *then* versus *now*. Stimulus discrimination is a technique derived from CT for posttraumatic stress disorder (PTSD; Ehlers & Clark, 2000) where it is used to help patients who have suffered a trauma discriminate between what happened in the past in their trauma and what is happening in the present. In the context of CT for PTSD, stimulus discrimination helps patients to recognize that their fear in the present is often linked to current cues, which have triggered their memories of their trauma. Patients learn that their fear is coming from their triggered memory rather than representing real threat in the present.

Turning to social anxiety disorder, patients also learn that their feelings in the present are linked to their past socially traumatic event. For example, Kelly had a fear of blushing and a negative self-image, in which she saw herself blushing as red as beetroot in front of people who then pointed and laughed at her. Her image of blushing was linked to an event at school when she blushed and her friends made fun of her. Kelly's memory is an event that happened in the past. Her image is what she is afraid will happen in the present. When Kelly feels anxious and experiences her distorted negative self-image, she believes that people will respond to her in the same way that they did in her memory. Another patient, Robert, who worried about coming across as incompetent and inadequate and in his image saw himself looking small and child-like, slumped in a corner with no one talking to him. Robert's image was linked to an experience he had at school when his friends made fun of him and called him a bookworm for reading instead of playing with them. A patient, Stan, believed that he was incompetent and that people would mock him if his speech was jumbled or had pauses. He did not have an image of how he would come across but he had an impression that he would come across poorly. His impression was linked to an event at school, in which his teacher criticized him for taking too much time to answer a difficult mathematics question.

Stimulus discrimination requires patients to identify the differences between what happened to them in the past and how people respond to them today. They are encouraged to look for differences between *then* and *now* whenever they have the same feeling that they experienced in their memory, which may include emotions such as shame, fear, sadness, disappointment, anxiety, and threat. When patients experience the feeling that they had in their memory, they are encouraged to see this as a golden opportunity to shift their attention from themselves to the outside world, so they may observe how others are really responding to them. They are encouraged to look at the differences between *then* (the memory) and *now* (themselves as an adult). The aim is to help patients process the present as it is actually happening and to help them to determine if their feeling is accurate or if it is linked to their memory of what happened to them. The more their attention is in the present and on what they know now, the less likely the past memory will color their present reality.

For example, Kelly could see three differences between her memory and how people respond to her now. In her memory, she was 16 years old and now she is 44 years old. In her memory, when she felt hot she believed that feeling hot was the same as blushing. Now she knows that there is a discrepancy between how she feels and how she looks and that she can feel hot without looking bright red as she previously feared. In her memory, her school friends humiliated her, but this is not how people respond to her now.

Robert saw two differences between his memory and now. In his memory he was 5 years old, now he is 36 years old. In his memory, four little boys made fun of him. Now, people listen to him, are friendly and responsive and never make fun of him. Stan also saw two differences between his memory and now. In his memory, he was 14 years old, now he is 38 years old. In his memory, his teacher was harsh and strict, only picking fault with his performance. Now, his colleagues value his work, thank him for his contributions, and have asked for his opinion on developing new company strategies.

Imagery Rescripting

In the context of social anxiety, imagery rescripting is an intervention with the primary aim of updating the earlier memory from which patients' negative imagery stems and the meaning linking the recurrent negative image and memory (Wild & Clark, 2011). Several cognitive-behavioral therapy (CBT) programs have successfully incorporated imagery rescripting techniques with therapeutic benefits, such as (CBT) programs for borderline personality disorder (Giesen-Bloo et al., 2006), bulimia (Cooper, Todd, & Turner, 2007), and PTSD arising from childhood sexual abuse (Smucker & Niederee, 1995).

A number of studies report the therapeutic effects of imagery rescripting for patients with social anxiety (Wild & Clark, 2011). Two studies (Wild et al., 2007, 2008) have demonstrated that imagery rescripting leads to change in negative beliefs and self-images in unselected populations of patients with social anxiety. Wild et al. (2007) reported pre- and postrescripting results in 14 patients with social anxiety with whom they developed this approach. Imagery rescripting alone was associated with significant improvement in patients' negative social beliefs, in the vividness and distress of their image and early memory, and in self-report measures of social anxiety. Wild et al. (2008) then compared a session of imagery rescripting with a control session in which images and memories were explored without being updated. Measures were taken before each session and 1 week later. The imagery-rescripting session was associated with significantly greater improvement in negative beliefs, image and memory distress and vividness, fear of negative evaluation, and anxiety in feared social situations (Wild & Clark, 2011).

Encapsulated Beliefs

Wild and Clark (2011) report that the recurrent negative images of patients with social anxiety appear to be memory images of past socially traumatic events, which are triggered in different social situations by cues that match the original event in some way. They suggest that like intrusive images in PTSD, the memory images heighten anxiety and remind the patient of past danger. The patient approaches social situations as if they hold the same contingencies as the past event, typically expecting people to respond to them in the same way as they did in their socially traumatic memory. Just as the memory images have similar cues to the past event, they also carry a similar meaning to the original memory, an "encapsulated belief" that captures the meaning of both (Wild et al., 2008). For example, one patient had a recurrent image of looking scarlet red with a sense that people were laughing and pointing at her, the way her ex-boyfriend did. This linked to a memory when she was an 18-year-old university student. Her boyfriend's friend used her toilet, clogged it with feces, and then implied that she had made the mess. She started blushing as her boyfriend accused her of lying, and he and his friend started to laugh and point at her. The encapsulated belief linking her image and memory was "I am inferior to other people. People will see this and reject me." Wild and Clark (2011) give an example of another patient who phrased the encapsulated belief linking her image and memory as "I'm an outsider and always will be. People will reject me or laugh at me because I'm not like them." Her recurrent image was of looking awkward, jittery, twitchy, and speaking in garbled sentences. This was linked to a memory when she was 13 years old and a group of children at her school cornered her against a wall and made fun of her and the way she was twitching and unable to speak. She thought she would be attacked in front of all the other children and it would be humiliating (Wild et al., 2008).

Emotions Linked to Encapsulated Beliefs

The encapsulated beliefs linking patients' recurrent negative imagery and past socially traumatic events are negative statements often characteristic of all-or-nothing thinking, such as "I am inferior to other people, people will see this and reject me." and "I'm an outsider and always will be. People will reject me or laugh at me because I'm not like them." Such beliefs are activated in feared social situations, particularly in situations with similar cues to past socially traumatic events. Patients' attention typically becomes self-focused when these beliefs are activated, when they notice internal signs of anxiety, or when they engage in behaviors to prevent their fears from happening. As a result, they may struggle to notice feedback from other people that is inconsistent with their beliefs. Common emotions linked to such beliefs include shame, sadness, despair, anger, fear, and anxiety. Some of these emotions, such as shame, cause people to withdraw in their feared situations and avoid thinking of the event that caused them shame. Therefore, imagery rescripting is the ideal intervention for such individuals since it gently helps patients to face their worst beliefs about themselves and with the help of cognitive restructuring and the memory rescripting process, to transform their beliefs and linked intense negative emotions.

The Imagery Rescripting Session

In this section, we discuss the imagery rescripting process in detail, including the theoretical basis for the intervention, patients' experience of emotions during the procedure, determining when to offer the procedure, and how to maintain gains.

Theoretical Basis

The theoretical basis for employing imagery rescripting in the treatment of patients with social anxiety lies in the link between their recurrent imagery in the present and their past socially traumatic events. Wild and Clark (2011) suggest that the negative self-beliefs and linked memory images of past socially traumatic events will continue to persist without intervention for two reasons. First, they become more negative over time because memory appears to be a process of continuous reconstruction as individuals recall and consider past events (Coles, Turk, & Heimberg, 2002), and therefore more negative interpretations are assimilated into the memory image over time. Postevent processing, which is common in patients with social anxiety, further supports the assimilation of more negative interpretations into the memory image and these remain in an unchanged form (Hirsch et al., 2006). Second, avoidance of the socially traumatic memory likely leads to the persistence of the negative images in the same way that thought suppression maintains intrusive imagery in PTSD. Avoiding the socially traumatic memory also prevents the opportunity to reflect on it in detail and to reconsider the accuracy of the original negative evaluations. Since patients with social anxiety tend to remember their negative interpretations as actually having happened even when they did not occur (e.g., Hertel, Brozovich, Joorman, & Gotlib, 2008), this likely causes them to persist (see Wild & Clark, 2011, for an extended discussion).

Engaging Emotion during the Imagery Rescripting Session

The imagery rescripting session in our CT for social anxiety begins with a 35–40 minute period of cognitive restructuring. Following cognitive restructuring, we then initiate the imagery rescripting procedure, which includes imaginal recreation and follows the three stages described by Arntz and Weertman (1999). In Stage 1, the patient relives the socially traumatic event from the age at which it occurred. In Stage 2, the patient relives the event again but from an adult observer perspective, observing her younger self as the event unfolds. In Stage 3, the patient relives the event again from the age at which it occurred. On this occasion, however, her adult self is with her and can intervene at any point, offer new information about how she comes across now, and provide compassion (Wild & Clark, 2011).

Patients appear to share common emotions during the three stages of imagery rescripting for social anxiety. In Stage 1, when patients relive their socially traumatic event, they may report experiencing fear, anxiety, trepidation, and threat. In Stage 2, when they relive the event again but from an adult observer perspective, observing their younger self enduring the event, they often describe an "aha" moment in which they start to notice that they were treated unkindly and that this carries negative meaning for the other people involved rather than for themselves. For example, Kelly was bullied by her boyfriend. When she relived the experience in Stage 2 of imagery rescripting, she could see from her adult perspective that her boyfriend and his friend had been particularly nasty, and that the experience meant they were immature, unkind people rather than that she was odd and different and that everyone would reject her like they had. Coupled with new realizations that appear to occur during Stage 2, patients may also experience sadness because they have held persistently negative beliefs for some time and have likely made life decisions, such as whether or not to go to university or to get involved with someone they are interested in, as a result of these self-perceptions. Stage 3 of the imagery rescripting procedure typically leads patients to feel satisfaction as they may intervene and impart corrective information to their younger selves as well as retribution to the other people involved in the event. They frequently report feeling relief when the intervention is completed and as though their memory no longer feels threatening.

Cognitive Restructuring and Imagery Rescripting

Cognitive restructuring aims to challenge the encapsulated belief and to ready an adult perspective that the patient can draw upon in the imagery with rescripting phase. Cognitive restructuring will often lead to an intellectual understanding that the negative event in the past carries a negative meaning about the other people involved, which can start to shift patients' own negative self-beliefs. However, we have found that incorporating this information into the memory image through imagery rescripting is often needed to produce emotional as well as intellectual change. This appears to be consistent with Arntz and Weertman (1999). They suggest that while verbal reasoning is important, more experiential methods, such as imagery rescripting, are necessary to update beliefs or schemas that were formed in childhood. They also suggest that activation of the affective memories is more effectively done with experiential methods than with "talking-about experiences." This fits with the idea that using as many senses as possible (as in imagery) results in better activation of implicational meaning representations necessary to change them (Teasdale, 1993). We would suggest that it is also necessary to insert the corrective information garnered from cognitive restructuring into the socially traumatic memory. This emerges from our work with PTSD, in which we have found that the intellectual shifts that occur with cognitive restructuring can be limited in their impact, and that it is necessary to insert this new information into the trauma memory during a planned reliving (see Ehlers, Hackmann, & Michael, 2004, for an extended discussion).

Thus, our imagery rescripting session includes a period of cognitive restructuring and then imagery rescripting, which involves repeated evocation of the trauma memory, corrective information inserted into the memory image, and compassionate imagery. Wild and Clark (2011) suggest that all these components are likely to be necessary for the procedure to be effective. The cognitive restructuring enables the patient to identify a convincing, intellectual argument against the encapsulated belief. Repeated evocation of the trauma memory in a planned and controlled way helps to lead to its reevaluation (Foa & Rothbaum, 1998). Wild and Clark (2011) suggest that corrective information inserted into the socially traumatic memory ensures that adaptive rather than negative interpretations are assimilated into the memory image. Compassionate imagery likely enhances the patient's feeling of being accepted, a central concept in social anxiety disorder. Finally, conducting much of the procedure in imagery may itself be beneficial since it may engender the sense of having had a concrete experience (Epstein, 1994) rather than simply having engaged in intellectual discourse.

Determining When to Offer Imagery Rescripting

Wild and Clark (2011) report that imagery rescripting for patients with social anxiety is intended for patients who experience negative imagery that is linked to a past socially traumatic event and whose response to standard, present-focused techniques to correct distorted self-images has been relatively modest. The authors note that while many patients with social anxiety report negative imagery linked to an identifiable event in the past (i.e., Hackmann et al., 2000), some patients experience negative imagery that appears to be unrelated to an earlier event. For these patients, the standard present-focused imagery modification techniques, such as videofeedback, behavioral experiments, and surveys, will likely be beneficial when offered as part of CBT programs for the disorder. Wild and Clark (2011) recommend offering imagery rescripting during an integrated CT program for social anxiety after patients have attended a minimum of around four sessions of therapy so they will have had time to experience the benefits of videofeedback and some behavioral experiments, which they may then draw upon in the cognitive restructuring phase of the procedure.

Maintaining Gains: Present-Focused and Imagery Rescripting CT Interventions for Social Anxiety

Following imagery rescripting, when patients experience the same feeling as in their memory, the therapist may encourage patients to see this feeling as a cue to remind themselves of what they have learned in their imagery rescripting session, the alternatives to their encapsulated belief, and their new image. After present-focused techniques, such as videofeedback and behavioral experiments, patients are typically encouraged to focus externally while carrying out more behavioral experiments in which they continue to drop safety behaviors and to recall the realistic image of how they come across, the image they may have seen on video.

Future Directions

In this chapter, we have presented an overview of CT for social anxiety disorder based on the Clark and Wells (1995) model of social anxiety, paying particular attention to experiential techniques aimed to update negative imagery and linked self-beliefs. For many patients, videofeedback, surveys, behavioral experiments, including decatastrophizing experiments, and stimulus discrimination are sufficient to update images and linked beliefs. However, for a subset of patients for whom these techniques lead to only modest improvement and for whom there is a clear link between their recurrent imagery and an earlier socially traumatic event, imagery rescripting appears to be an effective intervention to update imagery and linked memories and beliefs. For these patients, encapsulated beliefs capture the meaning of the negative imagery and past memory. While cognitive restructuring may help patients to experience an intellectual shift in how they interpret the past event, which can be helpful for modifying their beliefs, it is often necessary to incorporate corrective information into the memory image through imagery rescripting to produce emotional as well as cognitive change. Imagery rescripting is similar to reliving in PTSD in which patients engage in emotion while reliving their trauma and are then able to update the memory with information they have accessed since the trauma. Imagery rescripting appears to be effective because it evokes the earlier unpleasant memory similar to imaginal exposure in PTSD; it involves self-compassion, which may enhance patients' feeling of being accepted, a central concept in social anxiety; and it helps patients to update distorted maintaining images and beliefs with corrective information. However, to fully understand which components of imagery rescripting are most effective and whether all add value to the procedure, a component analysis study is needed. Future research is also needed to determine the long-term benefits of imagery rescripting. Although our initial research (Wild et al., 2007, 2008) has shown benefits at 1-week follow-up, it is necessary to determine that the gains with imagery rescripting are maintained for longer periods of time.

Further Resources

Articles

- For an excellent article about imagery rescripting of early traumatic memories in social anxiety disorder, see Wild and Clark (2011).
- For an excellent paper on the treatment of childhood traumatic memories, see Arntz and Weertman (1999).
- For a special issue of the journal *Memory* devoted to imagery and memory, see Volume 12, Number 4 (2004), edited by Emily A. Holmes and Ann Hackmann.

Books

- For an in-depth consideration of mental imagery in CT with some focus on social anxiety, see Stopa (2009).

Acknowledgments

This research was funded by Wellcome Trust Grant No. 069777.

References

Alden, L. E., & Taylor, C. T. (2004). Interpersonal processes in social phobia [Review]. *Clinical Psychology Review, 24*(7), 857–882.

Arntz, A., & Weertman, A. (1999). Treatment of childhood memories: Theory and practice. *Behaviour and Research Therapy, 37*(8), 715–740.

Bruce, S. E., Yonkers, K. A., Otto, M. W., Eisen, J. L., Weisberg, R. B., Pagano, M., et al. (2005). Influence of psychiatric comorbidity on recovery and recurrence in generalized anxiety disorder, social phobia, and panic disorder: A 12-year prospective study. *American Journal of Psychiatry, 162*(6), 1179–1187.

Cahill, L., Gorski, L., & Le, K. (2003). Enahnced human memory consolidation with post-learning stress: Interaction with the degree of arousal at encoding. *Learning and Memory, 10*, 270–274.

Clark, D. M. (1999). Anxiety disorders: Why they persist and how to treat them. *Behaviour Research and Therapy, 37*(Suppl.), S5–S27.

Clark, D. M. (2001). A cognitive perspective on social phobia. In W. R. Crozier & L. E. Alden (Eds.), *International handbook of social anxiety* (pp. 405–430). Chichester, UK: Wiley.

Clark, D. M. (2013). Psychodynamic therapy or cognitive therapy for social anxiety disorder [Letters to the editor]. *American Journal of Psychiatry, 170*, 1365.

Clark, D. M., Ehlers, A., Hackmann, A., McManus, F., Fennell, M. J. V., Waddington, L., et al. (2006). Cognitive therapy and exposure plus applied relaxation in social phobia: A randomised controlled trial. *Journal of Consulting and Clinical Psychology, 74*, 568–578.

Clark, D. M., Ehlers, A., McManus, F., Hackmann, A., Fennell, M., Campbell, H., et al. (2003). Cognitive therapy versus fluoxetine in generalized social phobia: A randomized placebo-controlled trial. *Journal of Consulting and Clinical Psychology, 71*(6), 1058–1067.

Clark, D. M., & Wells, A. (1995). A cognitive model of social phobia. In R. G. Heimberg, M. R. Liebowitz, D. A. Hope, & F. R. Schneier (Eds.), *Social phobia: Diagnosis, assessment and treatment* (pp. 69–93). New York: Guilford Press.

Coles, M. E., Turk, C. L., & Heimberg, R. G. (2002). The role of memory perspective in social phobia: Immediate and delayed memories for role-played situations. *Behavioral and Cognitive Psychotherapy, 30*, 415–425.

Cooper, M. J., Todd, G., & Turner, H. (2007). The effects of using imagery to modify core emotional beliefs in bulimia nervosa: An experimental study. *Journal of Cognitive Psychotherapy, 21*(2), 117–122.

Ehlers, A., & Clark, D. M. (2000). A cognitive model of posttraumatic stress disorder. *Behaviour Research and Therapy, 38*, 319–345.

Ehlers, A., Hackmann, A., & Michael, T. (2004). Intrusive re-experiencing in posttraumatic stress disorder: Phenomenology, theory, and therapy. *Memory, 12*(4), 403–415.

Epstein, S. (1994). Integration of the cognitive and the psychodynamic unconscious. *American Psychologist, 49*(8), 709–724.

Foa, E. B., & Rothbaum, B. O. (1998). *Treating the trauma of rape: Cognitive-behavior therapy for PTSD*. New York: Guilford Press.

Giesen-Bloo, J., van Dyck, R., Spinhoven, P., van Tilburg, W., Dirksen, C., van Asselt, T., et al. (2006). Outpatient psychotherapy for borderline personality disorder: Randomized trial of schema-focused therapy vs transference-focused psychotherapy. *Archives of General Psychiatry, 63*(6), 649–658.

Hackmann, A., Clark, D. M., & McManus, F. (2000). Recurrent images and memories in social phobia. *Behaviour Research and Therapy, 38*, 601–610.

Harvey, A. G., Clark, D. M., Ehlers, A., & Rapee, R. M. (2000). Social anxiety and self-impression: Cognitive preparation enhances the beneficial effects of video feedback following a stressful social task. *Behaviour Research and Therapy, 38*(12), 1183–1192.

Hertel, P. T., Brozovich, F., Joormann, J., & Gotlib, I. H. (2008). Biases in interpretation and memory in generalized social phobia. *Journal of Abnormal Psychology, 117*(2), 278–288.

Hirsch, C. R., Clark, D. M., & Mathews, A. (2006). Imagery and interpretations in social phobia: Support for the combined cognitive biases hypothesis. *Behavior Therapy, 37*(3), 223–236.

Hirsch, C. R., Clark, D. M., Mathews, A., & Williams, R. (2003). Self-images play a causal role in social phobia. *Behaviour Research and Therapy, 41* (8), 909–921.

Hirsch, C. R., Mathews, A., Clark, D. M., Williams, R., & Morrison, J. (2003). Negative self-imagery blocks inferences. *Behaviour Research and Therapy, 41*(12), 1383–1396.

Hoffart, A., Borge, F.-M., Sexton, H., & Clark, D. M. (2009). Change processes in residential cognitive and interpersonal psychotherapy for social phobia: A process–outcome study. *Behavior Therapy, 40*, 10–22.

Hofmann, S. G. (2004). Cognitive mediation of treatment change in social phobia. *Journal of Consulting and Clinical Psychology, 72*(3), 392–399.

Holmes, E., & Hackmann, A. (Eds.). (2004). Mental imagery and memory in psychopathology [Special issue]. *Memory, 12*(4).

Liechsenring, F., Salzer, S., Beutel, M., Herpertz, S., Hiller, W., Hoyer, J., et al. (2013). Psychodynamic therapy and cognitive-behavior therapy in social anxiety disorder: A multi-center randomised controlled trial. *American Journal of Psychiatry, 170*, 759–767.

McManus, F., Clark, D. M., Grey, N., Wild, J., Hirsch, C., Fennell, M., et al. (2009). A demonstration of the efficacy of two of the components of cognitive therapy for social phobia. *Journal of Anxiety Disorders, 23*(4), 496–503.

Mortberg, E., Clark, D. M., Sundin, O., & Wistedt, A. (2007). Intensive group cognitive treatment and individual cognitive therapy versus treatment as usual in social phobia: A randomised controlled trial. *Acta Psychiatrica Scandinavica, 115*, 142–154.

Mortberg, E., Hoffart, A., Boecking, B., & Clark, D. M. (2013). Shifting the focus of one's attention mediates improvement in cognitive therapy for social phobia. *Behavioral and Cognitive Psychotherapy*.

National Institute for Health and Care Excellence. (2013). Social anxiety disorder: Recognition, assessment and treatment of social anxiety disorder (Clinical guideline 159). Available at *http://guidance.nice.org.uk/CG159*.

Pilling, S., Mayo-Wilson, E., Mavranezouli, I., Kew, K., Taylor, C., & Clark, D. M. (2013). Recognition, assessment and treatment of social anxiety disorder: Summary of NICE guidance [Practice Guideline Research Support, Non-U.S. Gov't]. *British Medical Journal, 346*, f2541.

Rapee, R. M., & Heimberg, R. G. (1997). A cognitive-behavioral model of anxiety in social phobia. *Behaviour Research and Therapy, 35*, 741–756.

Smucker, M. R., & Niederee, J. (1995). Treating incest-related PTSD and pathogenic schemas through imaginal exposure and rescripting. *Cognitive and Behavioral Practice, 2*(1), 63–92.

Stangier, U., Heidenreich, T., Peitz, M., Lauterbach, W., & Clark, D. M. (2003). Cognitive therapy for social phobia: Individual versus group treatment. *Behaviour Research and Therapy, 41*(9), 991–1007.

Stangier, U., Schramm, E., Heidenreich, T., Berger, M., & Clark, D. M. (2011). Cognitive therapy versus interpersonal psychotherapy in social anxiety disorder. *Archives of General Psychiatry, 68*, 692–700.

Stopa, L. (Ed.). (2004). *Imagery and the threatened self: Perspectives on mental imagery and the self in cognitive therapy*. Hove, UK: Routledge.

Stopa, L., & Jenkins, A. (2007). Images of the self in social anxiety: Effects on the retrieval of autobiographical memories. *Journal of Behavior Therapy and Experimental Psychiatry, 38*(4), 459–473.

Teasdale, J. D. (1993). Emotion and two kinds of meaning: Cognitive therapy and applied cognitive science. *Behavior and Research Therapy, 31*, 339–354.

Wild, J., & Clark, D. M. (2011). Imagery rescripting of early traumatic memories in social phobia. *Cognitive and Behavioral Practice, 18*(4), 433–443.

Wild, J., Hackmann, A., & Clark, D. M. (2007). When the present visits the past: Updating traumatic memories in social phobia. *Journal of Behavior Therapy and Experimental Psychiatry, 38*(4), 386–401.

Wild, J., Hackmann, A., & Clark, D. M. (2008). Rescripting early memories linked to negative images in social phobia: A pilot study. *Behavior Therapy, 39*(1), 47–56.

Part IV

Emotion-Focused Approaches

Capturing and Enhancing In-Session Emotion as a Step toward Change

CHAPTER 11

Integrating Emotion-Focused Therapy into Cognitive-Behavioral Therapy

Nathan C. Thoma
Leslie S. Greenberg

Emotion-focused therapy (EFT) is a research-driven, time-limited psychotherapy that was developed within the humanistic tradition and which incorporates the contemporary science of emotion (Greenberg, 2002). Building upon the relationship conditions of client-centered therapy as a foundation (Rogers, 1951), EFT has added techniques from Gestalt therapy (Perls, 1973) and other experiential approaches (e.g., Gendlin, 1996) to form a comprehensive, integrated system of psychotherapy grounded in emotion theory and clinical evidence.

In EFT, emotion is viewed as fundamentally adaptive. From an evolutionary perspective, emotions are thought to have evolved to provide information, to orient, and to motivate an organism toward adaptive action (Frijda, 1986). Thus EFT therapists seek not only to facilitate emotional awareness, but also to deliberately increase the level of arousal of various kinds of client emotions during psychotherapy sessions. This approach stands in contrast to some other therapies, whose primary goal is to regulate or reduce emotion. Another important distinguishing feature of EFT is that it is process-oriented. This means that EFT therapists watch for the emergence of specific types of emotional processes in session to guide their interventions and to determine what to do when, based on what a client is experiencing in a given moment.

We view these two features—emotion conceptualization and if–then algorithms to guide the deployment of interventions—as making EFT a useful source of both theory and technique for a cognitive-behavioral therapy (CBT) context. Based on the empirical evidence, as well as on our own clinical experiences, we believe that an EFT approach can help CBT therapists engage their clients' in-session emotions more productively and that EFT techniques can also help overcome some common roadblocks that can arise in CBT. In this chapter we elaborate on EFT theory, discuss the empirical evidence for EFT, and describe some methods to successfully integrate EFT into CBT. Broadly speaking, the model of integration that we propose can be considered to be *assimilative integraton* (Messer, 1992), meaning that we propose that elements of EFT can be imported into a standard CBT framework in ways that enhance and extend the treatment.

Emotion Theory

According to a variety of contemporary emotion theorists, emotions can be seen as organizing processes that alert and motivate an organism toward action in pursuing important goals, needs, or values (Frijda, 1986). In humans, emotions are not only experienced physiologically in the body, but are also experienced in terms of core meanings that accompany these sensations. Such meanings can then be symbolized consciously in terms of thoughts and verbal expression, which can then go on to influence the experience of meaning itself, in a complex dialectic interplay. Due to the inextricable linkage between meaning and emotion, EFT sometimes refers to emotions as "affective-meaning states" and to the underlying neurobiological structures as "emotion schemes."

Emotion schemes have some elements in common with Aaron Beck's core beliefs (Beck, 1996), in that emotion schemes are seen as core mental structures that are inextricably linked to the sense of self and appraisal of interpersonal events. Emotion schemes include representations of self and expectations concerning others, yet go beyond the semantic, linguistically based construct of core beliefs in that emotion schemes are seen as emerging from prelinguistic processing that interconnects self–other representations with affects, physiological arousal, episodic memory, and action-oriented behavioral tendencies. Further, emotion is considered central to the structure, rather than an outgrowth, and is viewed as playing the role of a holistic organizing process for all elements.

Like Jeffery Young's schemas (Young, Klosko, & Weishaar, 2003), emotion schemes are seen as latent mental structures accrued through a personal learning history that can be triggered in the present through a wide variety of stimuli that tap into any of the emotion scheme's many facets. However, emotion schemes differ from Young's schemas through their emphasis on an idiographic nature, with a unique phenomenology for each individual, in contrast to Young's emphasis on a rationally derived taxonomy of 18 universal maladaptive schema prototypes (Young et al., 2003). This emphasis on uniqueness is important in that it sets up a process of codiscovery for both client and therapist.

Additionally, the term "scheme" is used rather than "schema" because a *scheme* is action-oriented (as in the phrase "to hatch a scheme"). In contrast, the more general term "schema," as commonly used in the cognitive science literature, often tends to denote a latent set of static traits or information-processing tendencies (Mineka, Rafaeli, & Yovel, 2003). In an activated emotion scheme, the live and evolving experience along with urges emerging from the body are considered an essential focus, such as "the feeling of sinking into the ground with shame" rather than restricting the focus to a belief of being unworthy.

In-Session Emotion Conceptualization

While emotion schemes are considered to be idiosyncratic and dependent upon the particular learning history of each individual, there are nevertheless several different important categories of emotion, based on functional differences, that are relevant to recognizing important in-session emotional processes. Recognizing the function of specific emotions helps EFT clinicians to understand what emotions to facilitate and enhance versus what emotions to target for transformation and change. We propose that this taxonomy of emotions can also be helpful for CBT therapists, providing a roadmap to be used when clients are experiencing strong emotion in session to help therapists answer the questions, "Do I want to see more of this emotion? Or less? Is this helping the client discover new meaning? Or is this more of a painful place where the client is just stuck and overwhelmed?"

Figure 11.1 shows the EFT schematic of types of emotions. The first distinction to be made is to determine whether an emotion is primary, secondary, or instrumental in nature. *Instrumental emotions* have an inauthentic quality and are used to try to manipulate or control the behavior of others. Common examples include histrionic crocodile tears that have a "put-on" sense to them or blustery anger meant to bully others into giving in to entitled demands when no real threat to the self is present. These emotions are unproductive in session, and therefore when instrumental emotions arise it is important to orient the client toward primary emotions that are more directly linked to core needs. Subtle reorienting of clients is done through empathic refocusing, empathizing with the authentic, vulnerable component of what the client is saying, rather than through confronting the inauthenticity directly.

Secondary emotions are emotional reactions to primary emotions. For

```
                    Adaptive
                   ↗        ↘
           Primary            Productive
                   ↘        ↗
                    Maladaptive
                              ↘
           Secondary ─────────→ Unproductive
                              ↗
           Instrumental ─────
```

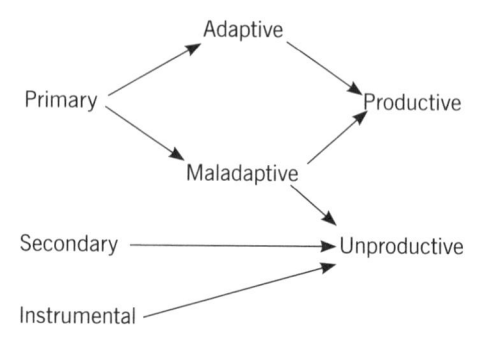

FIGURE 11.1. Types of in-session emotion.

example, anger is a common reaction to an initial feeling of being vulnerable or wounded, particularly among males. Additionally, feelings of depression, despair, and hopelessness can also be seen as secondary reactions to primary emotions such as shame, guilt, or fear. Feelings of despair and defeat tend to appear, especially when feelings such as shame, guilt, or fear arise consistently in the face of attempts to get interpersonal needs met. In EFT for depression, it is necessary to get past this initial layer of despair and hopelessness and into the primary emotions, even if the primary emotions are more acutely painful than the numbing effects of despair. Thus, feelings of despair are not considered to be productive in themselves, but are an attempt (usually unsuccessful) by clients to let go of or move away from more painful feelings.

Primary emotions are the initial, core reactions clients experience when emotion schemes are activated. There are two varieties. *Primary adaptive emotions* are those that alert clients to core needs of the self, orient them toward getting these needs met, and motivate them for action. The main primary adaptive emotions encountered in therapy are sadness over an important loss, anger over a personal violation, and hurt over a traumatic wound. Sadness allows for grieving, which is a necessary step in accepting a loss, making meaning of this experience, and moving on. Adaptive anger motivates healthy assertion and boundary drawing. Allowing oneself to fully experience the hurt of past traumas elicits self-compassion and social support, and through this reduces the sense of being alone and vulnerable to future harm. These emotions are considered productive, and therapists seek to help clients engage in each of these emotions as they arise. Clients benefit from deepening, differentiating, and making space for each.

Primary maladaptive emotions are initial reactions triggered by a current situation that are more related to past experiences than to the present.

They are "primary" because they are fast, automatic, and related to core issues that have come up again and again. They are "maladaptive" because these emotions do not motivate the client toward getting core needs met. These experiences have a familiar feeling to them, a place where the client may often find him- or herself stuck. As mentioned above, these are often feelings centering on fear (e.g., the anxiety of lonely abandonment or basic insecurity) and shame (e.g., a feeling of wretched worthlessness or inadequacy). Maladaptive emotions are typically overlearned feelings that arose repeatedly during the formative years when clients attempted to get their basic needs for safety, connection, and love met. Thus these emotions are frequently triggered in the present when clients feel those same basic needs.

While these emotions are *maladaptive* in clients' lives, in therapy these feelings can still be *productive*. In fact, it is seen as necessary to activate maladaptive emotion schemes in session so that clients are more open to transformation and change. To put it another way, it is necessary to fully arrive at a place before we can leave it (Greenberg, 2002). Maladaptive emotions are potentially productive to work with provided they are not totally overwhelming, such as may be seen when a client becomes highly dysregulated (e.g., sobbing uncontrollably or shrieking with anger). Additional characteristics of *unproductive* instances of primary maladaptive emotion can be seen when the client feels that he or she is the victim of the emotion, and is trapped by it, as though the emotion is having the client rather than the client having the emotion, and therefore the client is unable to take in information from the emotion and make new meaning by reflecting on it. When encountering overwhelming, unproductive, maladaptive emotion in session, therapists are advised to focus on emotion regulation, using diaphragmatic breathing, mindfulness, or other grounding exercises, even if momentarily, until the level of emotional arousal is again at a good working level.

A primary goal in EFT is to move past instrumental and secondary emotions in order to encounter primary maladaptive emotions. Subsequently going on to access adaptive emotion in the context of activated maladaptive emotion is the *central therapeutic process* that modifies the underlying emotion scheme, restructuring it in a lasting way. Thus the goals of EFT have some parallels with exposure therapy in that evocation of difficult affect is seen as a necessary step in providing a corrective emotional experience. However, EFT does not advocate for exposure to emotion across the board (cf. Barlow, Allen, & Choate, 2004), but rather promotes the activation of specific kinds of emotion and not, for example, symptomatic secondary emotions like anxiety. Instead, EFT therapists encourage client access to core fear and sadness related to attachment and core shame related to identity. Further, the proposed key mechanism of change in EFT is not habituation to repeated negative emotion, but rather the restructuring of maladaptive emotion schemes through the transformative effects of accessing adaptive emotion. In short, the idea is to use emotion to transform emotion.

In seeking to promote the restructuring of emotion schemes, EFT therapists use a warm, empathically attuned demeanor to make clients feel safe enough to encounter painful vulnerability, frequently using empathic reflection to help clients turn inward. This helps clients elaborate, differentiate, and verbally symbolize their experiences. Using empathic refocusing, EFT therapists continually guide clients toward their core emotional responses. This client-centered relational stance of empathic responding can itself provide substantial corrective emotional experience (Greenberg & Watson, 1998).

In addition to the ongoing provision of empathy and warmth, EFT therapists use a variety of active interventions to further facilitate emotional activation. Thus, the work involves a balance between leading and following. First, using empathic exploration and conjecture, therapists act as surrogate information processors by reaching into clients' inner worlds, offering them symbols to check against their internal experiences. This helps make the implicit explicit and to create new meaning. Notably, such expressions by the therapist are not interpretations of the client's internal conflicts or dynamics as might be used in psychodynamic therapy, but rather are statements meant to help elaborate that which already lies at the edge of a client's awareness.

Further interventions actively lead clients through emotion evocation and transformation, using a system of *markers* and *tasks* to guide therapists in knowing when to do what. *Markers* are spontaneously arising client in-session performances that indicate a particular kind of problem has come into the client's awareness and that the client is ready to work on this problem. *Tasks* are the affective goals the clients are aiming at and the interventions that are then employed to facilitate this aim. There are nearly a dozen different marker/task pairs that have been developed and systematically studied in EFT (see Elliott, Watson, Goldman, & Greenberg, 2004). We believe that a variety of EFT tasks could be productively integrated into a CBT context. For brevity, we have chosen to focus on two that CBT therapists are likely to find particularly valuable and which are also good "starter" EFT interventions for beginners. The first is the two-chair exercise for self-criticism. The second is the empty-chair exercise for unfinished business. These exercises are discussed in the "Clinical Application" section, p. 248.

Empirical Evidence

Several decades of programmatic research have helped to test and refine EFT interventions, with a number of controlled trials examining efficacy along with an extensive focus on process–outcome research. EFT for depression was tested in two randomized controlled trials (RCTs) against client-centered therapy (CCT) in a dismantling design to examine whether the active interventions of EFT add to the effects of client-centered relationship conditions (Goldman, Greenberg, & Angus, 2006; Greenberg & Watson, 1998). Combining the results meta-analytically (N = 72) shows a significant medium effect size[1] of d = 0.52 (Elliott et al., 2004), demonstrating that the active interventions contribute significantly to the effects of the therapy. This is also notable considering the rarity of finding significant differences between two bona fide treatments for depression (Cuijpers, van Straten, Andersson, & van Oppen, 2008). The CCT in these trials can be considered a bona fide active treatment because it meets Wampold, Minami, Baskin, and Tierney's (2002) criteria as a bona fide treatment, as well as the very large pre–post effect sizes in both treatment arms. Indeed, the EFT arms showed a combined pre–post effect size of d = 2.14 (Elliott et al., 2004), an effect size of relative rarity in psychotherapy research. Gains in the EFT group were well maintained at 18-month follow-up (Ellison, Greenberg, Goldman, & Angus, 2009). One RCT (N = 66) has compared EFT and CBT directly, showing substantial improvement in both groups with no difference in outcome on measures of depression, and with EFT showing a significant advantage on a measure of interpersonal problems (Watson, Gordon, Stermac, Kalogerakos, & Steckley, 2003). A controlled trial (N = 32) testing the efficacy of EFT for victims of early childhood abuse against a wait-list control found significant, large effects across a variety of outcomes at posttest and follow-up, including measures of general symptom distress, trauma, interpersonal problems, self-compassion, and a sense of resolution toward their abusers (Paivio & Nieuwenhuis, 2001). A randomized dismantling design (N = 45) was used to examine the incremental therapeutic advantages of using a two-chair technique in imaginally confronting clients' abusers in two versions of EFT for trauma (Paivio, Jarry, Chagigiorgis, Hall, & Ralston, 2010). While clients in both conditions saw large improvements across a variety of measures, significantly more clients in the imaginal confrontation arm were reliably improved (88% vs. 78%) or recovered (64% vs. 52%).

A number of trials have tested the efficacy of EFT for couples, which uses the same principles as EFT for individuals but additionally focuses on recognizing and reworking negative interactional cycles between the two partners that disrupt the meeting of healthy attachment and identity needs within the relationship. A meta-analysis has shown large effects on marital distress (d = 0.89) compared to other active treatments (including forms of CBT) and a very large effect (d = 1.93) compared to wait list (Elliott,

---

[1] By convention, an effect is considered small, medium, or large with d = 0.20, 0.50, and 0.80, respectively (Cohen, 1988).

Greenberg, & Lietaer 2004). A particular strength of the outcome data on EFT for couples is in the maintenance of gains at up to 2 and 3 years (e.g., Halchuk, Makinen, & Johnson, 2010).

The majority of the outcome trials of EFT have had relatively modest sample sizes and would benefit from further replication. However, confidence in their results is strengthened by the examinations of process–outcome relationships within the trials that are consistent with the predictions of EFT theory. As an experiential therapy, considerable focus is placed on enhancing client "experiencing." This has been operationalized by the Experiencing Scale (Klein, Mathieu, Gendlin, & Kiesler, 1969). In this seven-point scale, lower levels of experiencing are coded when clients are externally focused and see their problems as related to situational factors outside of themselves. Higher levels of experiencing are coded when clients are able to turn inward, focus on internal sensations and emotions, and then reflect upon them to derive new meanings, new ways of relating to oneself, and new resolutions to problems. Watson and Bedard (2006) found that in both CBT and EFT good outcome cases had higher levels of experiencing than poor outcome cases. In both treatments, experiencing was higher in mid- and late treatment than in early treatment, indicating treatment facilitated this process. Additionally, EFT clients experienced significantly higher mean and modal levels of experiencing than CBT clients, showing that the focus on experiencing in EFT enhances this variable more than CBT. Further supporting the importance of this variable, Pos, Greenberg, and Warwar (2009) used path analysis to show that client experiencing in midtreatment best predicted outcome in experiential therapy over and above the therapeutic alliance at early, mid-, and late treatment.

Several studies have found that not only is the process of turning inward to make new meaning important in EFT, but the level of emotional arousal is also related to outcome. Missirlian, Toukmanian, Warwar, and Greenberg (2005) found that increased emotional arousal in midtreatment, particularly when coupled with an internally focused style of perceptual processing (similar to high levels of experiencing), predicted reduced depressive symptoms in experiential therapy for depression. This relationship was significant even after controlling for the therapeutic alliance in early and midtreatment. Carryer and Greenberg (2010) refined this finding, showing that the relationship between arousal midtreatment and outcome is a nonlinear one, with an optimal, overall proportion of highly aroused emotion at 25% of the session. This proportion totaled up all of the emotionally aroused moments in the session, which in themselves may only last a matter of moments or minutes. More or less total time spent in a highly aroused emotional state in a 50-minute session was related to poorer outcome, thus showing a curvilinear relationship between arousal and outcome.

Auszra, Greenberg, and Herrmann (2013) found that in particular highly aroused *productive* emotions, as coded with the Productivity Scale

(Greenberg, Auszra, & Herrmann, 2007), are most related to positive outcomes in experiential therapy. Controlling for emotional arousal as well as the therapeutic alliance, ratings of the productivity of in-session emotion at midtreatment accounted for over 54% of the variance in depressive symptom reduction at posttreatment—one of the largest process–outcome relationships in psychotherapy research of which we are aware.

In keeping with EFT theory on the stage-like unfolding of types of emotion in the context of emotion scheme transformation, Pascual-Leone and Greenberg (2007) found that emotions emerged in the predicted sequential patterns, starting with secondary emotions in the form of global distress, moving into maladaptive emotions such as fear and shame, then accessing a positive emotional need, and finally adaptive emotions such as sadness/grief, assertive anger, or self-soothing, followed by an increased sense of agency (see Figure 11.2). These sequences have been found to occur repeatedly within a session. In sessions with good end-of-session outcome, Pascual-Leone (2009) found that clients spent increasing intervals of time experiencing adaptive emotions and progressively shorter emotional collapses into globalized distress over the course of a session.

At this point, it has yet to be demonstrated that the above emotional processes are the result of therapist intervention and not merely due to the natural unfolding of previously existing client capacities. However, the dismantling efficacy trials discussed above (Goldman et al., 2006; Greenberg & Watson, 1998) indicate that the active interventions of EFT add significantly to positive outcome over and above client-centered relationship

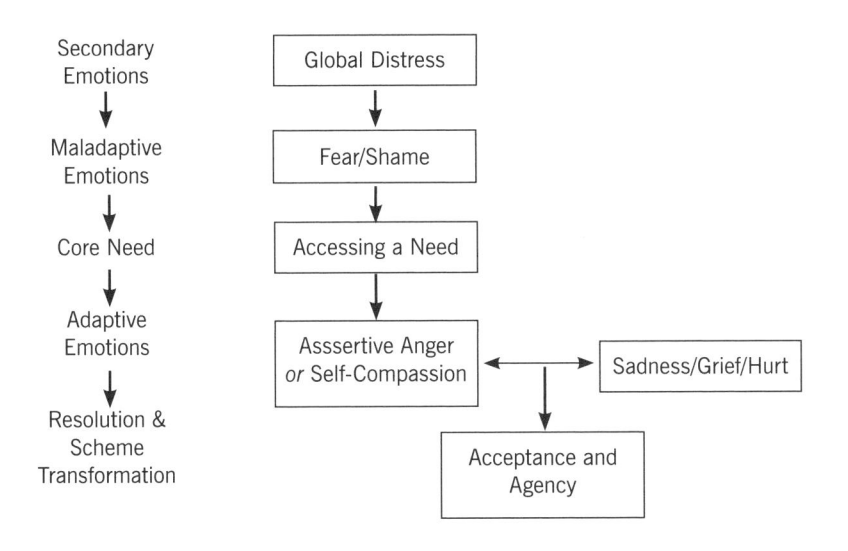

FIGURE 11.2. Sequential unfolding of types of emotion as in-session emotional processing progresses.

conditions at posttreatment and also show better maintenance of gains in responders at follow-up (Ellison et al., 2009). Additionally, there have been specific investigations aimed at understanding and refining many of the active interventions employed in EFT through empirical task analysis (see Pascual-Leone, Greenberg, & Pascual-Leone, 2009), including studies of the two-chair exercise for self-criticism (e.g., Greenberg, 1983) and the empty-chair exercise for unfinished business (e.g., Greenberg & Malcolm, 2002), among others. In summary, the evidence thus far for EFT is quite promising. Evidence from controlled trials demonstrates good efficacy for depression, trauma, and marital distress. Evidence from process–outcome research supports the proposed mechanisms of EFT, and indeed systematic study of these mechanisms has come to refine and enhance the therapy itself, guiding its developers to make ongoing changes and adjustments in the approach.

Clinical Application

The Two-Chair Exercise for Self-Criticism

In this chapter, we have selected two active interventions from EFT that we feel can be readily integrated into CBT to serve as exemplars of how EFT can enhance CBT. The first is the *two-chair exercise for self-criticism* (Greenberg, Rice, & Elliott, 1996). As the name of the intervention implies, the in-session marker that calls for this exercise is evident when the client expresses negative attitudes toward herself.[2] Common examples occur when a client labels herself incompetent, a failure, a loser, a freak, or otherwise inferior to other people. Another manifestation arises when a client is particularly demanding or holds unrelentingly high standards for her own behavior, habits, or accomplishments. In CBT, these ways of thinking would typically be addressed through cognitive restructuring (CR), helping the client to see the negative distortions in her view and to develop a more objective or rational way of evaluating herself. In my (N. C. T.) experience as a CBT therapist, CR is often quite helpful in this regard, and the client is able to see that her way of thinking is inaccurate and unhelpful. However, all too often, the client reaches a point where she may say something to the effect of "I get it rationally, but emotionally I still just feel like a loser." In a CBT context, this might be considered an additional part of the marker that calls for the use of this EFT intervention. Using a chair exercise to evoke and transform the maladaptive emotion schemes in an emotionally alive way can be quite a powerful experience, often taking the client much further than CR alone.

---

[2] For simplicity and clarity, the female pronoun will be used to refer to the client and the male pronoun will be used to refer to the therapist. This assignment was chosen arbitrarily.

In this exercise, the client will move back and forth between two chairs, and the therapist will facilitate a dialogue between two parts of the client that are at odds with each other. The goal is to use the process of sitting in two different chairs to highlight and differentiate two parts of the client's self, to bring them into further contact with each other, and then to reach a resolution. The two parts are the "critic," on the one hand, who makes demands of and criticizes the client and then punishes her when these demands are not met, and, on the other hand, the "experiencer," who feels all of the client's emotions (Greenberg, 2011; Greenberg et al., 1996). This part of the client is also the source of agency, in charge of making decisions and taking action in life, the part that ultimately mobilizes to meet the client's needs. Such a division could also be considered parallel to the client having a "thinking side" (in this case, a dysfunctional thinker of negative self-evaluations) and a concomitant "feeling side." As the therapist cues the client to move back and forth between the chairs, providing prompts, empathy, and coaching along the way, the process unfolds in a stage-like manner. First maladaptive emotions are evoked and activated by the self attack; next a basic need is contacted; then the client organizes around that need and contacts adaptive emotions. Engaging the adaptive emotions motivates the meeting of unmet needs (e.g., anger motivates assertive boundary setting; self-compassion motivates self-acceptance), and the client develops a new way of relating to herself on an emotional as well as a cognitive level.

Upon encountering the in-session marker, the therapist begins to set up the exercise by pointing out the client's mental behavior and framing it as one part of the self criticizing or demanding perfection from another part of the self. This should be stated in an empathic, concerned manner. Examples:

> "So it is kind of like you chastise yourself when that happens. You punish yourself in a way, beating yourself up."
> "Mmm, yes, here we have that again, where you end up calling yourself these harsh names, criticizing yourself when you don't do something just right."
> "Right, so you get it rationally that you are not a failure, but emotionally, it still feels like you are a failure. Mmm (*empathizing with the pain of that feeling*). And so you call yourself one, a failure, and as you said before also, things like 'a pathetic unemployed bum' and 'a crappy father.'"

The therapist then asks the client's permission to try something new. "You know what, we have a way of working with this that can be helpful, an exercise I'd like to do with you. Would you be willing to try it?" The client typically consents. We recommend getting permission to try "an exercise" rather than stating that the process will involve moving around and sitting in different chairs because in the latter case clients are more likely to say "no" out of unwarranted fear of embarrassment or to ask for intellectual explanations.

It is important to normalize the exercise by introducing it with both empathy and confidence. The therapist pulls up an additional chair and invites the client to sit in it. "Now I would like you to play that part of you that says those things. I'd like you to be that critical voice in your head, and to say the things to yourself that you hear in your mind." The therapist directs the client to speak directly to the chair she has just vacated.

Often clients feel foolish, and criticize the empty chair rather halfheartedly. The therapist further stimulates engagement by repeating some of the criticisms, particularly the harsh ones, and also by empathically summarizing or rephrasing them. "Yes, that's right, its like, 'You can't do anything right.'" The therapist sometimes asks the client to repeat a criticism when a core belief emerges. If clients speak directly to the therapist and want to discuss the process or complain that it feels "weird" to be talking to themselves this way, the therapist can point out, "That's true. But also, this is the voice you hear in your head, no? Right now, we want to get in contact with that, and amplify it, so we can see what goes on for you. So say those things to yourself now, the things that you so often hear in your head." The therapist redirects the client to speak to the empty chair if she is frequently engaging with the therapist rather than with the chair.

After an initial round of criticisms, the therapist asks the client to switch chairs, moving back to her original client chair. The therapist then asks, "What's that like for you, when you hear that?" The therapist focuses the client on current feelings in the body. This helps the client get in touch with primary maladaptive shame, really bringing the emotion scheme alive. The client is then directed to share her feelings with the critical chair.

It is important that the client recognize and make contact with her painful maladaptive emotions at this moment, rather than continuing to identify with the critical half of herself. For example, clients sometimes say, "I feel like it's true." In this case, the client remains fused with the critic in a state of collapse, immersed in secondary hopelessness. To help keep the client moving forward, it is important to help her get in touch with the critic's painful impact on the experiencing side's feelings. The therapist can respond with, "Right, and what's that *like* for you, in your body, when you hear it and think that it's true? What *feelings* does that bring up for you?" The therapist empathizes with the client's vulnerable feelings and helps the client express all aspects of her experience.

After the client expresses her emotional experience, the therapist asks the client to switch back to the critical chair. The critic often revs up the critique, now all the more dissatisfied with the client's experiencing side for being "weak" and struggling with difficult feelings rather than bucking up and getting things done. At this point, it is important to help the client contact specific criticisms as evidence for her shortcomings, and thus the notion that she deserves this kind of harsh treatment. This increasing harshness helps to show the client how unrelenting and unempathic the critical side of herself can be. Again the therapist assists the client in the criticism, helping the critic list the shortcomings and failures.

After helping the client get specific, calling upon memories and instances of falling short, the therapist asks the client to return to the experiencing chair and express what it is like to hear this. The goal is to assist the client in contacting her core maladaptive emotions, which are often related to fear and shame. Clients frequently cry once maladaptive fear and shame are fully present. Provided it is not overwhelming and dysregulated, this crying is a sign that maladaptive emotion schemes are activated in a productive manner.

At this juncture the therapist performs a key maneuver by asking the client, "What do you *need* right now? What do you *need* from that part of you?" Contacting a core need is the turning point in the intervention and has been shown to be crucial to positive outcome (Pascual-Leone & Greenberg, 2007). Clients need to feel they deserve the need to be met and this comes from having felt the pain of the maladaptive state and being motivated to stop the pain. Clients typically say one of two kinds of things. Either the client says she needs the criticism to stop or says she needs support, encouragement, or praise rather than demands and criticism. Often the former comes first. Clients often require validation of their need by the therapist and support in expressing it by assertively standing up to the critic. The goal in this context is to contact primary adaptive anger to motivate the assertion or primary adaptive sadness to promote a reaching out for comfort and/or an evocation of self-compassion. While the therapist knows that assertive anger is therapeutic, he needs to be careful to elicit the feeling from the client, to lead her to contact her own inner resources, rather than pushing the idea of anger upon the client. The therapist does this by noticing, repeating, and amplifying assertions that the client expresses. "Yeah, it's like, stop that. It really hurts me, and makes me totally shut down." Therapists can also attend to any modicum of assertive body language the client uses, such as a small hand gesture, and ask the client to magnify it as she repeats the assertive statement. Similarly, in evoking sadness, the therapist facilitates its emergence rather than engaging in instruction or psychoeducation (Greenberg et al., 1996).

After the client expresses a need, the therapist asks the client to change chairs to the critic again and asks the question, "How do you respond to this?" There are three basic possible outcomes. One is that the critic softens, empathizes with the client's pain, and expresses a willingness to try to meet the need of the experiencer. Self-compassion may be contacted, an adaptive emotion that undoes and transforms maladaptive shame. Another outcome is that the critic softens into its own protective stance of fear of the client's assertion of needs (this more often occurs with anxiety problems). The third possible outcome is that the critic remains harsh and unyielding in response to the expression of needs.

If at any point in the process of the exercise the critic softens, you can begin to try to facilitate a negotiation or integration between the two sides. As mentioned, there are several ways the critic softens: into fear, contrition, caring, or compassion. Often, softening comes in the form of a more benevolent stance such as "I want to protect you"—from criticism by others or from other external threats. With the critic softened, the client is better able to enter into a state of affective reorganization or into reflective negotiation and problem solving (Greenberg et al., 1996).

To facilitate negotiation the therapist can ask the critic what she needs from the experiencer. The critic often asks for the experiencer to work harder and to be more diligent. The critic's critique is often a misguided attempt to motivate the client into action. You can ask the experiencer to describe in further detail how the critic can help motivate her more effectively, such as by providing more encouragement. The critic can also function as a holder of values and standards or sometimes as a part of the client that looks out for threats, trying to protect the client against embarrassment in front of others. Again, the experiencer can give the critic feedback about what is helpful and what is hurtful about the way the critic goes about doing this. The therapist asks the client to continue to go back and forth between the two chairs, expressing the needs of each side, letting the two sides communicate openly, so that the client can reach a greater sense of integration as each side navigates toward greater adaptivity. The two parts of the client can become less conflicted and more symbiotic in their relationship, leading to a felt sense of integration and wholeness.

If the critic does not soften, and remains harshly critical, a positive outcome can still come about after facilitating the client's assertiveness in standing up to the critic. This can be particularly difficult for unassertive clients, who are typically hesitant or afraid to contact adaptive anger. Questions that elicit the client's needs and wants are helpful. "When you hear that said to you that way, what do you want?" "When you feel that way, and you tell that critical side about those vulnerable feelings, and this is the response you get, what does it make you want to say back?" A good question that can elicit anger is, "What do you *resent* about what that side is telling you?" Coaching the client to assume an assertive body posture when making a request or demand can help the client deepen her felt sense of anger and her entitlement to protect herself. "Try putting both of your feet firmly on the ground, and sit nice and upright, like this (*modeling for the client*). That's right, now say that again!" Standing up to the critic in session can be an empowering experience. Not only does it help the client practice responding to irrational negative thoughts with more adaptive responses, it does so in a way that builds emotional memories, enhancing self-efficacy and yielding a viscerally felt sense of agency.

If the client is overwhelmed by the intensity of her maladaptive shame, or perhaps becomes flooded with fear as a secondary reaction to contacting the beginnings of assertiveness, it is important to help the client regulate her emotion to tolerable levels. Ask the client to stop and breathe if she is unable to speak. If need be, use mindfulness and grounding exercises, such as asking the client to attend to what she feels physically in her feet, then legs, the belly, and so on, moving up the entire body in a body scan. Alternatively, the therapist can ask the client to describe what she sees around her in the room or to describe the expression she sees on the therapist's face. Notably, the two-chair exercise for self-criticism is not recommended for persons with severe borderline personality, for whom emotional lability is a chronic problem, unless they have been able to demonstrate the capacity to reregulate emotions in session with the assistance of the therapist (Pos & Greenberg, 2012).

Sometimes a full resolution—either assertively standing up to the critic and/or a softening of the critic—is reached within one session, but sometimes it takes several sessions. However, it is important to help clients contact their basic needs and also to begin to transform primary maladaptive shame with at least the beginnings of primary adaptive assertiveness and/or self-compassion in the first implementation of the exercise so that the client does not come away from the experience feeling completely defeated and further wounded. Therefore it is also important not to introduce the exercise for the first time with less than 25 minutes left in the session in order to give time for the process to unfold. Additionally, it is important for the therapist to express a warm and caring attitude throughout, empathizing especially with the experiencing side of the client. Part of the corrective emotional experience comes from the client experiencing herself as less alone in these difficult feelings, the sense of the therapist genuinely sharing her experiences (Elliott et al., 2004). Unconditional acceptance from the therapist in the context of feeling unacceptable can itself be powerfully healing, transforming the maladaptive emotion scheme by adding new information.

Even if substantial progress is made within one session, it is often helpful to revisit the exercise in future sessions. The in-session process markers discussed above can indicate whether there is more chair-work to be done in order to adequately strengthen the client's sense of agency in the face of her own criticism. In subsequent sessions, emphasis should be placed on further elaborating and exploring the nuances of the emotion schemes that are brought up, as well as any self-interruptions to adaptive emotion.

In exploring nuances of the emotion schemes, origins of the critic's harshness can also be explored, such as when the critic first came into the client's life or where the client learned to treat herself this way. Often the critic is an internalized version of the perceived criticism, threats, or standards for acceptability of an early caretaker, such as a parent. Sometimes asking the client "Does this voice remind you of anyone?" will bring forth the connection in the client's mind, activating her emotion schemes related to a parent. The client may then remark, "My god, it sounds like my mother!" If this kind of connection emerges, it can be a marker that there is "unfinished business" with the client's parent that would benefit from elaboration and resolution. The empty-chair exercise for unfinished business can be a helpful method of furthering this process.

The Empty-Chair Exercise for Unfinished Business

The empty-chair exercise is similar to the two-chair exercise for self-criticism, except that the dialogue is with an imagined other person rather than with a part of the client's self. The imagined other person is an internal representation of a real person from the client's life. While the client cannot change the past and cannot necessarily change the real person, the client can change their relationship to an internalized representation of that person, such as through holding the other accountable for past wrongs and de-blaming the self (Greenberg et al., 1996; Greenberg & Watson, 2006). Sometimes clients even change fundamental aspects of the representation itself, such as seeing the other as deeply flawed but well meaning rather than simply as punitive and uncaring. As with the two-chair exercise for self-criticism, the process moves in a stage-like manner from secondary emotional reactions, to primary maladaptive emotions, to primary adaptive emotions.

The in-session marker for this exercise, named "unfinished business," can be seen in statements by the client indicating that she experiences chronic anger or grief related to a significant person in her life. This is disruptive for the client because when specific emotion schemes associated with significant others are triggered, the client reexperiences elements of that past relationship in the present, often unconsciously. Such feelings qualify as unfinished business when they are more related to past interpersonal experiences rather than to current interpersonal conflict (e.g., marital distress).

Most typically, the early experiences were with a caretaker, such as a parent (Greenberg et al., 1996). Experiences of abuse or trauma may be related to a parent or to other persons from the client's life, such as another family member or family friend (Paivio & Pascual-Leone, 2010). Bringing the empty-chair exercise for unfinished business into CBT can be helpful in resolving "small 't' trauma," resulting from repeated, toxic, developmental experiences such as chronic criticism as a child, as well as facilitating the grieving process, such as with the death of a loved one. The technique has also been successfully applied with clients struggling with issues related to childhood physical and sexual abuse (Paivio & Pascual-Leone, 2010; Paivio & Nieuwenhuis, 2001), many of whom suffer from complex or chronic posttraumatic stress disorder (PTSD). Notably, the empty-chair exercise is typically not highly indicated for single experiences of trauma with a stranger (e.g., a sexual assault) or war trauma. When working in a CBT context, approaches such as prolonged exposure (Foa, Hembree, & Rothbaum, 2007) or imagery rescripting (Arntz, Chapter 8, this volume) may be applied. We should also note that because the exercise can be quite emotionally evocative, it is contraindicated in cases in which there is risk of self-injury, suicide, or violent acting out. In such cases, clients may not yet have sufficient ego strength for emotion-deepening exercises and may need more work on emotion regulation skills.

The following client statements could be examples of unfinished business:

> "My boss can be very intimidating and he makes me very anxious when I'm around him. It's like that same feeling I had growing up. You never knew when my father was going to explode about something."
>
> "My mother was all about her. Even when she showed caring for us, it was this big display, like she should be recognized for it."
>
> "After my parents divorced, I moved back and forth between my parents' houses. It was like it was my job to keep them connected somehow. And my mom got so busy with work, trying to support us. I just felt so alone sometimes."

With an in-session marker for unfinished business, typically resentment and disappointment are wrapped together into helpless complaint. There is also often a constricted quality to the emotions, the sense that the feelings are cut short with an incomplete attempt at acceptance. Part of the goal of the exercise is to unravel the complicated ball of feelings and give full voice to adaptive emotions such as anger, sadness, and hurt. When working with abuse or trauma and/or particularly fragile clients, it is important that the exercise not be introduced until there is a solid and stable bond between the therapist and the client that has helped to create a sense of safety and trust.

To introduce the exercise, it is often helpful to begin by offering an experiential formulation such as, "It sounds like you have a lot of pent-up anger and other feelings toward your mother." The therapist can go on to provide a rationale, "It seems like it would be helpful for us to get at these feelings and express them, so you don't feel as mired and tangled up in them. Are you willing to try that?" Next the therapist can introduce the task itself, "Let's start by bringing your mother in here, and placing her in this chair. What I'd like for us to do is have you talk to your mother, here, in the chair, and begin to tell her about some of these lingering feelings you were just mentioning to me." It is also important to make clear that this is not a role play or a practice exercise for things that the client should try to go and say to the significant other. "By doing this exercise in here, we can help you resolve some of these feelings. But, of course, we are not saying that you should necessarily go and actually say any of these things to her. This is mainly a way to get it out, and to speak to the version of your mother that lives in you. So you can feel safe in saying whatever you need to say."

It is crucial to get the client's permission to proceed. If clients express hesitation in proceeding, it is important to explore the nature of their reservations and address them. Sometimes clients feel that it is taboo to speak back to their parents or that doing so is a betrayal. Clients can be reminded that they are only speaking to the parent in their imagination. Clients can be afraid of encountering overwhelming emotion. In this case, several sessions may be needed to work up to the exercise, exploring the emotions and meanings that may arise for the client. Feelings of resignation and defeat—secondary emotional reactions—may inhibit the client's motivation to try, feeling that their parent will never change, and therefore talking about unresolved feelings is useless. The therapist can point toward the pain of the underlying maladaptive emotions, along with the potential benefits of resolving some of those feelings, regardless of whether the parent changes. In some cases, current conflicts with a parent become mixed and confused with past issues. The therapist may ask the client to "speak from the 6-year-old you." This helps to direct the client toward the core, original feelings.

Having obtained client consent, the therapist pulls up a chair and requests of the client, "I'd like you to picture your [significant other] sitting here in the chair." The therapist asks her to get a mental image and to briefly describe what she sees, such as the expression on the face of the other. It is important that the client make contact with the imagined other, perceptually as well as emotionally. Having activated the representation of the other, the therapist coaches the client to express her feelings to the other. The therapist empathizes continuously along the way, with brief affirmations, reflections, and summaries. The therapist uses "I" language, joining the client, and also bringing the client further into her own internal experience and process of meaning making. The client may start out with externally focused language, accusing the other of a litany of transgressions or of perpetrating a series of indignities. The therapist directs the client to get in touch with these experiences and express the impact they had on her. "Mmm, yes. And tell him what that was like for you when your father said those things to you." Sometimes the client will keep turning toward the therapist to tell stories about the other and to complain about various injustices. The therapist gently redirects the client back toward engagement in the dialogue. "Ah, yes, that was hard for you. Tell your father, tell him right now what that was like." Engagement with the empty chair allows for the greatest stimulation and activation of the underlying emotion schemes as it allows for the most direct interaction with the internalized representation of the other.

After the client has expressed some of her feelings to the other, for cases that do not involve trauma or abuse, the therapist asks the client to switch chairs, and to play the role of the other. "Now I'd like you to change chairs and sit over here. As your father, how do you respond to that?" Playing the other, the client will often start out by responding from an unempathic, blaming stance, or become defensive. This activates the negative representation of the other that is in need of transformation. (In cases of trauma and abuse, it is often advised to keep the client in her own chair for the whole exercise and not to ask her to try to play the role of her own abuser, which can be confusing and retraumatizing. The underlying emotion scheme is often sufficiently activated by imaginally confronting the negative other in the empty chair that the client does not need to take the role of the other, which clients sometime find aversive.) If the client has played the role of the negative other to heighten its stimulus value, the therapist directs the client to move back to her original chair and asks her to express to the other what it is like to hear the other's essentially rejecting response. This is likely to stir up the feelings that have always come up for the client in relation to this person. The therapist then seeks to deepen the activation of these maladaptive emotion schemes by helping the client access specific memories and instances in which these emotions were felt. The therapist helps the client move past secondary emotional reactions such as hopelessness, resignation, anxiety, complaint, and resentment in order to more fully access the core pain of the primary emotions underneath, such as shame, guilt, sadness, and anger. To access the sadness of loss, the therapist guides the client to her bodily felt sense of pain and encourages her to allow and accept her sense of lonely abandonment or loss. For the expression of anger, it becomes important to help the client get past secondary, generalized rage and to contact anger over specific violations. In cases of abuse, there is also often primary fear as well as disgust toward the other. Disgust is an emotion that compels the body to remove noxious materials. Contacting disgust toward an abuser is a way of experiencing an expulsion of the abuser from the body.

Having fully activated primary emotion, the therapist directs the client to tell the other what she *needs* from the other. Contacting the core needs associated with the primary emotions is a crucial step and a main turning point in the exercise. It deepens the sense of grief and/or assertive feelings of anger. This allows the client to feel entitled to her desire for such experiences as safety, consistency, appropriate boundaries, caring, warmth, praise, and love. This sets the stage for a sense of agency and self-worth as well as the possibility of a transformation in her internal representation of the other. The expression of unmet needs in itself can begin to expand the constricted view of the other.

Once needs and desires have been expressed, the therapist asks the client to play the role of the other. To help cue the possibility of a shift in the attitude of the other, the therapist may phrase his prompt, "Hearing that, what's that like for you? And how do you respond to that?" There are two possibilities. Often, the other may soften, become more empathic, and express regret over how the other has treated the client. Imagining the other really hearing such an authentic expression of needs, the client is able to contact imagined empathy and compassion in the other. The other also often is seen as separate, having his or her own problems, and possessing both good and bad qualities. Having transformed the inner representation of the other, the client no longer feels haunted by an uncaring other who is withholding or overwhelming and feels a sense of relief and resolve.

The other type of shift, common in cases of trauma and abuse, can involve the client seeing the other as less threatening, bullying, and dangerous. The other becomes weaker, with inner failings. Rather than being an unrelenting, powerful menace, the other becomes pathetic and flawed. The other is held accountable for her violations and is seen as deserving of the client's negative feelings. The self is deblamed, and flaws are attributed to the other. The self also becomes less threatened, no longer living in a dangerous world populated by such frightening figures.

These kinds of shifts in the other may begin immediately after the expression of needs and may lead to a sense of resolution within a single session. More commonly, a stage-like progression is started in a session, with collapses of the process along the way. The therapist asks the client to move back and forth between the chairs, facilitating forward movement and negotiation between the client and other, addressing blocks and stuck points, going over important turning points more than once. Several sessions are often needed to rework all important aspects of the relevant emotion schemes and for the client to feel safe in fully encountering both the fullness of her anger and the pain of her sadness over what she missed out on.

The highest level of resolution is achieved when the client has expressed all of her anger over past wrongs, her sadness over unmet needs and missed experiences, then sees the other as flawed but possessing fundamentally good intentions, and can go on to reach a point of forgiveness. Forgiveness does not happen in all cases and does not need to be emphasized or even suggested by the therapist—it can only happen when the client reaches this point on her own. The therapist's focus is on empathizing with the client's experiences and guiding her toward contacting and expressing core, adaptive emotion. In cases wherein the client is unable to see the other as forgivable, there is often a difficult stage of helping the client contact sadness over never being able to get what she wants from this other, and grieving this loss, in order to ultimately reach a place of acceptance. Short of forgiveness, there is often a sense of resolution simply in having a greater understanding of the other, along with a sense of entitlement to basic needs. As one might imagine, forgiveness is rare in cases of trauma and abuse. The sense of resolve in these cases resides primarily in the empowerment that comes from holding the other accountable for his or her wrongs and a letting go of the anger and sadness, that allows the client to move on.

Future Directions

We would like to note that the power and effectiveness of the chair exercises we have described is likely to be enhanced if additional EFT interventions are incorporated along the way. EFT was developed as an interrelated system of interventions, each of which can be called on to address stuck points with subtasks within tasks. For example, to help externally focused clients turn inward toward their emotions and their meanings, an intervention known as *focusing* is used. To help clients make deeper contact with blocked emotions, *the two-chair exercise for self-interruption* is employed. And to help clients develop self-compassion, a *two-chair exercise for self-soothing* can be used.

We would also like to emphasize the importance of therapist empathy, warmth, and genuineness throughout EFT implementation, as it is the reassuring presence of the therapist's unconditional acceptance and understanding, expressed through vocal quality, verbal affirmations, and empathic reflections, that help clients feel more safe, less alone, and more willing to encounter all aspects of their experience.

The effects of integrating EFT interventions into ongoing CBT has not been directly tested empirically. However, the EFT interventions discussed in this chapter have undergone testing as stand-alone interventions and have demonstrated positive outcomes on task-relevant measures, such as feelings of resolution and forgiveness toward a target person in the case of unfinished business (e.g., Greenberg & Malcolm, 2002) and increases in self-acceptance in the case of self-criticism (e.g., Greenberg, 1983). Additionally, Newman et al. (2011) added a treatment package that included EFT interventions to a standard CBT treatment package for generalized anxiety disorder (GAD) and found some indications of advantages for EFT + CBT versus supportive listening + CBT (see Erickson, Newman, & McGuire, Chapter 16, this volume, for further details). Thus further research on adding EFT to CBT for a variety of patient populations and problems is called for. Ongoing research indicates that the evidence for EFT as a stand-alone treatment package continues to accumulate. Preliminary results from trials currently under way show positive results with EFT for GAD as well as social anxiety, building on EFT's positive track record with depression, trauma, and couples work. The extent of process–outcome research on

EFT has been a model for programs of research on other psychotherapies. We look forward to further developments in process–outcome research in CBT, as well as in the integration of EFT into CBT, to help guide and validate which interventions to use with whom and when.

Further Resources

Books

- For more detailed discussion of EFT theory and techniques, see Greenberg (2002, 2011).
- Paivio and Pascual-Leone (2010) demonstrate how to tailor EFT in working with complex trauma.

Videos

- Two sessions of working with a depressed client are seen in *Emotion-Focused Therapy for Depression* (American Psychological Association, 2007). In the first session, the two-chair exercise for self-criticism is demonstrated. In the second session, the empty-chair exercise is demonstrated. See *www.apa.org/pubs/videos/4310798.aspx*.
- Six sessions with a single client can be seen in *Emotion-Focused Therapy over Time* (American Psychological Association, 2006). See *www.apa.org/pubs/videos/4310761.aspx*.

Websites

- For information on training in EFT at York University, Toronto, Ontario, Canada, go to *www.emotionfocusedclinic.org*.
- The International Center for Excellence in Emotionally Focused Couples Therapy offers training videos, books, research citations, and information on trainings in EFT for couples. Go to *www.iceeft.com*.

References

American Psychological Association. (2006). *Emotion-focused therapy for depression*. Available at *www.apa.org/pubs/videos/4310761.aspx*.
American Psychological Association. (2007). *Emotion-focused therapy over time*. Available at *www.apa.org/pubs/videos/4310798.aspx*.
Auszra, L., Greenberg, L. S., & Herrmann, I. (2013). Client emotional productivity—Optimal client in-session emotional processing in experiential therapy. *Psychotherapy Research*, 23(6), 732–746.
Barlow, D. H., Allen, L. B., & Choate, M. L. (2004). Toward a unified treatment for emotional disorders. *Behavior Therapy*, 35(2), 205–230.
Beck, A. T. (1996). Beyond belief: A theory of modes, personality, and psychopathology. In P. M. Salkovskis (Ed.), *Frontiers of cognitive therapy* (pp. 1–25). New York: Guilford Press.

Carryer, J. R., & Greenberg, L. S. (2010). Optimal levels of emotional arousal in experiential therapy of depression. *Journal of Consulting and Clinical Psychology*, 78(2), 190–199.

Cohen, J. (1988). *Statistical power analysis for the behavior sciences*. Hillsdale, NJ: Erlbaum.

Cuijpers, P., van Straten, A., Andersson, G., & van Oppen, P. (2008). Psychotherapy for depression in adults: A meta-analysis of comparative outcome studies. *Journal of Consulting and Clinical Psychology*, 76(6), 909–922.

Elliott, R., Greenberg, L. S., & Lietaer, G. (2004). Research on experiential psychotherapies. In M. J. Lambert (Ed.), *Bergin and Garfield's handbook of psychotherapy and behavior change* (5th ed., pp. 493–539). New York: Wiley.

Elliott, R., Watson, J. C., Goldman, R. N., & Greenberg, L. S. (2004). *Learning emotion-focused therapy: The process-experiential approach to change*. Washington, DC: American Psychological Association Press.

Ellison, J. A., Greenberg, L. S., Goldman, R. N., & Angus, L. (2009). Maintenance of gains following experiential therapies for depression. *Journal of Consulting and Clinical Psychology*, 77(1), 103–112.

Foa, E. B., Hembree, E. A., & Rothbaum, B. O. (2007). *Prolonged exposure therapy for PTSD: Emotional processing of traumatic experiences: Therapist guide*. New York: Oxford University Press.

Frijda, N. H. (1986). *The emotions*. New York: Cambridge University Press.

Gendlin, E. T. (1996). *Focusing-oriented psychotherapy: A manual of the experiential method*. New York: Guilford Press.

Goldman, R. N., Greenberg, L. S., & Angus, L. (2006). The effects of adding emotion-focused interventions to the client-centered relationship conditions in the treatment of depression. *Psychotherapy Research*, 16(5), 536–546.

Greenberg, L. S. (1983). Toward a task analysis of conflict resolution in gestalt therapy. *Psychotherapy: Theory, Research and Practice*, 20(2), 190–201.

Greenberg, L. S. (2002). *Emotion-focused therapy: Coaching clients to work through their feelings*. Washington, DC: American Psychological Association Press.

Greenberg, L. S. (2011). *Emotion-focused therapy*. Washington, DC: American Psychological Association Press.

Greenberg, L. S., Auszra, L., & Herrmann, I. R. (2007). The relationship among emotional productivity, emotional arousal and outcome in experiential therapy of depression. *Psychotherapy Research*, 17(4), 482–493.

Greenberg, L. S., & Malcolm, W. (2002). Resolving unfinished business: Relating process to outcome. *Journal of Consulting and Clinical Psychology*, 70(2), 406–416.

Greenberg, L. S., Rice, L. N., & Elliott, R. K. (1996). *Facilitating emotional change: The moment-by-moment process*. New York: Guilford Press.

Greenberg, L. S., & Watson, J. (1998). Experiential therapy of depression: Differential effects of client-centered relationship conditions and process experiential interventions. *Psychotherapy Research*, 8(2), 210–224.

Halchuk, R. E., Makinen, J. A., & Johnson, S. M. (2010). Resolving attachment injuries in couples using emotionally focused therapy: A three-year follow-up. *Journal of Couple and Relationship Therapy*, 9(1), 31–47.

Klein, M. H., Mathieu, P. L., Gendlin, E. T., & Kiesler, D. J. (1969). *The experiencing scale: A research and training manual* (Vol. 1). Madison: University of Wisconsin.

Messer, S. B. (1992). A critical examination of belief structures in integrative and eclectic psychotherapy. In J. C. Norcross & M. R. Goldfried (Eds.), *Handbook of psychotherapy integration* (pp. 130–165). New York: Basic Books.

Mineka, S., Rafaeli, E., & Yovel, I. (2003). Cognitive biases in emotional disorders: Information processing and social-cognitive perspectives. In R. J. Davidson, K. R.

Scherer, & H. H. Goldsmith (Eds.), *Handbook of affective sciences* (pp. 976–1009). New York: Oxford University Press.

Missirlian, T. M., Toukmanian, S. G., Warwar, S. H., & Greenberg, L. S. (2005). Emotional arousal, client perceptual processing, and the working alliance in experiential psychotherapy for depression. *Journal of Consulting and Clinical Psychology, 73*(5), 861–871.

Newman, M. G., Castonguay, L. G., Borkovec, T. D., Fisher, A. J., Boswell, J. F., Szodny, L. E., et al. (2011). A randomized controlled trial of cognitive-behavioral therapy for generalized anxiety disorder with integrated techniques from emotion-focused and interpersonal therapies. *Journal of Consulting and Clinical Psychology, 79*(2), 171–181.

Paivio, S. C., Jarry, J. L., Chagigiorgis, H., Hall, I., & Ralston, M. (2010). Efficacy of two versions of emotion-focused therapy for resolving child abuse trauma. *Psychotherapy Research, 20*(3), 353–366.

Paivio, S. C., & Nieuwenhuis, J. A. (2001). Efficacy of emotion focused therapy for adult survivors of child abuse: A preliminary study. *Journal of Traumatic Stress, 14*(1), 115–133.

Paivio, S. C., & Pascual-Leone, A. (2010). *Emotion-focused therapy for complex trauma: An integrative approach.* Washington, DC: American Psychological Association Press.

Pascual-Leone, A. (2009). Dynamic emotional processing in experiential therapy: Two steps forward, one step back. *Journal of Consulting and Clinical Psychology, 77*(1), 113–126.

Pascual-Leone, A., & Greenberg, L. S. (2007). Emotional processing in experiential therapy: Why "the only way out is through." *Journal of Consulting and Clinical Psychology, 75*(6), 875–887.

Pascual-Leone, A., Greenberg, L. S., & Pascual-Leone, J. (2009). Developments in task analysis: New methods to study change. *Psychotherapy Research, 19*(4–5), 527–542.

Perls, F. (1973). *The Gestalt approach and eye witness to therapy.* Oxford, UK: Science & Behavior Books.

Pos, A. E., & Greenberg, L. S. (2012). Organizing awareness and increasing emotion regulation: Revising chair work in emotion-focused therapy for borderline personality disorder. *Journal of Personality Disorders, 26*(1), 84–107.

Pos, A. E., Greenberg, L. S., & Warwar, S. H. (2009). Testing a model of change in the experiential treatment of depression. *Journal of Consulting and Clinical Psychology, 77*(6), 1055–1066.

Rogers, C. R. (1951). *Client-centered therapy: Its current practice, implications, and theory.* Oxford, UK: Houghton Mifflin.

Wampold, B. E., Minami, T., Baskin, T. W., & Tierney, S. C. (2002). A meta-(re)analysis of the effects of cognitive therapy versus "other therapies" for depression. *Journal of Affective Disorders, 68*(2–3), 159–165.

Watson, J. C., & Bedard, D. L. (2006). Clients' emotional processing in psychotherapy: A comparison between cognitive-behavioral and process-experiential therapies. *Journal of Consulting and Clinical Psychology, 74*(1), 152–159.

Watson, J. C., Gordon, L. B., Stermac, L., Kalogerakos, F., & Steckley, P. (2003). Comparing the effectiveness of process-experiential with cognitive-behavioral psychotherapy in the treatment of depression. *Journal of Consulting and Clinical Psychology, 71*(4), 773–781.

Young, J. E., Klosko, J. S., & Weishaar, M. E. (2003). *Schema therapy: A practitioner's guide.* New York: Guilford Press.

CHAPTER 12

Working with Modes in Schema Therapy

Eshkol Rafaeli
Offer Maurer
Nathan C. Thoma

> We do not have one mind, but many—at any one time, one of these minds may be dominant, and can be thought of as the current mind-in-place.
> —JOHN D. TEASDALE (1997, p. 70)

William James (1950) distinguished between the known self (*me*) and the knower self (*I*). This distinction has been complemented in recent years by the understanding that both the knower and the known are themselves multiple in nature, and not unitary. Though a monolithic conception of the self still permeates our culture and though we continue to refer to ourselves using the singular form, clinical theorists from diverse orientations (e.g., Berne, Bromberg, Greenberg, Perls, Young) recognize this multiplicity of the human self. This chapter describes an approach—schema therapy's mode model—that is based on a particular understanding of this multiple self.

Schema therapy (ST) is an integrative model of psychotherapy, and ST work based on the mode model (a.k.a. *mode work*) is a prime example of this integration. The etiological/developmental theory underling ST shares many of the assumptions of attachment theory as well as psychodynamic theories, such as object relations, self psychology, and relational psychoanalysis. Its pragmatism stems from Beck's cognitive therapy, from which it emerged. The experiential techniques that play a central role in mode work are rooted in gestalt and process–experiential approaches. Finally, the objectives of mode work are both experiential and cognitive, and it (like all of ST) makes extensive use of relational, cognitive, behavioral, and experiential tools.

This chapter begins with a theoretical introduction to the ST mode model. We explain how the mode concept has become central to the practice of ST, and present the taxonomy of modes, along with a developmental account of their etiology. We then review the extant evidence for the mode model. The greater part of the chapter illustrates the clinical work that stems from this model—that is, mode work. We conclude with a discussion of the limitations of this work and the future directions we hope it takes.

Background and Theory

ST and the Introduction of the Mode Concept

ST grew out of Beck's cognitive therapy, gradually developing into a unique integrative treatment for a spectrum of long-standing emotional/relational difficulties, most notably personality disorders. ST was developed by Young (1990) to address roadblocks to progress encountered when working within the Beckian model with clients suffering from chronic difficulties with mood (e.g., dysthymia) and chronic interpersonal problems (e.g., personality disorders). As Young discovered, cognitive therapy with nonresponders and relapse-prone clients required shifting the focus from surface-level cognitions or beliefs to deeper constructs—namely, *schemas*—as central to understanding psychopathology.

Schemas are considered to be enduring foundational mental structures, which go beyond being purely cognitive features of the mind to encompass emotions, bodily sensations, images, and memories. Young (1990) and his colleagues (Young, Klosko, & Weishaar, 2003) proposed a taxonomy of early maladaptive schemas that are thought to emerge when core emotional needs go unmet or are met inappropriately, usually by a child's caregivers.[1] These needs (e.g., for safety, security, validation, autonomy, spontaneity, and realistic limits) are seen as universal. In infancy and childhood, meeting these needs falls to the child's caregivers, and is considered necessary for a child to develop into psychological health as an adult. Young posited that enduring client problems often stem from present-day activation of early maladaptive schemas. At times, problems directly involve the distress felt when the schemas are activated. Quite often, however, they result from

---
[1]Though the formation of schemas is driven to a large degree by unmet needs, other factors such as temperamental vulnerability and cultural norms play major roles as well.

the characteristic behaviors enacted as a response to the schema—which Young referred to as "coping styles."

Starting in the mid-1990s, Young (e.g., McGinn & Young, 1996) began recognizing the necessity of revising ST to move beyond its predominant focus on universal *needs,* pervasive *schemas,* and characteristic *coping styles.* Needs, schemas, and coping styles are all *trait*-like, and therefore leave unexplained much of the phenomenology and symptomatology of the clients for whom ST was developed in the first place—individuals with borderline or narcissistic personality characteristics, who manifest quick and often intense fluctuation among various self-states or moods. This led to the development of the *mode* concept.

Young et al. (2003) defined *modes* as the predominant schemas and coping reactions active for an individual at a particular moment in time. Modes are transient, and at any given moment a person is thought to be predominantly in one mode. Though most individuals inhabit various modes over time, the manner in which they transition from one mode to another— that is, the degree of separation or dissociation between the modes—differs and lies on a spectrum. On the milder end of the spectrum, modes could be like moods (e.g., a woman may feel somewhat down and lonely for an afternoon, but gradually feel her mood lift by the evening). At the most extreme end, a total separation and dissociation could exist between modes (e.g., each mode may entail a complete and different personality, as is the case in dissociative identity disorder, formerly known as multiple personality disorder).

Individuals also differ in the specific identity of the modes they tend to inhabit. For example, persons suffering from borderline personality disorder (BPD) tend to experience abrupt transitions and a strong dissociation among a *specific* set of characteristic modes (Lobbestael, van Vreeswijk, & Arntz, 2008; Shafran et al., 2014). While the concepts of modes and of mode work are broad enough to describe any individual, recent efforts have been made to move from an abstract mode model to detailed, concrete, and disorder-specific mode models (cf. Arntz & Jacob, 2012).

Modes as Self-States

How does the structure of multiple modes develop, and how does it ultimately lead to an integrated, coherent person? Developmental theorists have suggested that a well-integrated self is the brittle outcome of tremendous integrative efforts made by the developing mind (cf. Putnam, 1989; Siegel, 1999). Human beings are born organized with a basic set of loosely interconnected "behavioral states," specific patterns of psychological and physiological variables that occur together and repeat themselves, often in highly predictable sequences, and that are relatively stable and enduring over time. Discrete behavioral states comprise particular affects, arousal and energy levels, motor activities, cognitive processing (e.g., abstractness of thought), access to knowledge and autobiographical memory, and a sense of self (Putnam, 1989). These states (or "states-of-mind"; Siegel, 1999) can be defined as the total pattern of activation in the brain at a particular moment in time. They serve as a clustering of functionally synergistic processes that allow the mind as a whole to form a cohesive state of activity. The benefit of such cohesion is quite clear: it maximizes the efficiency and efficacy of the processes needed in a given moment in time to deal with a current situation (Siegel, 1999).

States (or states-of-mind) start off as unique and ad-hoc combinations of mental faculties organized in response to discreet challenges or situations in the child's life. However, situations tend to repeat themselves and thus repeatedly activate the same states. Over time and with repeated activation, basic states of mind cluster together into self subsystems; as Siegel (1999) noted, the repeated reactivation of the same state of mind makes it evolve into an ingrained and separate "self-state." These self-states thus serve as the early prototypes of what ST refers to as "modes," which we continue to encounter throughout life. Below, we review the major categories of modes discussed by ST: (1) child modes, (2) coping modes, (3) internalized parental modes, and (4) the healthy adult mode. We also note the current thinking regarding these modes' etiology and briefly explain how ST works with each mode.

A Taxonomy of Modes and Their Etiology
Child Modes

When a child's needs are, on balance, appropriately met, the ensuing self-states tend to be flexible and adaptive. With repeated exposure to situations in which emotional needs are met, emotions can become regulated, distress is soothed, and the child (and later the adult) gains access to a *Happy Child mode*. In this mode, the person contacts capacities for closeness, trust, and contentment, and is able to draw on inner sources of vitality, spontaneity, and positive motivation. Toddlers, for example, are relentlessly curious and frequently joyful. Though their innate feelings and motivations may no longer be very accessible for adult (or even adolescent) clients whose parents failed to foster such curiosity and joy, ST seeks to reconnect clients with their Happy Child mode by removing barriers to these feelings or creating the opportunity to develop such feelings if no such opportunity existed in childhood.

When a child's needs do not get met in an adequate manner, a self-state referred to as the *Vulnerable Child (VC) mode* emerges. The VC mode is present for everyone to some degree, but its form and content differ from person to person, depending primarily on the unique profile of met and unmet needs. For example, when the childhood needs for safety and security were frequently met with frightening parental behaviors (e.g., anger or violence), the VC mode will be characterized by fear and anxiety about close relationships. When needs for empathy and validation were countered with no understanding or acknowledgment of the child, a client's VC mode will reflect a chronic sense of loneliness and of being unseen or easily misunderstood by others. When needs for praise and encouragement were met with frequent blame and criticism, the VC mode will contain feelings of shame, a lack of self-worth, and an expectation of further blame and criticism.

The VC mode, rooted in childhood experiences, can often be triggered in an adult's life. "Triggers" are situations that bear varying degrees of similarity to the originating experience (e.g., aversive or ambiguous interpersonal interactions). When these situations occur, clients essentially reexperience an earlier trauma, typically of a relational kind (Howell, 2013). The reexperiencing brings with it concomitant distress (e.g., fear, shame, loneliness). Typically, the client is not aware that the distress is linked to earlier experiences; instead, when in the VC mode, clients simply think and feel as they did as vulnerable or mistreated children and expect others to behave toward them the way people did at that age. In other words, the VC mode essentially embodies, in their purest form, most of the maladaptive schemas (with the exception of those characterized by acting out).

A primary goal of ST is to heal the relational trauma of unmet needs. To do so, ST aims to help clients make their VC mode present and visible, allow it to receive care (at first, from the therapists themselves), and, over time, learn how to internalize and generalize this care. This process, in which therapists identify and partially gratify the unmet needs of the VC, is the central therapeutic stance within ST, and is referred to as *limited reparenting*.

In addition to the Happy and Vulnerable child modes discussed above, early life experiences often give rise to two additional child modes. The first is the *Impulsive/Undisciplined Child (IUC) mode*, which often results from improper limit setting on the parents' part. It embodies those schemas characterized by externalizing behavior (e.g., entitlement and insufficient self-control schemas). The second is the *Angry Child (AC) mode*, which emerges in spontaneous angry, or even rageful, reactions to unmet needs. The AC mode can be thought of as an early manifestation of a coping reaction, and its function is a protective one. However, just like other coping reactions (and coping styles), it often fails to achieve its intended goal. When either the AC or the IUC modes are present, ST calls for empathic yet firm limit setting. It also calls for an empathic exploration to discover the unmet needs (which typically underlie the AC mode) or to distinguish whims and wishes from needs (if the IUC mode is present).

Coping Modes

Like the child modes described above, *maladaptive coping modes* also represent behavioral states that become full-blown modes owing to repeated activation. But, whereas child modes (and particularly the VC) capture the helpless and muted emotional reactions of the child, coping modes develop out of a child's basic survival operations: they are primarily automatic adaptation-promoting measures taken in order to survive in an emotionally negligent or otherwise noxious environment. At times, coping modes may emerge less in response to a depriving or abusive environment, and more as an internalization of it. For example, a child whose parents employ perfectionistic overcontrol in their own lives may herself learn to employ this coping style or mode—or more accurately, will fail to learn any alternative ways of being.

Maladaptive coping modes correspond to three coping styles (avoidance, overcompensation, or surrender), which parallel the basic organismic responses to threat: flight, fight, or freeze (Young et al., 2003). For different individuals, these modes may take on varied forms: avoidance may come across as emotional (and sometimes dissociative) detachment or as behavioral inhibition; overcompensation as grandiose self-aggrandizement or as perfectionistic overcontrol; and surrender as compliance and/or dependence.

A prominent avoidant coping mode is known as the *Detached Protector*. This mode disconnects clients from emotions—painful ones, but also adaptive ones such as sadness over a loss, assertive anger over a violation, feelings of closeness to others, or a sense of vitality and motivation. The Detached Protector can take the form of feeling numb, cut off from others and/or oneself, or feeling nothing at all. Clients in this mode may also engage in various behaviors aimed at distracting from or avoiding emotion: self-isolation, emotional eating, or excessive drinking or drug use. A goal of ST is to bypass the Detached Protector so that the therapist may make contact with the VC mode.

The Detached Protector is often present in individuals prone to dissociation and avoidance (e.g., ones with BPD). Other clinical groups are characterized by other coping modes. For example, the *Self-Aggrandizer*, often seen in narcissistic personality disorder, is an overcompensating coping mode meant to bolster the fragile self-esteem of a shame-filled VC. The *Bully/Attack Mode*, often seen in individuals with antisocial traits, is a more extreme adult version of the Angry Child mode. The *Compliant Surrenderer*, typical of individuals with dependent personality traits, is an example of a surrender coping mode.

Once established, coping modes continue to be deployed when schemas are triggered, as a way of coping with the ensuing distress. Paradoxically, though, coping modes lead to schema maintenance by blocking the opportunity for new corrective emotional learning. Thus, they are considered, by definition, maladaptive, and are typically seen as a cause of much, if not most, present-day problems. It is important to note, however, that coping modes involve behaviors that were, at some point, adaptive responses to difficult (or even impossible) interpersonal environments. For example, a young child of verbally brutal and physically abusive parents has little choice but to switch into a detached self-state, which may at least minimize the pain and reduce additional confrontations with the abusers. The resultant Detached Protector (i.e., avoidant) mode was essential for survival under those harsh circumstances. Still, when this mode becomes the main tool for coping with stressful situations later in life, it ceases to be adaptive (for similar ideas stemming from a relational psychoanalytic perspective, see Bromberg, 1998). In ST, the therapist uses *empathic confrontation* to help clients recognize the costs involved in the inflexible use of such modes and to reduce their reliance on these modes.

Parental Modes

A third and more pernicious class of modes, are the *internalized dysfunctional parental modes*. Through the process of introjection, which incorporates principles of implicit learning through modeling (e.g., Bandura, 2006), children learn to treat themselves the way their parents treated them—ways that are often quite dysfunctional. Internalized parental modes represent distinct ways in which individuals may be their own worst enemies—a phenomenon recognized by many clinicians, with terms such as punitive super-egos (Freud, 1940), internalized bad objects (Klein, 1946), malevolent introjects (Chessick, 1996), perpetrator parts (van der Hart, Nijenhuis, & Steele, 2006), or internal critics (Greenberg & Watson, 2006).[2]

ST recognizes two prototypical forms of internalized parental modes: a *Punitive Parent (PP)* and a *Demanding Parent (DP)*. In a PP mode, the client becomes aggressive, intolerant, impatient, and unforgiving toward himself (or others), usually due to the perceived inability to meet the mode's standards. When in a DP Mode, he might feel as if he must fulfill rigid

---

[2] Although the titles chosen by Young to label these modes point directly to the parents as their source, neither we (nor Young himself) took it to imply that all critical, punitive, or demanding self-states are indeed the result of direct internalization of parental figures. At times, it is the broader society's messages regarding some aspect of the self, present in the child, that are internalized to create a vicious self-deprecating self-state (e.g., an internal homophobic self-state). At other times it might be a harmful non-parental person or a peer group with whom the child had some direct contact (e.g., sexual abuse perpetrated by a stranger; ostracism within one's social milieu). Still, good-enough parental support in such adverse circumstances tends to mitigate their long-term negative impact dramatically, resulting in much weaker internal influence of malevolent self-states.

rules, norms, and values and must be extremely efficient in meeting all of these standards. In either mode, he might become very critical of self or of others, and, as a result of the VC mode's coactivation, may also feel guilty and ashamed of his shortcomings or mistakes, believing he should be severely punished for them (Arntz & Jacob, 2012). The goal in ST is to help the client recognize these modes, come to view them as ego-alien voices, assertively stand up to their punitiveness or criticism, and learn to protect and shield the VC mode from their destructive effects.

Healthy Adult Mode

Alongside painful child modes, maladaptive coping modes, and dysfunctional parental modes, most people also have self-states that are healthy and positive. We discussed one (the Happy Child mode) earlier. The other, referred to as the *Healthy Adult (HA) mode*, is the part of the self that is capable, strong, and well functioning. When parents do an adequate job of meeting the child's basic needs, they model a healthy adult approach (instead of a punitive, demanding, or neglectful one). Indeed, for many clients, the HA mode is modeled after these positive aspects of their caregivers. For others, who lacked such models, the task of constructing such a mode is more challenging, yet not impossible. In fact, a major aim of ST is to have the therapists' behaviors, and particularly their limited reparenting efforts, serve as a model for the development or reinforcement of this mode. The Healthy Adult mode, like an internalized therapist, has to respond flexibly to the various other modes. It nurtures, protects, and validates the VC mode, sets limits on the impulsivity and the angry outbursts of the AC and IUC modes, negotiates with maladaptive coping modes so as to limit their presence, and combats the effects of dysfunctional parent modes.

Modes become activated in response to environmental triggers, but also in response to each other. For example (see Figure 12.1), a friend's cancellation of a date (abandonment schema cue) (1) triggers the VC mode (feeling lonely and sad), leading to (2) the activation of a PP mode (feeling it's all my fault and also that feeling so sad about it is a terrible sign of weakness or stupidity). This, in turn, might lead to (3) even stronger activation of the VC mode, culminating either in (4a) an impulsive or rageful gesture, such as lashing out at the friend, or in (4b) an emotional shutdown using alcohol or drugs (Detached Protector coping mode).

Research Evidence

ST as a whole has undergone several recent empirical tests. Since the mode model is now the primary organizing framework for ST, these tests offer promising though indirect evidence for the effectiveness of the model in

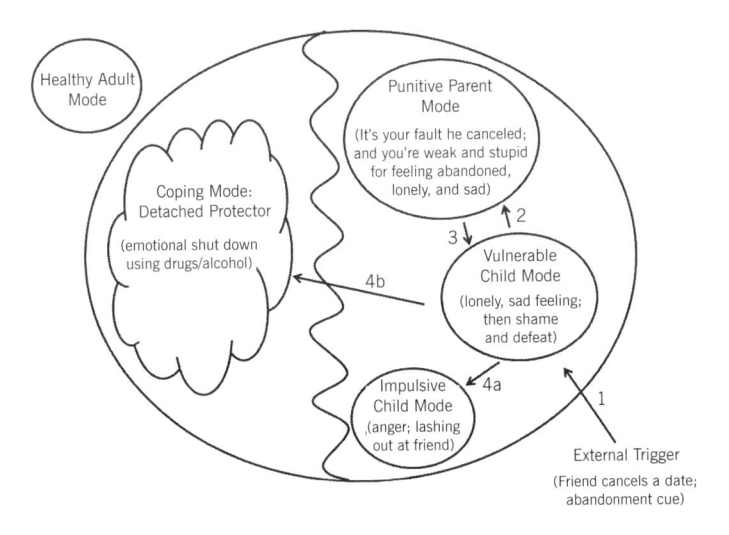

[Diagram: Illustrative mode activation model with Healthy Adult Mode, Punitive Parent Mode ("It's your fault he canceled; and you're weak and stupid for feeling abandoned, lonely, and sad"), Coping Mode: Detached Protector (emotional shut down using drugs/alcohol), Vulnerable Child Mode (lonely, sad feeling; then shame and defeat), Impulsive Child Mode (anger; lashing out at friend), and External Trigger (Friend cancels a date; abandonment cue), with arrows labeled 1, 2, 3, 4a, 4b.]

FIGURE 12.1. Illustrative model of a client's characteristic mode activation sequence.

clinical work. In the first major test of ST, Giesen-Bloo et al. (2006) conducted a multicenter randomized controlled trial of ST versus transference-focused therapy (TFP), a psychodynamic therapy, in the treatment of 86 patients with BPD, treated twice weekly for a period of 3 years. A significantly greater proportion of patients were found to be recovered or reliably improved in BPD symptoms at the end of treatment in the ST arm (45.5% recovered and 65.9% improved) than in the TFP arm (23.8% recovered and 42.9% improved). Given that patient retention is notoriously difficult in the treatment of PDs, it is important to note that dropout rates were considerably lower in ST (25%) than in TFP (50%). Among those who dropped out, ST patients had a median of 98 sessions (close to 1 year), while TFP patients had a median of 34 sessions (roughly 4 months).

These findings are notable as it is relatively rare for one active treatment to do significantly better than another in head-to-head trials (e.g., Baardseth et al., 2013). Extending the generalizability of these findings, Nadort et al. (2009) conducted a feasibility study with 62 patients with BPD in which the patients were randomly assigned to two conditions, with or without between-session phone contact with the therapist. There was no difference in outcome, indicating that it was the within-session work that contributed to outcome. Overall, the treatment was found to be feasible and effective when delivered in the community, with 42% of patients reaching recovery from BPD after 1.5 years of treatment.

In another multicenter RCT, Bamelis, Evers, Spinhoven, and Arntz

(2014) extended the mode model to patients with avoidant, dependent, obsessive–compulsive, paranoid, histrionic, and/or narcissistic PD. A total of 300 patients were randomized to either ST, psychodynamically oriented treatment-as-usual (TAU) in the community, or clarification-oriented psychotherapy (COP). At the end of 2 years of treatment ST had significantly better outcomes than TAU and COP, with PD recovery rates of 81.4%, 51.8%, and 60.0%, respectively. Interestingly, a moderator effect showed that the second of two cohorts of schema therapists drove the positive findings. This second cohort was trained more extensively in implementation of various ST techniques, including experiential ones. Preliminary process ratings validate that these therapists did use more of the ST techniques than the earlier cohort. This provides initial evidence that it is methods of actively evoking modes (which allow working with emotion) that serve as key active ingredients. Several other trials of ST are under way, focusing on forensic populations, chronic depression, and posttraumatic stress disorder (PTSD). Preliminary analyses from each of these suggest results that are quite positive. Additionally, very promising results emerged for the use of ST in a group format with patients with BPD (Farrell, Shaw, & Webber, 2009), and preliminary results from an international multicenter replication study of group ST bolster the excitement about the group modality. Finally, some additional (though smaller) effectiveness studies have also yielded positive results (see Bamelis, Giesen-Bloo, Bernstein, & Arntz, 2012). Overall, the evidence for the efficacy of ST can be considered promising but preliminary, as there have not yet been any direct replications of the RCTs reviewed above.

Though tests of ST as a complete intervention package provide indirect support for the utility of the mode model, more research is needed to further validate it as a model of pathology. Some research into the reliability and validity of modes has been conducted (see Lobbestael, 2012, for a review), mainly centering on the development of the Schema Mode Inventory (Lobbestael, van Vresswijk, Spinhoven, Schouten, & Arntz, 2010), a measure of 14 clinically relevant schema modes. This measure taps the main modes discussed in the present chapter but offers further differentiation of some modes (e.g., differentiating the Angry Child and the Enraged Child). Using this measure, modes have largely been found to relate to personality disorders in theoretically coherent ways. For example, patients with BPD have been found to be higher in the frequency of the Abandoned/Abused Child, the Punitive Parent, the Detached Protector, and the Angry Child than both healthy controls and Cluster C PD patients. Experimental studies involving watching a traumatic film clip (Arntz, Klokman, & Sieswerda, 2005) as well as anger induction experiments (Lobbestael, Arntz, Cima, & Chakhssi, 2009) have begun to validate the theory that modes are state-like experiences that occur in response to triggers in the environment, and much more so for patients with PD. More work is needed to show that in addition to activated emotion, modes also involve characteristic ways of thinking and behaving. Finally, a clear priority for empirical investigation of the mode model lies in the area of process–outcome research, to demonstrate that in-session mode states can be reliably recognized, and further, that working actively with modes transforms underlying schemas and leads to lasting mental health.

Application of Mode Work

Overview

Mode work—and a conceptualization based on modes—has become central to ST in the last two decades. This is obviously the case when clients are characterized by strong fluctuations among various modes, but is also true with clients for whom modes are less volatile. In either case, when schema therapists engage in mode work, they attend to the specific modes present in the therapy room—and those that appear in "real life." In collaboration with the client, the therapist labels these modes, explores their origin, and links them to current problems. Over time, the client is encouraged to consider and experiment with the possibility of modifying or even giving up some modes.

A unique aspect of ST is its emphasis on deliberately inviting or activating all of a client's modes, including the maladaptive ones, in session. Schema therapists seek to give voice to various modes, to differentiate them, and to use experiential techniques to set up deliberate interactions between these normally dissociated self-states. This "hot" emotional activation of the client's neural and cognitive circuitry is seen as essential for affecting change for deeply rooted, long-standing problems.

Conceptualization

ST begins with an initial period of assessment that typically requires four or five sessions but at times may be much longer (cf. Rafaeli, Bernstein, & Young, 2011). Assessment often involves informal history taking, administration of questionnaires (such as the Young Schema Questionnaire; see Rafaeli et al., 2011, for more details), assignment of thought and mood monitoring to obtain examples from daily life, as well as the use of imagery techniques for assessment (described below). At the conclusion of the assessment phase, and as a guide to the intervention phase, a case conceptualization, which is developed collaboratively by therapist and client, is created. In it, the problems and symptoms reported by the client or identified by the therapist are recast using the concepts of needs, schemas, coping responses, and (most pertinently) modes. The process of jointly conceptualizing the problems provides considerable psychoeducation (e.g., about the universality of needs, about the ways in which schemas get maintained throughout life). It involves exploring the origins of the schemas and modes, as well as the ways in which they are tied to present-day problems. A good conceptualization "fits well"—it eschews jargon and instead labels schemas and modes using terms that are understandable, even familiar, to the client—and may indeed come *from* the client. Several recent books and chapters (e.g., Rafaeli et al., 2011; Arntz & Jacob, 2012) discuss the conceptualization process in detail.

The conceptualization helps both the client and the therapist differentiate, identify, and name the relevant modes that play a part in the client's experience. Differentiation is key to mode work, as ST prescribes very different responses to modes of various types. Vulnerable, Impulsive, Angry, and Happy child modes are responded to with relevant forms of *limited reparenting* (appropriate nurturance and protection; limit setting; encouragement for ventilation along with limit setting; and playful joining, respectively). Maladaptive coping modes are responded to with *empathic confrontation* (empathy for the difficulty or distress that prompted the coping response, and for the typical feeling that "there's no other choice," along with confrontation toward the maladaptive behavior itself). Internalized dysfunctional parental modes are confronted so that they become *externalized* and ego-dystonic. Finally, the Healthy Adult mode is responded to with recognition and mirroring, along with modeling of additional adaptive parental responses. At first, the differential response to modes may be the therapist's purview. However, over time, the therapist models this differential response and the client's Healthy Adult internalizes and practices it.

Mode Work as a Form of Structural Therapy

The ST conceptualization culminates in a treatment strategy, which usually centers on the client's modes. The strategy suggests ways of altering the overall configuration of modes and the relative dominance or power of specific modes. We use the metaphor of structural therapy here, as it emphasizes the idea that in ST, we view the person as a system, comprising multiple and mutually interacting modes. Our aim is to change the way these parts work together. In broad terms, this requires three key processes: clarifying what the modes are, giving voice to adaptive and vulnerable modes, and creating adaptive boundaries between the modes. One technique often used in ST to facilitate all three of these processes is chairwork (Kellogg, 2004), and in particular, two-chair dialogues.

Shifting the Balance between Modes: Two-Chair Dialogues

Chairwork began as a technique within psychodrama and Gestalt therapies (e.g., Carstenson, 1955; Perls, 1973) and has been adopted by several therapy models influenced by Gestalt, including ST (Young et al., 2003). In ST chairwork, the client is encouraged to conduct dialogues (or broader conversations) among different parts of the self (internal conversations) or between the self and a meaningful external figure (external conversations), while actively moving between different chairs; modes, figures, or parts are situated in different chairs. The client is encouraged to take on each chair (i.e., each mode or figure) fully—expressing that mode's views wholeheartedly and responding to the other present modes forcefully from that mode's perspective. Once one mode's views and responses are clear, the client moves to another chair and takes on that chair's (i.e., that mode's) viewpoint.

A typical example of such work may involve a two-chair (internal) dialogue between the Vulnerable Child mode and the Demanding Parent mode for a client who has a prominent defectiveness schema related to her sexual orientation and obesity. In it, the client may be invited at first to voice the internalized parent's criticism and demands. In the parental seat, she will verbalize the harsh and demeaning messages she received (and still receives) from her father. Once these are voiced, the client would switch to the child seat, and respond to these messages. The therapist would encourage the client to express her emotional reactions to the parental voice, rather than argue the facts with it. The client may switch back and forth several times, until both modes' viewpoints are fully expressed. The therapist ensures that the child mode ultimately asserts its needs and confronts the parental mode. However, it is essential to also ensure that the parental mode is not permitted to "hide its cards"—we want to confront it in its fullest and strongest form.

Two-chair dialogues emphasize direct contact between modes. When in one mode, the client is asked to speak directly to the mode "sitting" in the opposite chair. To do so, the therapist may instruct the client to imagine the look, sound, and feel of the mode as it "sits" in the opposite chair, assigning person-like qualities to it. For example, a Demanding Parent mode could have a stern, contemptuous look with a crinkled brow. Should a client have difficulty staying with a particular mode, the therapist may help clarify that mode's voice. For example, the therapist may suggest certain phrases that seem consistent with the mode's viewpoint, or help name feelings as they arise, so that they become verbalized. Additionally, when the client seems to begin voicing another mode's position, the therapist may motion for her to change seats (thus avoiding "cross-talk").

The simplest and most common use of chair dialogues involves two chairs, but ST mode work may at times involve three, four, or even more chairs. For example, a therapist may find it useful to pull in a separate chair on which the client's coping mode would sit. In it, the client might be encouraged to voice his typical behavioral coping reaction to the parental punishment or criticism (e.g., disengagement, surrender, escape). Dialogues between this mode and the child mode (and/or the therapist) can be very informative, especially among avoidant, compliant, or dependent clients. Once the coping mode's voice is made clearer, the therapist may use empathic confrontation with it, so that it steps aside to allow the key drama between the child and parent modes to play out. Other modes that may warrant their own chair at times are the Angry Child mode, the Healthy Adult, or the internalized representation of another parent or significant other who was experienced as psychologically different. In our earlier example, this may involve pulling in a chair for the client's helpless and passively neglectful mother, in addition to the chair representing the abusive and critical father.

Chairwork is inherently psychodramatic. This dramatic nature can be further enhanced by attending to the dramaturgy of the chairs' physical placement. The confrontation of maladaptive modes versus healthy or vulnerable ones is easier to see when these chairs are placed oppositely. Therapists can convey their support and encouragement for certain modes (e.g., the vulnerable child or the healthy adult) by situating themselves closer to these chairs. Finally, the buffering (and interfering) role of coping modes can be illustrated well by placing their chair(s) in awkward middle spaces (e.g., at 90° to the other chairs).

Common Mode Work Interventions

ST resembles structural therapy in its systemic outlook on the multiplicity of self-states or modes and on the need to create systemic change that would be reflected in a changed structure. Unlike systemic approaches, however, ST does not shy away from seeing particular units within the broader structure as needing specific interventions. Below, we illustrate three types of mode work interventions, which center respectively on coping, parental, and child modes.

Overcoming and Bypassing Coping Modes: Imagery for Assessment

Coping modes emerge early in life to protect or shield the vulnerable child. Over time, they become ingrained and inflexible, and often begin to serve as the client's "greeting card." For example, a narcissistic client with a lonely/inferior child mode may find it almost inconceivable to allow this mode to be seen by anyone, including his new therapist. Instead, he is likely to spend the majority of time, especially early in therapy, in a compensatory Self-Aggrandizer mode. The keys to the sports car would be prominently displayed; the therapist's education and credentials would be arrogantly questioned; and sessions would often feel like bouts of verbal sparring. These behaviors interfere with the most basic tasks of therapy—building rapport and trust, clarifying the client's needs and distress, and formulating a plan of action.

To address such maladaptive coping behaviors, ST advocates empathic confrontation. Often, such confrontation utilizes cognitive or behavioral methods (cf. Arntz & Jacob, 2012). For example, the therapist might encourage the client to identify and label the coping mode or to draw up a list of pros and cons for maintaining it. However, emotion-focused interventions can be a part of empathic confrontations. One such intervention—the inclusion of a separate chair for the coping mode within multiple-chair dialogues—was described above. Here, we will present a second emotion-focused technique, *imagery for assessment*, used early in therapy to bypass coping modes. (This technique is also mentioned, briefly, by Arntz in Chapter 8, this volume, where it is referred to as *diagnostic imagery*).

When therapists use imagery as an assessment tool, they invite the client to shut his or her eyes and to visualize certain scenes, memories, or experiences in a vivid way. The client is asked to verbalize what he or she sees, hears, and feels, and to do so as if the client is present in the scene (thus, speaking in the first person and in the present tense). The purpose is for the client to become absorbed in the scene—to "be" in it, rather than to relate to it from a distanced perspective.

With the narcissistic client described earlier, as with most clients, imagery for assessment might be introduced early (by Sessions 5–6). The therapist begins by presenting the rationale for using this technique, emphasizing its utility: identifying and triggering the client's needs and schemas, clarifying the childhood origins of these needs and schemas, and helping tie the client's presenting problems to his needs and schemas. After presenting the rationale, the client is invited to imagine a safe place. This allows the client to experience imagery first within a nonthreatening scene and also creates a safe haven to which the client can return at the completion of the imagery exercise, or at any intermediate point in which he feels too activated. The therapist may help the client construct a safe image if one is not forthcoming (e.g., by suggesting calm natural scenes that often work well). At times, the client may simply be encouraged to close his eyes and simply imagine the therapy room itself.

Once the safe place is sufficiently experienced, the therapist asks the client to let an image of an upsetting childhood situation enter his mind. Little guidance is given, other than asking that this be an image of a time or place from before the age of 9–10, and that it involve the client with at least one of his parents or another significant person. The client is invited to immerse himself in the image, noticing his own thoughts, feelings, and bodily sensations. He is then invited to speak to the other people in the image, expressing his needs, thoughts, or feelings to the extent possible. He is asked to attend to the other person's verbal and nonverbal responses, and to carry out a dialogue between himself (as a child) and the other figure. This dialogue continues until the affect, need, or wish of the child are made very clear; often, the other person's response (limited or deficient in many cases) also becomes clear.

After the childhood scene is sufficiently explored, the therapist asks the client to focus on the emotions or physical sensations that are most salient and to amplify them while allowing the actual scene to fade away. In its place, the client is asked to imagine a scene from his present-day life, in which the same emotions and physical sensations are felt. Once again, the client is asked to enter the imagined scene, immerse himself in it, and ultimately carry out a dialogue with whatever figures are present in this scene. Like in the childhood scene, this dialogue's objective is to activate and clarify the client's affect, needs, and wishes, and to get a sense of the other's responses. There's no expectation that resolution would occur. After the present-day scene is sufficiently explored, the therapist invites the client to return to the safe place image, which helps regulate elevated negative affect that usually arises during the imagined scenes.

We would like to note that when clients are summoning images from childhood, therapists should take care not to suggest elements in the imagery that were not present (e.g., abuse that did not take place), and thus lead the client to "create" false memories (cf. McNally, 2003). Additionally, while therapists offer considerable validation to the emotions felt during imagined scenes or memories, they should be mindful not to assume automatically the veracity of these memories (nor to inculcate such an assumption in their clients). At this point in the work, what is most important is not finding out exactly what happened in the past, but rather how it felt for the client and what meanings he took from his past experience.

Arntz (Chapter 8, this volume) discusses many of the general practical issues related to the use of imagery techniques at various times. Though we focus specifically on imagery for assessment as a technique used to bypass coping modes, it should be said that other forms of imagery work (including imagery rescripting, detailed by Arntz and noted below) and can also be used with the same purpose, at any stage of the therapy. Certainly, coping modes continue to exert their influence long after the assessment phase. Nonetheless, the basic architecture of an assessment imagery exercise is a useful one to keep in mind; it can serve as the template around which future imagery exercises are improvised.

Imagery for assessment can (and should) be repeated, so as to access affect and memories tied to all parents or caregivers. One benefit of doing so several times early in the course of therapy is that it sets the stage for future emotion-focused work. In a way, introducing imagery exercises early in the assessment phase socializes clients to the rhythm and style of a therapy focused on experience, rather than on cerebral discussion. This, in its own right, is a challenge for the avoidant coping modes of many.

Confronting Parental Modes: Imagery with Rescripting (ImRs)

Dysfunctional Parental modes are the echoed voices of key external figures. These figures, typically caregivers, can be the father who denigrates his daughter; the mother who conveys a sense of conditional regard (*You are worthy only if you fulfill* my *needs or expectations*); the peer group who ostracize or bully a newcomer. Tragically, the damage done by these figures at an early impressionable age is perpetuated by those parts, within the adult client, that learned or internalized the lessons too well. An important ST goal is to help clients recognize these pernicious voices of self-criticism and self-punishment as ego-alien in nature and to help them fight and (if possible) even banish these voices.

To do so, schema therapists place themselves squarely on the side of compassion and self-acceptance—that is, on the side of the (sometimes barely nascent) Healthy Adult. Together with the Healthy Adult, they attempt to dislodge internalized voices that purport to have a monopoly on "truth," "values," or "standards," but in fact use these to oppress, devalue, or torment the client (and particularly the client's VC).

A variety of tools can be deployed in ST for this purpose. They include cognitive and psychoeducational efforts to identify and label these modes, help understand their origin, and begin building the case *against* them and *for* an alternative view of truth, values, and standards; behavioral techniques aimed at changing specific habits tied to these modes (e.g., working with a self-critical client to deliberately schedule more leisure time or to engage in pleasurable activities); and the use of the therapy relationship as a source of (limited) reparenting that models the antithesis of dysfunctional parenting. Yet ST's most powerful tools for combating the Dysfunctional Parental modes are experiential techniques, particularly chairwork (described elsewhere in this chapter) and ImRs (described in detail by Arntz, Chapter 8, this volume; see also Arntz & Jacob, 2012). We will therefore limit our discussion of this technique to a few general points that may help to situate it as part of the broad ST mode-work strategy, and to distinguish between ImRs and assessment imagery (described above).

1. When describing imagery for assessment, we noted that a typical sequence begins with an upsetting image from childhood and proceeds to an upsetting image from current life, linked through the affect experienced in the two scenes (the "affect bridge"). This progression reinforces an important ST lesson regarding the childhood origins of present-day distress, unmet needs, and maladaptive schemas. This sequence, however, is not set in stone, and in ImRs is often reversed or not followed in full. For example, if a client enters a session already upset about a current situation, we would use imagery of this situation as the starting place and then work

back in time, asking the client to get an image from childhood that feels the same. We could also use images of specific symptoms or of hard-to-understand feelings as starting points. For example, we might say, "Can you focus on the tears that are coming up now? What could these tears be saying?"

2. Imagery in general, and ImRs in particular, may exert its effects through several mechanisms (e.g., reattribution and emotional processing, reviewed by Arntz, Chapter 8, this volume). One additional potential mechanism noted by many schema therapists is that imagery activates affect in both the client and the therapist, simultaneously. The importance of "hot" versus "cold" cognitive processing by the client is well documented (see Thoma & Greenberg, Chapter 11, this volume). However, the evocation of affect in the therapist may also play an important role in increasing the empathy and attunement he or she provides. Moreover, the activation of a shared emotion (e.g., the client's and the therapist's anger) regarding a shared focus (e.g., the dysfunctional parent's behaviors in the scene) may play an important ameliorative part, in providing patently evident validation for the client.

3. When therapists request permission and enter an image, they typically do so with two purposes: to nurture the VC and to confront or combat the internalized parent or perpetrator. ImRs does not always entail the latter: in some instances, the gentle care and attention given to the client's VC is key. It is important to note, however, that imagery is *never* focused only on the perpetrator, and *always* requires care and attention to the child; when confrontation is called for, we must stay cognizant of the experience—sometime terrifying, sometimes ambivalent—of the child who is witnessing it as it unfolds.

Giving Voice to the Angry or Vulnerable Child Modes: The Empty-Chair Technique

Among many clients, even those with ample reasons for hurt or angry feelings, the Vulnerable and Angry Child modes often sound very muffled or cannot be heard at all. These modes hold most of the client's distress and negative affect, but are often buffered or obscured by coping modes, or overpowered by internalized parental modes. When schema therapists recognize this silencing, they strive to give these modes greater voice: their hurt or angry feelings are the most direct expression of the client's unmet needs, and ST revolves around recognizing and validating these needs and finding ways to meet them inside and outside the therapy room. Few therapeutic aims are more important than this.

Like all ST aims, this can be achieved in a variety of ways. Therapists' care and validation (key parts of the limited reparenting stance) are expressly directed at the client's vulnerable parts. Two-chair and imagery techniques aimed at strengthening the HA, curtailing the effects of coping modes, or combating Internalized Parental modes also carry an empowering message to the hurt VC. Various cognitive tools (e.g., schema flashcards) can help convey the psychoeducational message that vulnerabilities (and the unmet needs that underlie them) are themselves a healthy, if painful, response. But a key emotion-focused way of empowering the child modes is the *empty-chair technique*.

In empty-chair work, therapists help clients express their hurt or angry feelings towards an external person, while imagining this person to be present and sitting in another chair in the room. The imagined other here is typically a real person—a neglectful or punitive caregiver, an uncaring authority figure, or a vicious perpetrator. Inviting clients to confront such a person (even if only in imagined form) tends to activate very strong affect. This activation is of course essential for the salutary effects of this work, but the invitation to experience it may not be met with great enthusiasm from many clients. Clients are often aware cognitively of the hurt or anger, but shy away from experiencing them strongly or from expressing them. They may be terrified of the emotions or hopeless about the prospect that letting them out would lead to anything but more grief. Moreover, the dramatic and performative aspects of this technique may make some clients balk at using it. These are formidable concerns and should be carefully addressed; chair-work of this sort should be preceded with a clear presentation of the rationale for this work, and requires the client's consent before proceeding with it.

Early in this work, the therapist strives to ensure that the client vividly and directly experiences the other person—in Gestalt terms, that *contact* was established (cf. Elliott, Watson, Goldman, & Greenberg, 2004). This may be done with brief imagery instructions (e.g., "Close your eyes and imagine your mother there. What does she look like? What expression do you see on her face? What can you tell from her body language?"). It could also involve having the client alternate seats, expressing his own needs and feelings from one seat, and responding to them as the other person (e.g., the mother) would respond. Hearing the imagined other's responses tends to imbue the work with more affect, which usually facilitates the process.[3]

Once the imagined other is evoked, the client is encouraged to express his feelings directly toward this person. The therapist gently directs the

---

[3] When the imagined other is the perpetrator of severe abuse, empty-chair work must be undertaken with great caution, and the therapist would be unlikely to suggest that the client alternate into the empty chair. Instead, the work may first tackle different significant others (e.g., a passive mother who did not shield the child from the perpetrator's actions). Additionally, while the client may need to express pain, hurt, and anger at the abuser, it would rarely be useful to express sadness (or a need for nurturance) to an abuser.

client away from abstract or experience-distant statements (e.g., "She wouldn't have agreed to have this conversation") and refocuses him on concrete, present-focused conversation (e.g., "Can you tell her what it's like for you to see that expression on her face right now?"). The main objective is to activate pent-up emotion in the client, and not to engage in a logical or factual argument with the imagined other. Additionally, the therapist emphasizes that this work will typically not culminate with any "real-world" change—that is, in the client's need suddenly being met by the other person. Such change is unlikely; instead, clients will benefit from learning (on an emotional level) that it *was their right* to have this need met. Helping clients disentangle what should have been (i.e., the need's validity) from what couldn't happen (i.e., the impossibility of getting it met) is a step toward accepting and mourning what cannot change.

In EFT, Greenberg and his colleagues (cf., Elliott et al., 2004; see also Thoma & Greenberg, Chapter 11, this volume) describe the use of chairwork in addressing "unfinished business," a broad category that includes unexpressed hurt and anger. They note the therapist's role in facilitating this process, and in particular, in ensuring that the feelings expressed are primary emotions (e.g., anger, fear, shame, and sadness), and not secondary ones (hopelessness, anxiety, complaint, or blame). Despite the difference in terms, the EFT formulation is similar to that of ST. Specifically, schema therapists encourage the activation and expression of the basic emotions felt by the (vulnerable or angry) child, which are tied directly to the child's unmet needs, rather than the processed secondary emotions that emerge from coping modes, which are tied more to these modes' maladaptive coping attempts.

In a review of chairwork techniques across several integrative approaches, Kellogg (2004) noted that some (e.g., Gestalt therapists) use them primarily for facilitative purposes (i.e., to increase awareness of unresolved difficulties), while others (e.g., CBT therapists) use them primarily for corrective purposes (i.e., to catalyze cognitive shifts). As Kellogg notes, ST pursues both purposes and has a third, confrontational purpose: of directly combating maladaptive self-states. Young et al. (2003) place the greatest emphasis on this third purpose, and advocate using empty-chair dialogues to completely vanquish the Internalized Parental modes. Our experience is that at times, this technique can be followed with other aims in mind. This is particularly true with clients from more interdependent cultures, as well as with clients for whom the child mode is more mature and capable of holding on to an integrated (good *and* bad) image of the internalized parent. In particular, like Greenberg and his colleagues (cf. Elliott et al., 2004) we see many clients modify their view of the parental figure. At times, this leads to the shrinking presence of this figure or its impact (as Young et al., 2003, suggest); at other times, it opens the road for forgiveness or resolution.

Whereas the empty-chair technique is focused on an external other, opportunities ("markers," an EFT term) for this work often present themselves when using internal, two-chair dialogues. For example, when speaking as their own Perfectionistic Overcontroller mode, the client may come across as demanding and rigid. The therapist could inquire whether the tone or content of that message sounds like someone else—maybe the client's overbearing and critical father—and suggest placing the father in a chair. Alternatively, when a client comes into contact with her own vulnerability (e.g., her sense of defectiveness and shame), she may spontaneously associate it with the person who was the source of this shame (e.g., the ballet instructor who shamed her repeatedly).

Though empty-chair work is useful for facilitating both hurt *and* angry feelings, we should note that ST views the VC and the AC modes as requiring different therapist responses. Limited reparenting used with a VC is typically characterized by warmth, care, and nurturance. Empty-chair work with this mode primarily gives voice to the very fragile, hurt, and needy parts; through it, the client learns to recruit compassion, first and foremost from himself. In contrast, the therapeutic stance with the AC often requires a balance of validation and limit setting. If this mode is underregulated, the client may act out in rage and place himself and/or others at risk. If the mode is overregulated, the client loses out on the adaptive use of anger as a response to violations or boundary transgressions. Empty-chair work with this mode helps a client ventilate anger in safe and effective ways; through it, the client learns to assert himself and establish safe and adaptive boundaries with other people.

Coda: The Integrated Self

We are often asked whether the emphasis on differentiating modes and responding to them differentially carries a risk of leading to a fragmented, nonunified self. The truth is quite the opposite. We see the distress that brings clients into therapy as a clear indication that their current self-organization is not working well for them. Typically, their coping modes are working overtime but do not fully block the negative messages of the Internalized Parental modes; the child modes do not receive adequate response, and the HA, if it exists at all, is fighting an uphill battle. By recognizing these modes and the ways in which they are at odds with each other, we try to help clients attain a better integration. The experiential, emotion-focused techniques outlined above, along with cognitive, behavioral, and relational techniques, are all embedded within a therapeutic relationship characterized by the ideal of limited reparenting. This package of interventions aims to strengthen the client's own HA mode, so that it provides the ultimate integration.

Giving Voice to the Integrated Self: Letter Writing

One last emotion-focused technique, *letter writing,* can aid in this integration process. In this technique, usually employed late in the therapy, clients are invited to write (though usually not send) a letter to their parents or other significant others who have hurt them when they were young. These letters help clients summarize what they had learned, and typically reflect many of the emotional insights gained in imagery and chairwork exercises, as well as the effects of the corrective emotional experience of the therapeutic relationship. Once written, the client is invited to read these aloud with the therapist, sometimes during a two-chair dialogue with the letter's addressee. The careful crafting of these letters (in or out of session) helps clients see the arc of the work they have done. It usually touches on the hurt itself, gives the clients a chance to voice their needs and assert their rights, and at times culminates with the modified view of the other (as guilty, damaged, limited; but at times, also as worthy of forgiveness or compassion). The subsequent reading of the letter in session is usually experienced as very cathartic, and gives the client and the therapist an opportunity to review and integrate many of the gains from the course of therapy.

Future Directions

The mode model includes both a theoretical developmental account and a pragmatic approach for addressing modes in the therapy. Above, we reviewed the growing evidence for the clinical utility of ST employing the mode model. In contrast, the empirical (and theoretical) foundation for the developmental account undergirding ST or the mode model is far from complete. We hope to see future work tackling this lacuna, and believe that it will further improve the treatment itself. For example, better understanding of the process through which internalized parental modes come into being may help resolve clinical dilemmas regarding the most appropriate course of intervention vis-à-vis these modes (i.e., outright confrontation vs. efforts at dialogical integration of these modes into the client's healthy adult).

Thus far, very little research that we are aware of has focused on process–outcome relationships. Such research is essential if we are to validate the proposed mechanisms of change in ST and particularly the causal role of specific emotion-focused or experiential therapist interventions thought to facilitate change. We view this as a priority in future research on ST, and are actively pursuing such work ourselves. Such research would need to further validate the existence of schema modes (e.g., Shafran et al., 2014); to demonstrate the possibility of reliable in-session recognition of modes by trained clinicians; and to demonstrate whether specific interventions aimed at specific modes lead to positive changes both within session and over the course of treatment.

The integrative nature of ST and its flexible framework are both strengths and potential limitations. The multiple toolboxes at the disposal of schema therapists reflect many influences and include varied techniques—emotion-focused, relational, cognitive, and behavioral. This plenitude may lead to substantial variability between therapists in the actual application of the approach: the same agreed-upon theoretical principles can lead to very different clinical choices by different therapists. We believe further research will lead to more detailed and nuanced models, which will improve our ability to approach particular clients (e.g., ones with a certain diagnosis or with certain characteristic needs or modes) with appropriate versions of the mode model, and with the specific interventions most likely to generate effective, efficient, and powerful change.

Further Resources

Articles/Chapters

- For a review of chairwork, see Kellogg (2004).
- For further reading on imagery and rescripting, see Holmes and Matthews (2010) and Arntz (Chapter 8, this volume).

Books

- See Young, Klosko, and Weishaar (2003) for a comprehensive practitioner's guide to ST.
- See Rafaeli, Bernstein, and Young (2011) for a more concise introduction to ST.
- See Arntz and van Genderen (2009) for the use of ST in treating BPD and Arntz and Jacob (2013) for broader guidance regarding mode work in ST.

Training Materials

- An American Psychological Association training video by Young is available at *www.apa.org/pubs/videos/4310804.aspx*.
- Videos illustrating specific ST techniques are available from *www.schematherapy.nl*.

References

Arntz, A., & Jacob, G. (2012). *Schema therapy in practice: an introductory guide to the schema mode approach*. New York: Wiley.

Arntz, A., Klokman, J., & Sieswerda, S. (2005). An experimental test of the schema mode model of borderline personality disorder. *Journal of Behavior Therapy and Experimental Psychiatry*, 36(3), 226–239.

Arntz, A., & Van Genderen, H. (2009). *Schema therapy for borderline personality disorder.* New York: Wiley.

Baardseth, T. P., Goldberg, S. B., Pace, B. T., Minami, T., Wislocki, A. P., Frost, N. D., et al. (2013). Cognitive-behavioral therapy versus other therapies: Redux. *Clinical Psychology Review, 33*(3), 395–405.

Bandura, A. (Ed.). (2006). *Psychological modeling: Conflicting theories.* Piscataway, NJ: Transaction.

Bamelis, L., Giesen-Bloo, J., Bernstein, D., & Arntz, A. (2012). Effectiveness studies of schema therapy. In M. Vreeswijk, J. Broersen, & M. Nadort (Eds.), *The Wiley–Blackwell handbook of schema therapy: Theory, research and practice* (pp. 495–510). New York: Wiley.

Bamelis, L. L. M., Evers, S. M. A. A., Spinhoven, P., & Arntz, A. (2014). Results of a multicentered randomized controlled trial on the clinical effectiveness of schema therapy for personality disorders. *American Journal of Psychiatry, 171,* 305–322.

Bromberg, P. M. (1998). *Standing in the spaces: Essays on clinical process, trauma, and dissociation.* Hillsdale, NJ: Analytic Press.

Carstenson, B. (1955). The auxiliary chair technique—A case study. *Group Psychotherapy, 8,* 50–56.

Chessick, R. D. (1996). Archaic sadism. *Journal of the American Academy of Psychoanalysis, 24,* 605–618.

Elliott, R., Watson, J. C., Goldman, R. N., & Greenberg, L. S. (2004). *Learning emotion-focused therapy: The process–experiential approach to change.* Washington, DC: American Psychological Association Press.

Farrell, J. M., Shaw, I. A., & Webber, M. A. (2009). A schema-focused approach to group psychotherapy for outpatients with borderline personality disorder: A randomized controlled trial. *Journal of Behavior Therapy and Experimental Psychiatry, 40,* 317–328.

Freud, S. (1940). An outline of psycho-analysis. *International Journal of Psychoanalysis, 21,* 27–84.

Giesen-Bloo, J., Van Dyck, R., Spinhoven, P., Van Tilburg, W., Dirksen, C., Van Asselt, T., et al. (2006). Outpatient psychotherapy for borderline personality disorder: A randomized trial of schema-focused therapy vs transference-focused psychotherapy. *Archives of General Psychiatry, 63,* 649–658.

Greenberg, L. S., & Watson, J. C. (2006). *Emotion focused therapy for depression.* Washington, DC: .American Psychological Association Press.

Holmes, E. A., & Mathews, A. (2010). Mental imagery in emotion and emotional disorders. *Clinical Psychology Review, 30,* 349–362.

Howell, E. F. (2013). *The dissociative mind.* New York: Routledge.

James, W. (1950). *The principles of psychology.* Cambridge, MA: Harvard University Press. (Original work published 1890)

Kellogg, S. (2004). Dialogical encounters: Contemporary perspectives on "chairwork" in psychotherapy. *Psychotherapy: Theory, Research, Practice, Training, 41,* 310–320.

Klein, M. (1946). *"Envy and gratitude" and other works, 1946–1963.* London: Hogarth Press.

Lobbestael, J. (2012). Validation of the schema mode inventory. In M. Vreeswijk, J. Broersen, & M. Nadort (Eds.), *The Wiley–Blackwell handbook of schema therapy: Theory, research, and practice* (pp. 541–551). New York: Wiley.

Lobbestael, J., Arntz, A., Cima, M., & Chakhssi, F. (2009). Effects of induced anger in patients with antisocial personality disorder. *Psychological Medicine, 39,* 557–568.

Lobbestael, J., van Vreeswijk, M. F., & Arntz, A. (2008). An empirical test of schema

mode conceptualizations in personality disorders. *Behaviour Research and Therapy, 46*(7), 854–860.
Lobbestael, J., van Vreeswijk, M., Spinhoven, P., Schouten, E., & Arntz, A. (2010). Reliability and validity of the short Schema Mode Inventory (SMI). *Behavioural and Cognitive Psychotherapy, 38*(4), 437–458.
McGinn, L. K., & Young, J. E. (1996). Schema-focused therapy. In P. Salkovskis (Ed.), *Frontiers of cognitive therapy* (pp. 182–207). New York: Guilford Press.
McNally, R. J. (2003). *Remembering trauma*. Cambridge, MA: Harvard University Press.
Nadort, M., Arntz, A., Smit, J. H., Giesen-Bloo, J., Eikelenboom, M., Spinhoven, P., et al. (2009). Implementation of outpatient schema therapy for borderline personality disorder with versus without crisis support by the therapist outside office hours: A randomized trial. *Behaviour Research and Therapy, 47*(11), 961–973.
Perls, F. S. (1973). *The Gestalt approach and Eye witness to therapy*. Oxford, UK: Science and Behavior Books.
Putnam, F. W. (1989). *Diagnosis and treatment of multiple personality disorder*. New York: Guilford Press.
Rafaeli, E., Bernstein, D. P., & Young, J. (2011). *Schema therapy: Distinctive features*. New York: Routledge.
Shafran, R., Rafaeli, E., Gadassi, R., Papamarkou, S., Berenson, K., Downey, G., et al.. (2014). *Examining the schema-mode model in borderline and avoidant personality disorders using experience-sampling methods*. Manuscript in preparation.
Siegel, D. J. (1999). *The developing mind: How relationships and the brain interact to shape who we are.*. New York: Guilford Press.
Teasdale, J. D. (1997). The relationship between cognition and emotion: The mind-in-place in mood disorders. In D. M. Clark & C. G. Fairburn (Eds.), *Science and practice of cognitive behaviour therapy* (pp. 67–94). Oxford, UK: Oxford University Press.
van der Hart, O., Nijenhuis, E. R. S., & Steele, K. (2006). *The haunted self*. New York: Norton.
Young, J. E. (1990). *Cognitive therapy for personality disorders: A schema-focused approach*. Sarasota, FL: Professional Resource Exchange.
Young, J. E., Klosko, J. S., & Weishaar, M. E. (2003). *Schema therapy: A practitioner's guide*. New York: Guilford Press.

CHAPTER 13

Emotional Schema Therapy

Robert L. Leahy

Social Construction of Emotion

Fritz Heider proposed that individuals maintain beliefs about themselves and others regarding the nature of causes of behavior, intentionality, and the organization of the self (Heider, 1958). Heider observed that the ordinary person is a "psychologist" in his or her own right, utilizing models of attribution and evaluation and inferring traits and personal qualities. This "naïve psychology," as it was called, became the basis of the field of social cognition. In this chapter, I describe how "naïve psychology" may be extended to a model of how individuals conceptualize emotions in the self and others and how these specific models of emotion may lead to problematic strategies of emotion regulation. I also propose ways of helping psychotherapy clients address such problems, using an approach I have come to call emotional schema therapy (EST), which is an approach that calls attention to and reworks clients' attitudes toward and reactions to emotion.

Although Darwin proposed a universal evolutionary basis of emotion and the expression of emotion, there is considerable evidence that individuals differ in their interpretation and rules for display of emotion. There are significant historical and cultural differences in the social construction of emotion, giving rise to a new area of historical scholarship alternately called "emotion history" or "emotionology." Max Weber (1930), in *The Protestant Ethic and the Spirit of Capitalism*, proposed that the personal qualities that underlie capitalism (emphasis on hard work, delay of gratification, savings, success as a sign of moral worth) were facilitated by the Protestant values of internalization, guilt, personal responsibility, and the emphasis on "the elect." In *The Civilizing Process: Sociogenetic and*

Psychogenetic Investigations (2000), Norbert Elias traces the development of rules for internalization and the control of sexual and aggressive behavior that occurred with the rise of courtly society, increased concentration of population, and the rise of social control. Manners, courtly etiquette, and an emphasis on internalized models of self led to a rise in guilt, shame, and conscientiousness. Within American and British society between the 19th and 20th centuries there was an increased emphasis on self-control—the rise of "cool"—and the protection of the young. Whereas in 19th-century childrearing literature parents were urged to have their children (especially boys) face the fear that they felt, in 20th-century childrearing, after the influence of Benjamin Spock, the emphasis was on protecting and comforting the child and avoiding upsetting situations (Stearns, 1994). The change in emotional models was from teaching courage to avoiding discomfort.

One can see the cultural and historical differences in popular conceptions of emotion by examining the change in how crying is viewed. In the 18th century in Britain, men who followed the Sentimentalism movement believed that the expression of intense emotion, accompanied by crying, signified sincerity in claims of love or even in attempts to advocate in Parliament. Crying was viewed as a sign of commitment and veracity. However, with the rise of self-control strong overt expressions of emotion were viewed as inappropriate. Thus, in contrast to the Sentimentalists who viewed strong expression as desirable, Lord Chesterton counseled his son to show no intensity of emotion—to avoid crying and laughing. The ideal, according to Chesterton, was that the other person would never know how you truly felt. Crying has a long history of ups and downs, and there is considerable cultural diversity in its "legitimacy" (Lutz, 2001). Indeed, cultural and historical factors are important in a variety of cultures—for example, there is reduced emphasis on emotional expression and emotional labeling in Asian cultures (Yeh, Draper, & Yu, 2007).

As Heider suggested, individuals conceptualize emotions on the basis of their theories of causes, duration, and impact. Emotion theory and social cognitive theory have converged to identify several factors that affect how individuals view the emotional impact of events. "Affect forecasting" refers to the tendency to predict emotional responses in the future without sufficient attention to factors that might affect one in the future, leading to overpredicting or underpredicting the impact of events on one's emotions (Gilbert & Wilson, 2009; Wilson & Gilbert, 2003, 2005; Wilson, Wheatley, Meyers, Gilbert, & Axsom, 2000). Thus, individuals predict how they will feel in the event of losing their job based on limited information. Five processes have been identified that have direct relevance to affect forecasting:

1. *Focalism*—an overemphasis on specific details to the exclusion of other information (Kahneman, 2011; Kahneman, Krueger, Schkade, Schwarz, & Stone, 2006; Schkade & Kahneman, 1998;

Wilson, Wheatley, Meyers, Gilbert, & Axsom, 2000). Thus, the individual may focus on the image of being alone after a divorce without recognizing other possible events and experiences.
2. *Impact bias*—the tendency to predict that an emotion will be more extremely negative (or positive) than it turns out to be (Wilson & Gilbert, 2003). Thus, individuals may believe that the consequences of divorce will be extremely negative and the consequences of a promotion will be extremely positive (Gilbert & Wilson, 2009).
3. *Durability*—a form of impact bias wherein the individual believes that an emotion will continue for a long time. Thus, the individual who achieves a promotion may believe that she will be happy for years.
4. *Immune neglect*—the tendency to ignore one's ability to cope with negative events and to consider other factors that might mitigate the emotional impact of an event. For example, the individual anticipating the effects of divorce may not consider the effects of new relationships.
5. *Time discounting*—an emphasis on present events or emotions in predicting the future, such that current emotions become an anchor or a basis on which future emotions are predicted (Frederick, Loewenstein, & O'Donoghue, 2002).

The emotional schema model draws on these social cognitive factors as they are related to how individuals may differ in their prediction of the durability, negative impact, and intensity of emotion, while ignoring factors that might moderate emotional responses.

As the foregoing implies, the expression, perception, and evaluation of emotion is not a reflexive or hard-wired process. Like other "naïve theories" of self and others, these beliefs are affected by socialization and cultural mores. In this chapter I outline a model of how individuals conceptualize and evaluate emotions and how these naïve theories of emotion may contribute to vulnerability to psychopathology.

Theory

The stress-appraisal theory proposes that individuals experience "stress" (anxiety, emotional difficulty) when a "stressor" (an external force) is viewed as too difficult to handle (Lazarus, 1999; Lazarus & Folkman, 1984). Thus, if I am able to lift 100 pounds, but you present me with 120 pounds, my appraisal is that I will be unable to lift this amount and I will experience stress. Stress is further related to core values and goals and the degree to which I view these issues as central in my life (Lazarus, 1999). This cognitive-behavioral model of stress can be elaborated further to examine how one evaluates the *internal experience* of stress. The model described in this chapter—emotional schema theory—proposes that individuals have appraisals of their stress—of their emotion, sensations, and thoughts—and that these appraisals either reduce or magnify the experience of stress. One can be *stressed about the stress*.

Consider two individuals who recently experienced a breakup in their intimate relationship. Neurotic Ned has received a text-message from Becky that she is no longer interested in continuing their rocky 4-month relationship and, further, that he should not contact her because there is nothing to discuss. Neurotic Ned is stunned and goes through a kaleidoscope of feelings: anxiety, sadness, anger, hopelessness, confusion, and even a tinge of relief. These feelings seem to hang over his confused and conflicted mind as he believes that a "real man" would not be so upset, that he should only feel one way, and he worries that his feelings will go out of control and he won't be able to function. He ruminates on his emotions and on what happened, tossing in bed at night unable to let go, and he believes that he will never get over this breakup. He subsequently sleeps in, misses work, stops exercising, and avoids his friends because he believes that he will be a burden. Neurotic Ned is characteristically stuck in his depression.

As a remarkable coincidence, Michael the Mensch has also received a text message from his soon to become ex-girlfriend, Sally, claiming in similar terse language that it is all over. Similar to Neurotic Ned, Michael has a range of feelings—he is confused, sad, anxious, angry, hopeless, and even relieved—but he steps back for a few moments and recognizes that his apparently conflicting feelings make sense, since he is confused that she would break off in such a callous manner, sad that a relationship that did matter is over, anxious because he is just beginning to process this breakup, angry because he doesn't think he should be treated this way, hopeless because he has a momentary thought that he will never be happy again and relieved because Sally was a high-maintenance partner and now he can pursue possibly better alternatives. Michael is determined to normalize his life, while acknowledging that he is upset, to seek validation and support from his friends, and to keep himself busy with productive action. He understands that the breakup was unfortunate, but not a catastrophe, and that painful feelings dissipate with time.

These two individuals began with similar emotions, but followed with different appraisals, which led to either maladaptive or adaptive emotion regulation strategies. Individuals have appraisals of their emotions and theories about emotion regulation. These appraisals and theories of regulation exacerbate emotional disorder. For example, individuals with negative emotional schemas believe that their emotions will have long duration, are out of control, will escalate, are dangerous, do not make sense, are unique to the self, cannot be expressed or validated, and that "contradictory" emotions cannot be tolerated. These beliefs lead to guilt, avoidance, withdrawal, attempts to suppress emotion, rumination and worry, substance abuse, and the sense that emotions are out of control. The schematic in Figure 13.1 illustrates the emotional schema model.

The emotional schema model draws on other theoretical models in the cognitive-behavioral therapy (CBT) tradition. For example, Wells has advanced the metacognitive model that focuses on the process of responding to thoughts rather than to the content of thoughts (Wells, 2009). According to this model, individuals have both positive ("I need to worry to be prepared") and negative beliefs about worry ("My worry is going to make me sick"), focus excessively on their thinking, distrust their memory, and—as a consequence—are locked into threat appraisals driven by their thinking. Wells views worry and rumination as part of the cognitive attentional syndrome, which is characterized by excessive focus or attention on the content and meaning of cognition (Wells, 2002, 2004). Thought

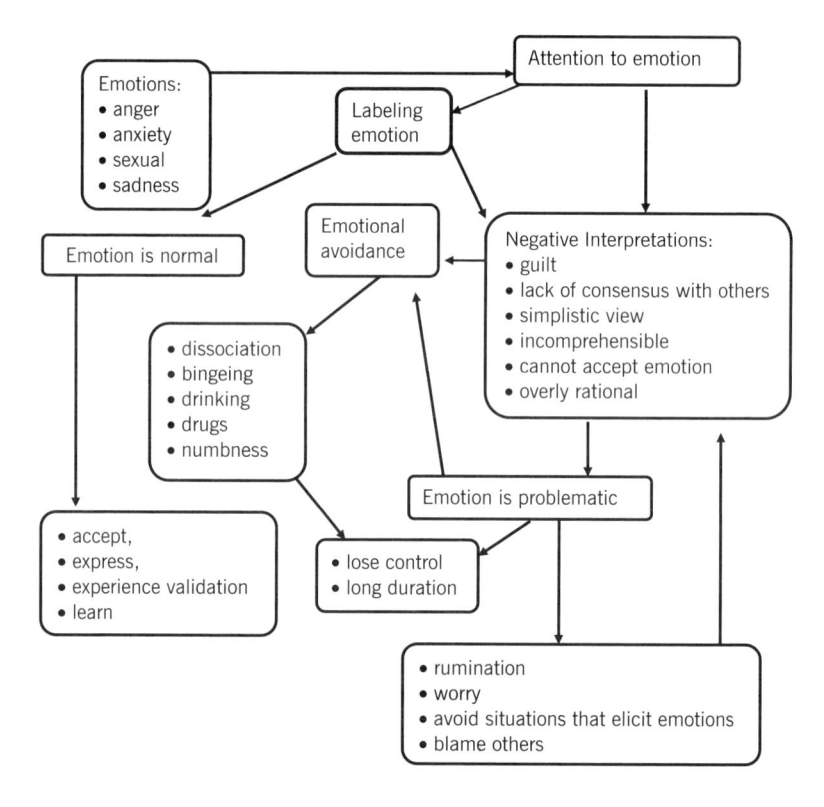

FIGURE 13.1. The emotional schema model. From Leahy, Tirch, and Napolitano (2011). Copyright by the authors. Reprinted with permission from The Guilford Press.

monitoring, thought suppression, and excessive mental control keep the individual locked in a struggle with the content of his or her thinking rather than follow productive action. The emotional schema model draws on the metacognitive model, stressing the negative interpretation of internal experience (e.g., emotions), but differs from the metacognitive model in a variety of ways. First, emotions are different from thoughts and involve physical sensations, action tendencies, and interpersonal functioning. Second, the emotional schema model (and the associated treatment, EST) focuses on the relationship between emotions and core values, such that painful emotions may often be the direct result of important values that the patient maintains. Third, EST places considerable emphasis on the role of validation and the therapeutic relationship as important factors in the attachment issues that arise in the sharing of emotion. Fourth, EST draws directly on evolutionary psychology and the adaptive function of emotion to help patients normalize their experience. Finally, EST relates current maladaptive interpretations of emotion to the patient's socialization experiences and to current interpersonal relations.

Empirical Support for the Emotional Schema Model

Thus far, research on the emotional schema model has centered on the development and validation of a measure of the proposed types of emotion-related schemas, the Leahy Emotional Schema Scale (LESS). Measurement development and the establishment of construct validity can be considered a first step in programmatic research (Anastasi & Urbina, 1997), and thus empirical validation of the model can be considered to be in its initial stages. The LESS-I consists of 50 questions divided into 14 dimensions that assess beliefs and strategies about emotion. The 14 dimensions were rationally derived. These 14 dimensions are Validation ("Others understand and accept my feelings"), Expression ("I feel I can express my feelings openly"), Duration ("I sometimes fear that if I allowed myself to have a strong feeling, it would not go away"), Control ("I worry that I won't be able to control my feelings"), Comprehensibility ("My feelings don't make sense to me"), Guilt ("Some feelings are wrong to have"), Simplistic View ("I like being absolutely definite about the way I feel about someone else"), Consensus ("I often think that I respond with feelings that others would not have"), Values ("There are higher values that I aspire to"), Numbness ("I often feel 'numb' emotionally—like I have no feelings"), Overemphasis on Rationality ("I think it is important to be rational and logical in almost everything"), Acceptance ("You have to guard against having certain feelings"), Rumination ("When I feel down, I sit by myself and think a lot about how bad I feel"), and Blame ("Other people cause me to have unpleasant feelings").

A series of correlational studies using clinical samples have examined the associations between emotional schemas and anxiety, depression, metacognitive factors in worry, psychological flexibility, risk aversion, mindfulness, personality disorders, and relationship satisfaction. In an early study of emotional schemas, most of the 14 emotional schema dimensions were significantly correlated with the Beck Depression Inventory (BDI) and the Beck Anxiety Inventory (BAI) (Leahy, 2002). In a separate study a stepwise multiple regression analysis indicated the following order of predictors of depression on the BDI: guilt, rumination, control, and validation (Leahy, Tirch, & Melwani, 2012). In another study of the relationship between anxiety, psychological flexibility, and emotional schemas, multiple regression analysis indicated that psychological flexibility and duration predicted anxiety (Tirch, Leahy, Silberstein, & Melwani, 2012). In a study of the relationship between a derived measure of negative beliefs about emotion (summing across LESS dimensions), each of the metacognitive factors in the Wells model (Metacognitive Questionnaire [MCQ]) were significantly correlated with Negative Beliefs about Emotions, adding to the construct validity of the scale (Leahy, 2011b). These findings on the relationship among the LESS, MCQ, and depression suggest that metacognitive factors of worry may partly be activated because of negative beliefs about emotion. The pattern of predictors in a stepwise multiple regression on anxiety (BAI) also reflect this integrative metaemotion/metacognitive integrative model: Control, Uncontrollability and Danger of Worry (MCQ), Positive Worry (MCQ) (neg), Cognitive Self-Consciousness (MCQ), Comprehensibility, Expression (neg), and Validation. In a study on satisfaction in intimate relationships, every one of the 14 LESS scores is significantly correlated with marital satisfaction (Dyadic Adjustment Scale [DAS]). Even when controlling for depression (BDI), most emotional schema dimensions that were perceived to be held by partners were predictive of relationship dysfunction on the DAS. Specifically, these were Comprehensibility, Validation, Guilt, Simplistic View of Emotion, Duration, Expression, and Consensus (Leahy, 2012). These data indicate that validation may modify other emotional schemas, thereby assisting in emotional regulation. This may be why patients who are emotionally overwhelmed seek out validation.

An examination of the predictors of higher scores on the Borderline Personality Dimension of the Millon Clinical Multiaxial Inventory–III (MCMI-III) revealed the following predictors: Comprehensibility, Rumination, Validation, Numbness, Blame, Simplistic View of Emotion, Control, Higher Values, and Rational (lower) (Leahy & Tirch, 2011). These data strongly suggest the importance of emotional schemas in psychopathology. Emotional schemas are differentially related to personality disorders. Adult patients completed the LESS and personality disorder dimensions on the MMCI-III. Individuals scoring higher on Avoidant, Dependent, and Borderline Personality had overly negative views of their emotions, while individuals scoring higher on Narcissistic and Histrionic personality had overly positive views of their emotions. Unexpectedly, individuals scoring higher on Compulsive personality also had positive views of their emotions. The latter finding may reflect the possibility that compulsive individuals do not distinguish between thoughts and emotions on this measure, believing that what they think or feel makes sense to them. In a separate study of the emotional schemas endorsed by individuals scoring higher on Borderline Personality, multiple regression analysis of the specific dimensions on borderline personality disorder indicated that the most predictive were comprehensibility, validation, rumination, blame, numbness, and control, reflecting the fact that borderline individuals believe that their emotions do not make sense, they are not validated, they ruminate about their feelings, they blame others, they experience numbness, and they feel out of control. Contrast this with the multiple regression for individuals scoring higher on Narcissistic personality: lower scores on guilt, expression, rumination, and higher values. These data suggest that Narcissistic individuals have less guilt about their emotions, believe that they can express their feelings, ruminate less about how they feel, and believe that their emotions are related to their higher values.

Application of the Model

The emotional schema therapist follows a structured approach to assessing current beliefs about emotions, developing a case conceptualization of how these beliefs maintain negative mood, how these emotional schemas are related to maladaptive styles of coping, and how emotional schemas can be modified. In this section I examine the assessment of emotional schemas, beliefs about duration, beliefs about incomprehensibility, guilt over emotions, and linking emotions to higher values.

Identifying Problematic Coping Strategies
Adaptive and Maladaptive Strategies

A key element of EST is the relationship between beliefs about emotion and emotion regulation strategies. Patients who are likely to become or remain depressed often respond to sadness with passivity and isolation, further cutting themselves off from the possibility of positive experiences and a sense of self-efficacy (Martell, Dimidjian, & Herman-Dunn, 2010). Others may believe that they need to rely on friends or family to regulate their emotion, thereby turning to others with a desperate search for support. Of course, this response may backfire and lead to further rejection if the patient perseverates on negativity while rejecting the help that is offered (Joiner, Brown, & Kistner, 2006). Adaptive strategies of emotion regulation have been identified, including problem solving, acceptance, cognitive restructuring, mindfulness, distraction, and behavioral activation (Aldao, Nolen-Hoeksema, & Schweizer, 2010; Leahy et al., 2011). However, many patients will utilize maladaptive strategies, such as thought suppression, emotion suppression, avoidance, excessive reassurance seeking, substance abuse, complaining, ruminating, blaming, and other unhelpful behaviors. These problematic strategies further add to the sense of hopelessness, ironically confirming the negative beliefs about emotion, and thereby encourage the patient to intensify these strategies.

Often the most effective way of helping patients modify their emotion beliefs is to address their problematic strategies of coping with emotion. The therapist can inquire, "When you are feeling upset (anxious, sad, lonely, empty) what do you do next to cope with that feeling?" Figure 13.2 illustrates a range of adaptive and maladaptive strategies, including cognitive restructuring, acceptance, problem solving, and behavioral activation as adaptive strategies, and rumination, worry, substance abuse, avoidance, and bingeing as maladaptive strategies. Some patients may utilize reassurance seeking that may be helpful, but—if perseverative—can alienate members of their support network.

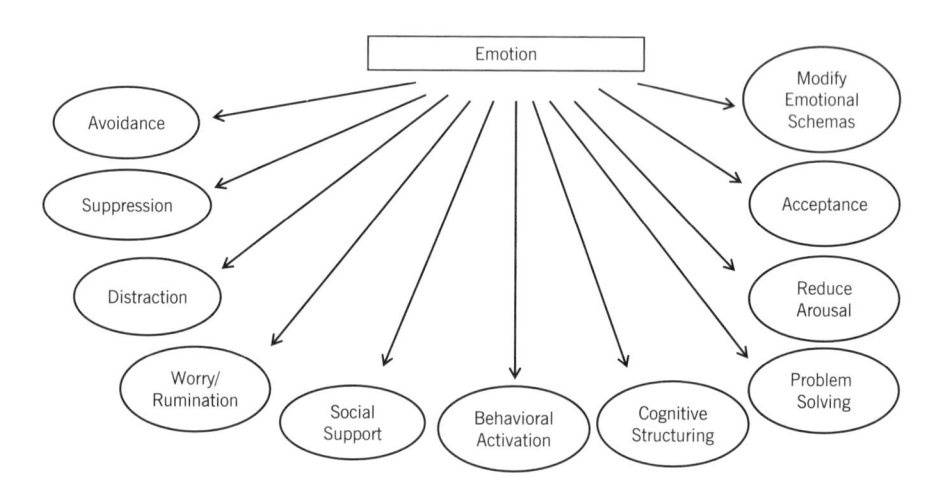

FIGURE 13.2. Maladaptive and adaptive strategies. From Leahy, Tirch, and Napolitano (2011). Copyright by the authors. Reprinted with permission from The Guilford Press.

Examining the Costs and Benefits of Coping Style

The therapist can help the patient examine the tradeoffs of their coping strategy. "What are the costs and benefits of bingeing at the time you feel anxious and you are alone?" One patient described the benefits as distraction from feeling anxious, feeling in control of getting what she wanted, and getting short-term relief. The costs were feeling out of control, self-criticism, gaining weight, and still having to deal with her problems. "So the benefits are short term. I wonder if we could find other ways of coping with your emotion that might have longer term benefits?"

Recognizing That There Are Alternative Ways to Cope

Patients who have habitually relied on maladaptive strategies may not recognize that responding to an emotion is a choice, not a reflex. For example, the patient who ruminates about why he or she feels bad may believe that this is an automatic response that is not affected by willful intention. "I just dwell on things" is a common response. The therapist can indicate that there is a choice: "If your boss called you on the phone, would you tell her you can't speak right now because you are ruminating?" Suggesting that there are alternative ways to cope—including improving the moment, problem solving, and accepting that things are difficult but committing to productive behavior—may provide greater hope.

Linking Emotional Schemas to Maladaptive Coping

The therapist can suggest that beliefs about emotion may lead to problematic coping. "I noticed that you indicated on the LESS that you believe that your emotions will go out of control, last a long time, and that you cannot accept your emotions. If you didn't have these beliefs about your emotion, I wonder if you would be less likely to use these emotion control strategies." This may be the first time that the patient will recognize that maladaptive coping is a direct consequence of his or her beliefs about emotion. "If you believed that your emotions were temporary and you could accept some discomfort, would you be more likely to tolerate the emotion and be able to go through it to get past it?"

Assessing Emotion and Emotional Schemas

Patients often experience their emotions as internal sensations and feelings that seem to come over them—or, alternatively, are caused by events outside of them. They seldom have the meta-awareness that their interpretations of their emotions may prolong, exacerbate, or reduce emotional intensity and that these interpretations may lead to maladaptive coping strategies. The initial sessions in therapy often are experienced as a new way of looking at one's emotions, suggesting that there may be new strategies and interpretations that may be employed.

The Leahy Emotional Schema Scale–II

The initial assessment involves having the patient complete the Leahy Emotional Schema Scale–II (LESS-II), a 28-item questionnaire that addresses the 14 emotional schema dimensions. Reviewing the patient's response, the therapist may note which emotional schema dimensions are elevated. For example, one patient indicated that she believed that her emotions did not make sense, that they would last a long time, and that they would go out of control. She also believed that others did not understand how she felt. The therapist followed up by asking which emotions would go out of control and last indefinitely. She responded that her anxiety and sadness would go out of control. The therapist asked if she became anxious and sad about the idea that her emotions would last indefinitely and go out of control—that is, that she was anxious about her anxiety.

The therapist can also inquire about specific emotions as related to specific emotional schemas. For example, the questionnaire can be modified to inquire about sadness, anger, anxiety, and loneliness. Some patients may have very negative views of certain emotions (e.g., anxiety), but not anger. This can lead to a discussion of emotion myths, such that certain emotions are labeled as "bad" while others are labeled as "legitimate." The patient may have secondary appraisals such that bad emotions must be eliminated (e.g., using alcohol, food, or sex) while good emotions can be tolerated—or even indulged. Thus the patient may have a mixed motive about decreasing anger and hostility if this emotion is not seen as problematic.

A further elaboration of the evaluation is the patient's beliefs about positive emotion. For example, does the patient believe that positive emotions will not last very long or that he is trivial and shallow? Does the patient believe that he has no control over feeling positive emotions, and therefore it is pointless to try to feel better? Some patients may believe that positive emotions are illusory or undeserved. They may even believe that to be sad, anxious, and resentful is a sign of depth or sophistication. In other cases, individuals may become sad about having a "happy feeling" since it exemplifies even more what is missing. Just as some individuals may believe that their negative emotions are out of control, they may also believe that their positive emotions are simply fortuitous and cannot be repeated.

Nonverbal Emotion

The therapist should also be attentive to any nonverbal signs of emotion—especially attempts of the patient to hold back an emotion. For example, a young woman described her long history of depression, self-defeating relationships, an earlier suicide attempt, and feelings of loneliness, while maintaining a smile on her face. The therapist reflected to her that she was describing painful memories while apparently treating them as trivial, given her smile and lack of emotion. This led to a discussion of how she believed that her emotions could never be validated, that emotions were viewed as inconsistent with the family image that everything is fine, and that she did not want to humiliate herself in front of the therapist. As a result she felt alone with her emotion, unable to seek out support, and distrustful of anyone who might get close to her—including the therapist (see also Safran & Kraus, Chapter 15, and Tsai, Fleming, Cruz, Hitch, & Kohlenberg, Chapter 17, this volume).

One aspect of emotional schemas is the patient's beliefs about touch—touching others and being touched. Research indicates that touch therapy—being touched, eceiving a massage, and so forth—can significantly reduce stress, anxiety, and pain and, in premature infants, increase weight gain, mobility, and strength (Field, 2001). Harlow's early research on surrogate infant mothers strongly supports the idea that touch can help infants cope with threat and to strive. The therapist can inquire about the patient's experience as a child with physical affection—were the parents warm, did they hug and kiss the child, did they offer physical touch? One patient observed that he thought that other people thought he was "untouchable"—that he was overly intellectualized, aloof, and cold, although he believed that he wanted to be hugged. He observed that he must give off signals that others should not get near him. This added to his sense of being defective and unlovable. Another patient described how her mother would physically and mentally abuse her and then call to her feigning an apology. She recalled that when she went to her mother to "make up" her mother slapped her.

Beliefs about Duration

Affect forecasting is a general tendency to overpredict one's emotional response to situations, and is often characterized as the belief that either positive or negative emotions will last much longer than they actually do. Many individuals predict their future emotions dependent on their current emotion—a process called *emotional anchoring*. Our research indicated that one of the primary predictors of depression and anxiety is the belief that negative feelings will last a long time. Some patients treat emotions as if they are "experiential traits" that are independent of situation and time. Yet the nature of emotions is that they are often ephemeral, changing with the situation, the people with whom one interacts, the goals that one focuses on, and even the time of day.

Costs and Benefits of Believing in Durability

Since beliefs in durability of emotion are key for anxiety and depression, it is important to examine the motivational tradeoffs for this belief. The therapist can suggest that there may be costs and benefits of believing that one's emotion will be long lasting. One patient indicated the following tradeoffs of the belief in durability: Costs—feeling hopeless, helpless, depressed, immobilized. Benefits—I won't get my hopes up. I can have realistic expectations. I can avoid situations that will make me feel worse. Evaluating the benefits can be helpful in examining the patient's willingness to change. For example, lowering expectations so that one does not get his or her hopes up can lead to helplessness, hopelessness, and the unwillingness to test out one's beliefs. This will perpetuate the negative mood. Indeed, the anticipated benefits of durability actually maintain depression since they lead to passivity and avoidance. The therapist can suggest that there is little risk in attempting to disconfirm the belief that emotions can change.

Self-Monitoring

One of the most widely used techniques in CBT is self-monitoring. Self-monitoring allows the patient and therapist to collect information, evaluate which behaviors or situations are associated with specific feelings, how behaviors may or may not impact the individual, and collect data to evaluate progress. Self-monitoring is helpful in EST for similar reasons. For example, a patient with borderline personality disorder believed that her anxious and lonely feelings would last indefinitely—and that there was no escaping them. The therapist suggested that the patient keep an activity schedule and monitor every hour the intensity of the anxiety along with other "pleasurable" feelings. Examination of this self-monitoring record indicated that the feelings of anxiety were strongest when the patient was alone at night ruminating about being alone at night. During the day she observed that she had some feelings of pleasure while talking to people at school, walking through the city, working on her assignments, exercising, and watching the news on television.

Eliciting Predictions about Durability

Many patients who utilize passivity and avoidance as coping strategies believe that taking action and confronting reality will make matters worse. The therapist can suggest some activities that the patient might consider and elicit predictions about the intensity and duration of negative feelings that will ensue. "How unpleasant do you think it will feel for you if you go to the health club? How long will that negative feeling last? Will the intensity remain the same? Will it get worse?" Eliciting specific predictions for exposure exercises can be quite illuminating. One patient predicted that if he touched a "contaminated" surface that he would have intense anxiety and that the anxiety would last throughout the day—and maybe for days after. The therapist further inquired, "How will this affect you? Will you be able to function in any way?" The patient answered, "I won't be able to think, I won't be able to work." These dire predictions were noted and the patient indicated a willingness to try some exposure. As he progressed with the exposure he noted that his anxiety was less than he thought it would be. He tried further exposure. The anxiety was less. At the following session, 3 days later, he indicated that he had a good day after the exposure session and, on his own, did more exposure. He noted that his next day at work was also very positive.

The therapist inquired what the consequence was of overpredicting that negative moods would last indefinitely and possibly get worse. The patient acknowledged that his beliefs in the durability of emotion kept him trapped in avoidance, further maintaining his obsessive–compulsive disorder and confirming his hopelessness.

Past History of Duration

Recent research on affect forecasting indicates that individuals prone to depression actually derive a similar degree of pleasure from activities but that they falsely recall and falsely predict past and future pleasure. This bias has been linked to serotogenic processes in the brain.

This demotivational bias in affect memory and forecasting may account for the reluctance of depressed individuals to try new activities. If they do not recall pleasure and do not predict pleasure, then it is logical for them to be reluctant to exert effort to acquire pleasure. This may be a key factor in the passivity and avoidance of depressed individual—that is, their negative response to negative emotion may be a biochemically based bias in cognition. Since the patient may falsely recall that past behaviors were not pleasurable, he may conclude that new behaviors cannot affect his mood—and that it makes no sense to try.

Some patients who experience intense anxiety believe that their anxiety will last indefinitely, thereby leading to more anxiety. This belief in the durability of an emotion can lead to avoidance of situations that elicit the emotion and escalating anxiety about having the emotion. The patient described above believed that her intense anxiety would last a long time. The therapist addressed this belief by asking her if she had these emotions in the past and if they had decreased in intensity. Why did they decrease in intensity?

Intervening Mitigation of Mood

One reason why people may believe that their future affect will be negative for a long time is that they underestimate intervening experiences that might mitigate their mood. For example, a patient experiencing a breakup in a relationship may be anchored to his or her current negative mood of loneliness, sadness, hopelessness, and anxiety. They predict the future through the lens of the current mood. However, future experiences may distract the patient from this mood and provide new rewarding experiences for the patient. These possible new experiences are often unforeseen by the individual who feels trapped in his or her current mood.

The therapist can suggest that "we often predict our future mood based on our current mood. If we are feeling sad and lonely, we expect that we will feel that way in the future. We often do not anticipate many of the positive experiences that might change our mood. What could be some experiences that might be rewarding or pleasurable in the future that could possibly happen to you?" Sometimes patients have difficulty imagining these positive experiences and stay trapped in their current mood. The therapist can ask if they had beliefs in the past about negative moods lasting indefinitely but found out, subsequently, that these moods did change. Why did they change? The therapist can ask if it is possible to imagine the patient experiencing positive emotions at work or with friends, doing activities, learning, exercising, traveling, forming new relationships, or having new experiences.

Some patients are better able to see malleability of moods in others. "Do you have any friends who have gone through a difficult time—the death of a close relative, loss of a job, breakup of a relationship, financial setback—but subsequently had positive experiences? "Yes, I recall that my sister lost her job and felt really hopeless and depressed, but she eventually got a new job and actually started a new relationship." The therapist can ask, "Is it possible that you are better able to see the positive experiences that others have, but have a difficult time anticipating these for yourself? If so, wouldn't that make you likely to maintain beliefs in hopelessness? Is it possible that you really don't know for sure what positive things could happen for you?"

Incomprehensibility

Many patients believe that their emotions do not make sense—they may describe themselves as being overcome by an emotion or that an emotion took over. "I don't know why I was feeling so sad at the office today. There was nothing going on. I just felt this sad feeling and I felt tired and I had no interest in doing anything." The consequence of believing that one's emotions do not make sense is that there is little that one can do to predict or control emotions. Furthermore, when emotions do not make sense individuals may believe that their emotions are distinct to them and that no one would understand them. There are a number of techniques to use that can address this issue of incomprehensibility.

Linking Emotion to Thoughts and Events

The activity schedule illustrates that emotions come and go depending on what you are thinking and what you are doing. For example, a patient who described himself as sad and lethargic kept an activity schedule for the following week. He noted that his feelings of sadness, pleasure, and competence changed dependent on what he was doing. For example, he rated several activities or interactions as positive for pleasure—talking to his wife, playing with his son, listening to music, reading, and talking with colleagues at the office. He rated working on a project as high in competence. He noted that his "down" feeling seemed to be limited to sitting in his office thinking "I have nothing to do," or sitting at home on the weekend thinking "There is nothing going on." He was able to recognize that his down feeling was related to "having nothing to do." The therapist suggested using the "downward arrow" technique: "Let's imagine you had nothing to do. Why would that bother you?" This led to the following string of thoughts: "If I have nothing to do, I am not productive. If I am not productive, then I am not successful. If I am not successful, then I am ordinary. If I am ordinary, then I am inferior." The therapist could utilize a number of traditional cognitive therapy techniques to address these thoughts, such as the costs and benefits of needing to be productive 100% of the time, examination of evidence of success, normalizing having time with nothing to do, and reframing this time as "free time" as opposed to "wasted time."

Linking Emotion to Rumination and Worry

Emotional schemas often result in unhelpful coping strategies that further maintain or augment the emotion. Rather than focus on the content of the thinking, the therapist can direct the patient to his or her response to the occurrence of negative thoughts. For example, in the example above, the individual activated rumination as a coping strategy to "deal with his emotion." He indicated, "If I think about why I am feeling sad, then I will be able to solve the problem." The nature of self-directed ruminations is that they were geared toward negativity: "What's wrong with me? I have nothing to feel bad about. I must have some deep-seated issues." The therapist was able to indicate that one of his major vulnerabilities was that he responded to a negative mood with rumination, passivity, and isolation—which were the ingredients of depression. Making sense of emotion involved recognizing that a response to a negative emotion could perpetuate it. Alternatively, he could utilize other techniques that might be more helpful. For example, he could normalize having "down time," recognize that he was overly focused on productivity, use the down time in ways that might be constructive or pleasurable (e.g., reading, problem solving, planning ahead, reviewing past work, taking a walk, exercising), and reframe down time as free time. Replacing rumination and worry with constructive action or normalization and acceptance helped him understand that different ways of responding to a mood led to different emotions.

Making Sense by Knowing What Would Make a Difference

Some patients believe that their emotions are a mystery to them, but they may harbor a clear idea of what would lead to a change in their emotion. Patients could make sense of their emotion if they can identify what would lead to a change in their emotion. For example, in the example above the therapist asked, "What could happen at that moment that might have changed the way you feel?" He replied: "If my boss came in and said, "I have a new exciting project for you." "Why would that make you feel better?" "Because then I would feel productive—like I had something to do." This line of inquiry further supported the overly conscientious style and demanding standards that he maintained. He felt sad and lethargic because he did not have a goal at that moment.

Another patient complained of fatigue and the desire to curl up on the couch and do nothing. She said, "I don't know why I felt so tired, like I had no energy. I hadn't been doing anything. I had no reason to feel this way." Bewildered by her fatigue and lack of interest in anything she began to think that her emotions "came out of nowhere." This sense of incomprehensibility led to her belief that her emotions were not within her control and that there was nothing that she could do to feel better. She would often sleep late on weekends, alternating with binging on junk food. The therapist suggested that her emotions might make sense if she recognized that she had a biological predisposition toward depression, that her mood was worse in the morning (diurnal variation), that passivity and rumination were depressive responses to a negative mood, and that it would be hard to imagine not feeling depressed if she responded to negative moods with the strategies that she utilized. "Are there times during the week when you wake up in a negative mood, but force yourself to go to work?" "Yes, almost every morning." "And when you are at work does your mood change?" "I actually feel better because I am distracted." "Any other reason for feeling better when you are at work?" "I guess I am busy feeling like I am doing my job and I get into what I am doing."

Guilt and Shame

Many patients feel ashamed about describing their emotions in therapy. They may believe that their sexual fantasies will be judged negatively, that describing their fears will make them appear weak, or that admitting to their envy and jealousy will be humiliating. Guilt and shame about emotion may lead to isolation, rumination, worry about losing control, attempts to suppress the emotion, and self-critical depression. The therapist can address these issues directly.

Normalizing Emotion

Recognizing that others may have the same feelings may help reduce the sense of shame or guilt about an emotion. The patient can list the specific emotions that he or she considers "abnormal" and list the advantages and disadvantages of thinking that these are "normal" feelings. The patient can conduct a survey and ask friends if they or anyone they knew had ever had a specific emotion that the patient views as abnormal (e.g., envy, jealousy, anger). The patient can list any songs, poems, stories, or novels that depict these emotions. For example, if the patient has feelings of jealousy, then he or she can identify songs about jealousy or literature that depicts jealousy. If others have the same feelings—and, indeed, if these feelings are universal—why should you feel ashamed or guilty about feeling what is human?

Challenging Self-Critical Thoughts about Emotion

Some patients ruminate about their self-critical thoughts, believing that they should not feel the way they do. "I shouldn't have these fantasies about other women, I am married," one man claimed. His underlying belief about sexual attraction was that he should only find his wife appealing enough to fantasize about. The therapist indicated that it would be more adaptive for the species if humans were capable of desire for a wide range of other people, rather than for one person. Further, he indicated that a fantasy is different from an action—it is actions that constitute choices. Fantasies come and go, they cannot be controlled or eliminated, and attempting to suppress them only makes them more powerful. "Why not thank the fantasy as a reminder that you are alive?" Similar to thought suppression, suppression of emotion and fantasy may only add to the negative beliefs that feelings and imagination are dangerous.

Distinguishing Emotions from Actions

Many people who have powerful emotions fear that their feelings will result in action. This "thought–action" fusion leads to further monitoring of feelings, fear of feelings, and attempts to suppress them (Rachman & Shafran, 1999). The married patient just described feared that he would act on his fantasy and destroy his marriage and humiliate himself in front of his children. The therapist inquired, "Let's imagine that this happened. You pick up a woman, take her to a hotel, have sex, then start an intense affair. This goes on for weeks and months, and then your wife finds out, she throws you out, and you end up getting divorced. Why hasn't this happened?" The patient indicated that he would never act out like this because he feared losing his marriage. "In other words, you see attractive women every day and decide not to act out every day. Does this show that you can have a fantasy without acting on it?" Further, the therapist indicated that making a moral choice involved confronting "temptation" and choosing to act in accord with your principles. "So, rather than feeling guilty about your fantasy you might feel proud that you have not acted on a wish."

Linking Emotions to Higher Values

Emotions Point to Core Values

People have emotions because they find something important to care about. Emotions are about something, they have an "intentionality" to them. Thus, a woman feels anxious because she is concerned with getting her work done correctly. The conscientious value is that she wants to do a good job. A man worries about his wife's recurrence of cancer—his anxiety points to the value of caring for the woman he loves. A woman describes her jealousy that her boyfriend has dinner with an ex-girlfriend. Her feelings reflect the value of commitment and fidelity in a relationship. Assisting patients in realizing that emotions have a reason and a value or goal toward which they aim helps validate and make sense of their emotion and reduce the sense of shame and guilt. "The reason that you are feeling jealous is that you value this relationship, you value love and commitment and honesty, and you feel, on some level, that this might be threatened. Those are good values—commitment and honesty—and, so, we have to examine how this is affecting you. Does his behavior really indicate that he is not committed to you? We both know that commitment is important, but we might want to see if this is a sign of lack of commitment or something else?" On closer inspection, the patient observed that her boyfriend was committed to the relationship but that he was insensitive at times to her vulnerabilities, an issue that was important but different from jealousy.

Climbing a Ladder of Higher Meaning

Typically in CBT the therapist may ask the patient a series of questions about the implication of a negative thought: "If you ended up alone, that would bother you because it would mean . . . ?" Further questions following this form attempt to get to the core fear or issue: "It would bother me because I would be miserable. I would be miserable because I would have no one. If I had no one it would mean I am unlovable. Then, life would not be worth living." This valuable technique, however, necessarily ends up on a negative note—even if it points to an irrational premise. The alternative in EST is to identify higher values. For example, a widow complained that when she returned home to her empty apartment she felt alone. The therapist asked her to climb a ladder of higher meaning, pointing to the positive values that would follow if things were different. "If you had someone there it would be better because . . . ?" The string of implications were: "I would have someone to share my life with. That would be good because then I would have someone to love. I am a loving person." The ladder of higher meaning points to the values that she may want to keep, even if there is a painful emptiness in her life at present. "I think that these are excellent values—loving and giving—and I know that it is hard not to have your husband with you since you are a loving person. Let's not lose those values of love. Are there other people that you can care for, love, get to know, and connect with? Then you would be pursuing your values." She was able to identify friends and her daughter, with whom she had difficulties. Rather than viewing herself as a burden to these people, acting on her values of love and kindness directed her to understanding and forgiving them. The therapist observed, "It's important that you not lose your values after losing someone you love. Showing love is something that you might continue to do."

Future Directions

As noted earlier in this chapter, a growing body of data indicates a direct link between emotional schemas and a wide range of psychopathology. However, these data are correlational and are open to interpretation. For example, perhaps the painful emotions arise and lead to negative beliefs about emotion. Or negative beliefs about emotion interact in a reciprocal, reflexive manner to spiral emotions out of control. It would be helpful to have data that manipulate beliefs about emotion and then assess emotional responses and problematic coping. In addition, it would be helpful to assess which emotions are more amenable to changes in emotional schemas. For example, some patients may enjoy their anger and may be reluctant to modify their emotional responses. They may believe that their emotions make sense and point to higher values. These positive emotional schemas may lead to resistance to change. Finally, there have yet to be any studies applying the techniques and strategies of EST to evaluate its effectiveness. It would be helpful to determine if an emotional schema conceptualization, along with the use of a wide range of techniques, is as effective as other empirically supported treatments.

Further Resources

Articles

- See Leahy (2002) for a description of the emotional schema model.
- See Leahy (2011a) for a description of how the model can be applied.
- See Leahy (in press) for a description of the emotional schema model applied to treatment of a patient.

Books

- See Leahy, Tirch, and Napolitano (2011) for a description of how other forms of CBT can be integrated into an emotional schema model.

References

Aldao, A., Nolen-Hoeksema, S., & Schweizer, S. (2010). Emotion-regulation strategies across psychopathology: A meta-analytic review. *Clinical Psychology Review, 30*(2), 217–237.

Anastasi, A., & Urbina, S. (1997). *Psychological testing.* Upper Saddle River, NJ: Prentice Hall.

Elias, N. (2000). *The civilizing process: Sociogenetic and psychogenetic investigations* (E. Jephcott, Trans.). Oxford, UK: Blackwell. (Original work published 1939)

Field, T. (2001). Massage therapy facilitates weight gain in preterm infants. *Current Directions in Psychological Science, 10*(2), 51–54.

Frederick, S., Loewenstein, G., & O'Donoghue, T. (2002). Time discounting and time preference: A critical review. *Journal of Economic Literature, 40,* 351–401.

Gilbert, D. T., & Wilson, T. D. (2009). Why the brain talks to itself: Sources of error in emotional prediction. *Philosophical Transactions of the Royal Society B, 364,* 1335–1341.

Heider, F. (1958). *The psychology of interpersonal relations.* Hoboken, NJ: Wiley.

Joiner, T. E. Jr., Brown, J. S., & Kistner, J. (Eds.). (2006). *The interpersonal, cognitive, and social nature of depression.* Mahwah, NJ: Erlbaum.

Kahneman, D. (2011). *Thinking, fast and slow.* New York: Farrar, Straus & Giroux.

Kahneman, D., Krueger, A. B., Schkade, D., Schwarz, N., & Stone, A. A. (2006). Would you be happier if you were richer?: A focusing illusion. *Science, 312*(5782), 1908–1910.

Lazarus, R. S. (1999). *Stress and emotion: A new synthesis.* New York: Springer.

Lazarus, R. S., & Folkman, S. (1984). *Stress, appraisal, and coping.* New York: Springer.

Leahy, R. L. (2002). A model of emotional schemas. *Cognitive and Behavioral Practice, 9*(3), 177–190.

Leahy, R. L. (2011a). Emotional schema therapy: A bridge over troubled waters. In J. Herbert & E. Forman (Eds.), *Acceptance and mindfulness in cognitive behavior therapy: Understanding and applying the new therapies* (pp. 109–131). New York: Wiley.

Leahy, R. L. (2011b, April). *Emotional schemas and implicit theory of emotion: Overcoming fear of feeling.* Keynote presented at the International Conference of Metacognitive Therapy, Manchester, UK.

Leahy, R. L. (2012). *Emotional schemas as predictors of relationship dissatisfaction.* Unpublished manuscript, American Institute for Cognitive Therapy, New York, NY.

Leahy, R. L. (in press). Emotional schema therapy. In W. J. Livesley, G. Dimaggio, & J. F. Clarkin (Eds.), *Integrated treatment for personality disorders.* New York: Guilford Press.

Leahy, R. L., & Tirch, D. D. (2011, June). *Emotional schemas, psychological flexibility and borderline personality.* Paper presented at the International Congress on Cognitive Psychotherapy, Istanbul, Turkey.

Leahy, R. L., Tirch, D. D., & Melwani, P. S. (2012). Processes underlying depression: Risk aversion, emotional schemas, and psychological flexibility. *International Journal of Cognitive Therapy, 5*(4), 362–379.

Leahy, R. L., Tirch, D. D., & Napolitano, L. A. (2011). *Emotion regulation in psychotherapy: A practitioner's guide.* New York: Guilford Press.

Lutz, T. (2001). *Crying: A natural and cultural history of tears.* New York: Norton.

Martell, C. R., Dimidjian, S., & Herman-Dunn, R. (2010). *Behavioral activation for depression: A clinician's guide.* New York: Guilford Press.

Rachman, S., & Shafran, R. (1999). Cognitive distortions: Thought–action fusion [Special issue]. *Clinical Psychology and Psychotherapy: Metacognition and Cognitive Behaviour Therapy, 6*(2), 80–85.

Schkade, D. A., & Kahneman, D. (1998). Does living in California make people happy?: A focusing illusion in judgments of life satisfaction. *Psychological Science, 9*(5), 340–346.

Stearns, P. N. (1994). *American cool: Constructing a twentieth-century emotional style.* New York: New York University Press.

Tirch, D. D., Leahy, R. L., Silberstein, L. R., & Melwani, P. S. (2012). Emotional schemas, psychological flexibility, and anxiety: The role of flexible response patterns to anxious arousal. *International Journal of Cognitive Therapy, 5*(4), 380–391.

Weber, M. (1930). *The Protestant ethic and the spirit of capitalism.* London: Unwin Hyman.

Wells, A. (2002). Worry, metacognition and GAD: Nature, consequences and treatment. *Journal of Cognitive Psychotherapy, 16,* 179–192.

Wells, A. (2004). A cognitive model of GAD: Metacognitions and pathological worry. In R. G. Heimberg, C. L. Turk, & D. S. Mennin (Eds.), *Generalized anxiety disorder: Advances in research and practice* (pp. 164–186). New York: Guilford Press.

Wells, A. (2009). *Metacognitive therapy for anxiety and depression.* New York: Guilford Press.

Wilson, T. D., & Gilbert, D. T. (2003). Affective forecasting. *Advances in Experimental Social Psychology, 35,* 345–411.

Wilson, T. D., & Gilbert, D. T. (2005). Affective forecasting: Knowing what to want. *Current Directions in Psychological Science, 14*(3), 131–134.

Wilson, T. D., Wheatley, T., Meyers, J. M., Gilbert, D. T., & Axsom, D. (2000). Focalism: A source of durability bias in affective forecasting. *Journal of Personality and Social Psychology, 78*(5), 821–836.

Yeh, Y.-Y., Draper, M. R., & Yu, L. (2007, August). *Alexithymia, somatization, positive and negative affect: A cross-cultural study* Paper presented at the American Psychological Association Conference, San Francisco, CA.

CHAPTER 14

Emotion Regulation Therapy

An Experiential Approach to Chronic Anxiety and Recurring Depression

Mia Skytte O'Toole
Douglas S. Mennin
David M. Fresco

Chronic anxiety and recurring depression (i.e., generalized anxiety disorder [GAD]; major depressive disorder [MDD]; American Psychiatric Association, 2013) are commonly co-occurring conditions that are sometimes referred to as "distress disorders" because they share a component of negative affect, or subjective emotional distress (Krueger & Markon, 2006; Watson, 2005). Clinical research has shown that distress disorders in particular pose a challenge to our available treatment in that a sizeable subgroup of individuals with these disorders fail to make sufficient treatment gains. For example, in a meta-analysis of cognitive-behavioral therapy (CBT) for GAD, Borkovec and Ruscio (2001) found that only 50–60% of treated individuals demonstrated clinically meaningful change. Although psychological treatments for MDD may be overall more efficacious, the difference between these treatments and nondirective supportive therapy is small (Cuijpers, van Straten, Andersson, & van Oppen, 2008). For individuals with GAD and comorbid MDD, gains in treating depression are not very durable (Newman, Przeworski, Fisher, & Borkovec, 2010). Finally, in the recently concluded Sequenced Treatment Alternatives to Relieve Depression Study, funded by the National Institute of Mental Health (NIMH), the subgroup of individuals with mixed anxiety-depressive disorder was most treatment-refractory (Farabaugh et al., 2010).

More so than other conditions, distress disorders have been found to be characterized by temperamental features that reflect heightened emotional experience (often referred to as "emotionality," "neuroticism," or "emotional intensity"; see Barlow, 2002; Krueger & Markon, 2006; Watson, 2005; Mennin, Holaway, Fresco, Moore, & Heimberg, 2007) and a heightened sensitivity to underlying motivational systems related to threat/safety and reward/loss (Chorpita, Albano, & Barlow, 1998; Klenk, Strauman, & Higgins, 2011; Woody & Rachman, 1994). In order to dampen the emotional experience, and as an effort to obtain safety, individuals with distress disorders may engage in reactive, compensatory strategies such as negative self-referential processing (i.e., worry, rumination, and self-criticism), behavioral avoidance, and reassurance seeking (Cougle et al., 2012; Mennin & Fresco, 2013; Michelson, Lee, Orsillo, & Roemer, 2011). However, such strategies may prevent the experience or awareness of the motivational messages that are being conveyed through emotions (Klenk et al., 2011).

Taken together, there is an increasing interest in understanding the role of emotions and how this knowledge might generate new targets for intervention, particularly in treatment-resistant cases such as those with distress disorders. Congruent with current directions in affect science, we have developed an emotion regulation therapy (ERT; Mennin & Fresco, 2009, 2014) to improve treatment of chronic anxiety and recurring depression. In the remainder of this chapter, we review the conceptual model underlying ERT, demonstrate how ERT reflects an experiential approach to distress conditions such as chronic anxiety and recurring depression, and present data in support of this approach.

Background and Theory

We see ERT as a member of the CBT family. Traditional and contemporary CBTs reflect two overarching principles. First, CBT works by teaching clients *skills* to overcome deficits in emotional and cognitive processing. Second, as clients show some facility with new skills, treatment then focuses on creating opportunities for exposure and new learning to extinguish fear/anxiety responses while increasing approach behavior and reward activation. ERT represents our effort to simultaneously remain true to these core principles in CBT while also incorporating theory and evidence from the burgeoning basic and translational science of emotions in the hopes of improving our understanding and treatment of GAD. As compared to more traditional CBTs, ERT conceptualizes and treats chronic anxiety and recurring depression via a greater delineation of the functional role of emotions and underlying motivations (Mennin & Farach, 2007). Recent advances in the basic affect sciences stress the notion that emotional responses have developed for the purpose of security in the face of threat, and gain in the face of rewards (Gray & McNaughton, 2000; Lang, 1995). Thus, although not always productive, emotions serve as signals to an individual's pull toward both security and reward motivations. As an experientially oriented therapy, ERT considers the full experience of emotions and underlying motivations a mechanism of change. We define *experience* in a manner consistent with Greenberg (2002a, 2002b), who sees an experience as being the result of attention to and awareness of ongoing events in mind and body. Accordingly, an *experiential* method or technique refers to the means by which the individual's full experience is engendered in the therapeutic context, just as he or she would experience the same events in the world. Put in other words, the individual is invited to pay attention to and become aware of all the constituents of the full experience.

ERT stands on the shoulders of both emotion-focused therapies (Greenberg, 2002a), which explicitly have a functional view of emotions and contemporary CBT packages that are increasingly incorporating an emphasis on the experience of emotion. These include dialectical behavior therapy (DBT; Linehan, 1993); compassion-focused therapy (Gilbert, 2010); mindfulness-based cognitive therapy (MBCT; Segal, Williams, & Teasdale, 2002); acceptance and commitment therapy (ACT; Hayes, Strosahl, & Wilson, 1999); acceptance-based behavior therapy (Roemer, Orsillo, & Salters-Pedneault, 2008); and behavioral activation (Jacobson, Martell, & Dimidjian, 2001). The net effect is an integrated, mechanism-targeted, experientially oriented CBT that strives to improve the acute and enduring treatment efficacy for patients suffering from chronic anxiety and recurring depression.

Target Mechanisms: Motivational, Emotion Regulation, and Contextual Learning Systems

ERT is organized around three core target mechanisms and specifically seeks to (1) increase motivational awareness, (2) develop regulatory capacities, and (3) engage new contextual learning repertoires. We describe these mechanisms from a normative perspective that is then contrasted with how these processes can become dysfunctional in chronic anxiety and recurring depression.

Motivational Mechanisms

The functionality of emotions is evidenced when understood as sources of information about what our motivational orientations are and how we should prepare or act accordingly (Keltner & Gross, 1999). Although we have evolved over time, humans remain pushed and pulled by very basic motivations of security and reward (Mennin & Fresco, 2009, 2014). The security system instigates avoidance of threats and safety-seeking behaviors, while the reward system mobilizes behavioral approach and minimization of loss. The security and reward systems are relatively independent and can be activated alone or in unison in response to a prompt (Stein & Paulus, 2009). All individuals are subject to conflicting pulls from safety and reward motivational systems. Normatively, the two motivational pulls are balanced, bringing both safety and reward to human lives through effective behavioral actions. Individuals with chronic anxiety and recurring depression, however, may evidence a primary concern of safety, often at the expense of reward (Klenk et al., 2011), and consequently be relatively less effective in resolving motivational conflicts (Aupperle & Paulus, 2010). ERT aims at restoring a motivational balance.

Regulatory Mechanisms

Expanding on Gross's temporal model of emotion regulation (for an extensive review, see Gross & Thompson, 2007), we see emotions unfolding over time, and they can be regulated at different points. Over the course of emotional unfolding, the amount of cognitive elaboration can differentiate these regulatory strategies. "Elaboration," in this sense, refers to the degree to which verbal mediation is required to engage a particular capacity. Greater elaboration requires greater mental effort and can result in greater cognitive resource depletion (Joorman, Nee, Berman, Jonides, & Gotlib, 2010; Keng, Robins, Smoski, Dagenbach, & Leary, 2013; MacNamara & Hajcak, 2010; Muraven & Baumeister, 2000). Therefore, optimal emotion regulation may begin with engaging less elaborative strategies and become increasingly elaborative as needed. Emotion regulation flexibility concerns the individual's ability to choose contextually appropriate regulatory strategies. Correspondingly, emotional dysfunction can occur at varying points of an unfolding emotional response. In the case of chronic anxiety and recurring depression, emotion dysregulation includes *attentional rigidity* by either fixating on or avoiding both interoceptive and exteroceptive emotional stimuli (Mogg & Bradley, 2005). These individuals likely fail to spontaneously direct their attention as demanded by the motivationally salient emotional stimulus (Etkin, Prater, Hoeft, Menon, & Schatzberg, 2010; Etkin & Schatzberg, 2011). Therefore, they may resort to more elaborative and oftentimes depleting strategies, such as negative self-referential processes (e.g., worry, rumination, and self-criticism; Mennin & Fresco, 2013). Such responses reduce clarity in understanding and optimally responding to the emotion (Schultz, Izard, Ackerman, & Youngstrom, 2001), and therefore are an important target in ERT.

Contextual Learning Mechanisms

Knowing and providing contextually adaptive behavioral responses is key to optimal functioning of an individual. Adaptive and flexible behavioral responses are dependent on the ability to increase awareness of cues and contingencies in the environment, and to respond in ways that promote both survival and success. Adaptive motivational responses and regulatory capacities provide a foundation for behavioral flexibility by helping us attain maximal emotional clarity (e.g., Gohm & Clore, 2002) and subsequently implement effective and goal-relevant responses for optimal behavioral outcomes. Individuals with distress disorders show behavioral inflexibility in multiple ways. As we noted, attentional rigidity likely prevents them from properly attending to other cues than threat/safety cues in their environment, thereby making them miss important information that could otherwise foster more adaptive responses. Likewise, elaborative regulatory capacities, when inflexibly employed, generate cognitive load and hinder emotional processing (Borkovec & Sharpless, 2004; Newman & Llera, 2011), diminish the ability to discriminate stimuli and learning contingencies (Salters-Pedneault, Roemer, Tull, Rucker, & Mennin, 2006), and decrease the likelihood of new reward-based learning (Bar, 2009; Joorman & Tran, 2009).

Preliminary Evidence

ERT is a manualized treatment developed for the treatment of chronic anxiety and recurring depression. To date, the efficacy of ERT has been demonstrated in a recently concluded NIMH-funded open trial (OT; $N = 19$; Mennin, Fresco, Heimberg, & Ritter, 2014) and a randomized clinical trial (RCT; $N = 60$) (Mennin & Fresco, 2011; Mennin, Fresco, Heimberg, & Ciesla, 2012). ERT was well tolerated by clients as evidenced by low rates of attrition in the course of treatment. In terms of clinical outcomes, OT patients evidenced reductions in both clinician-assessed and self-report measures of GAD severity, worry, trait anxious, and depression symptoms, and corresponding improvements in quality of life, with within-subject effect sizes well exceeding conventions for large effects (Cohen's $d = 1.5$–4.5). These gains were maintained for 9 months following the end of treatment. The RCT patients receiving immediate ERT, as compared to a modified attention control condition, evidenced significantly greater reductions in GAD severity, worry, trait anxious, and depression symptoms, and corresponding improvements in functionality and quality of life, with between-subject effect sizes in the medium-to-large range ($d = .50$–2.0). These gains were maintained for 9 months following the end of treatment. A sizable subgroup of GAD patients with comorbid MDD ($N = 30$) were enrolled and treated. Within-subject effect sizes in both clinician-assessed and self-report measures of GAD severity, worry, trait anxious, and depression symptoms, and corresponding improvements in functionality and quality of life were comparable to the overall trial findings, thereby suggesting that MDD comorbidity did not interfere with treatment efficacy ($d = 1.5$–4.0).

Furthermore, depression-related outcomes such as rumination and anhedonia were reduced considerably (d = 1.5–2.0).

We are currently examining whether these treatment outcomes are the result of changes in the outlined target mechanisms. One promising preliminary finding is related to emotional conflict adaptation (Etkin & Schatzberg, 2011). A subset of our ERT clients (N = 15) completed the Etkin Emotional Conflict Task at pretreatment and at the midpoint of ERT. Findings indicate that by midtreatment, clients had improved their ability to shift their attention in the face of emotional conflict (pretreatment to midtreatment d = 0.74) to levels comparable to healthy controls (Etkin et al., 2010). Furthermore, clients who showed the greatest gains in conflict adaptation by midtreatment also showed the greatest pre- to posttreatment change in anxiety, anhedonic depression, and worry. We have also examined responses to more complex emotional stimuli, which likely require more effort and elaboration to manage. Specifically, we assessed heart rate variability (HRV; an index of parasympathetic flexibility; Porges, 2001; Thayer, Åhs, Fredrikson, Sollers, & Wager, 2012) during a fearful film paradigm at pretreatment and midtreatment (N = 18). At pretreatment, clients displayed a flattened response throughout the experimental period, suggesting reduced flexibility. At midtreatment, clients displayed a quadratic pattern of vagal withdrawal (i.e., reactivity) and vagal rebound (pretreatment to midtreatment d= 0.81) reflecting a more normative response to these changing emotional contexts. Period-averaged HRV levels at midtreatment also increased to within 1 SD of levels in a healthy control sample. Finally, clients who showed the greatest increases in parasympathetic flexibility from pretreatment to midtreatment showed the greatest pre- to posttreatment gains in diagnostic severity, anxiety, worry, anhedonic depression, impairment, and life quality. Taken together, these preliminary data are supportive of our hypotheses that ERT may, in part, exert its therapeutic impact through normalization of emotion regulatory mechanisms.

Application

ERT consists of 16 weekly sessions organized into two parts. The flow of ERT draws on Gross's (2002) emotion regulation model, which distinguishes between efforts to regulate emotions earlier (i.e., antecedent-focused strategies) and later (i.e., response-focused strategies) in the emotion generative process. Clients first progress through ERT by learning skills to enhance their emotional experience. Then, through experiential exposure exercises, they are invited to increase values-informed behavioral actions that strike a balance between security and reward motivational pulls. Figure 14.1 depicts the flow of therapy and the core therapeutic processes.

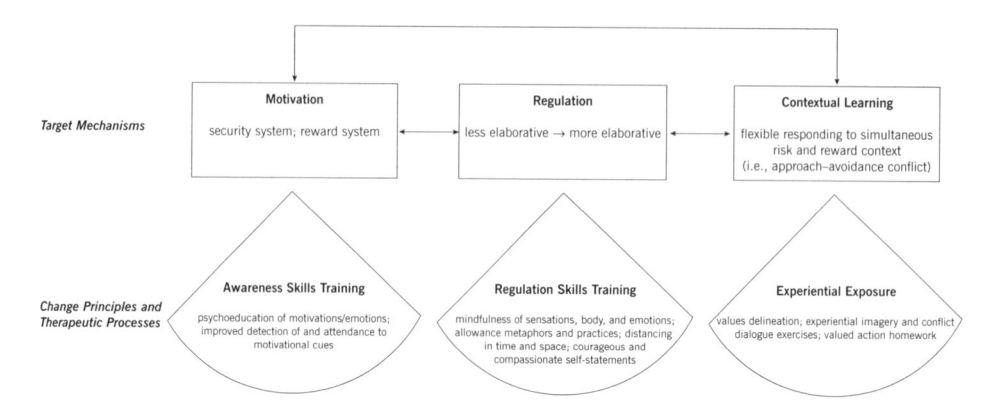

FIGURE 14.1. Conceptual model of target mechanisms, change principles, and therapeutic processes in emotion regulation therapy. From Mennin and Fresco (2014). Copyright 2014 by The Guilford Press. Reprinted by permission.

ERT Part 1: Skills Building

The overarching theme for this first half of ERT is building and expanding the client's experiential skill repertoires that over the course of treatment become increasingly more elaborative. All the skills are aimed at developing alternatives to the reactive response-focused emotion regulation that has characterized their lives. Thus, clients are taught how to approach their lives "counteractively" by learning emotion regulation skills. These skills include a set of antecedent-focused emotion regulation strategies (e.g., psychoeducation, cue detection/self-monitoring, and mindfulness exercises), all relevant at different time points in the unfolding of emotion.

Psychoeducation

Initially, normative functioning related to the three target mechanisms in ERT is contrasted with the characteristics of chronic anxiety and recurring depression. Clients are encouraged to give personally relevant examples that depict their struggles concerning these mechanisms as a way for them to begin to see both past and current patterns through the lenses of ERT. At this introductory stage of therapy, clients are encouraged to adopt an open perspective and to start noticing the way they are swayed by emotions and motivations.

Clients are presented with two metaphors that help foster this open perspective. The first metaphor illustrates the temporal unfolding of emotions and is meant to illustrate that it requires less effort when emotions are handled via less elaborative regulation strategies earlier on, than with more elaborative strategies after the full-blown emotional responses are present. Clients are asked to imagine a fluffy white snowball, consisting of pristine snow free of any dirt or blemishes. Then clients are asked to picture this snowball rolling down a hill, and in the course of its travel, picking up dirt and twigs and becoming increasingly hard and icy. In effect, the snowball's tumble down the hill has obscured the primacy and purity of the original snowball with extra and unwanted elements. The travel of the snowball down the hill alludes to the unfolding of our emotional experience when engaging increasingly more elaborative and maladaptive emotion regulation. Individuals with chronic anxiety and recurring depression are likely to be reactive instead of counteractive, and oftentimes notice the snowball only after it has rolled all the way down the hill, that is, when they have engaged reactive responding (e.g., worry, rumination, self-criticism, behavioral avoidance, and reassurance seeking). Through various practices, clients are invited to pay attention to the emotion in its purest form, as the fluffy white snowball.

The second metaphor speaks to the motivational configuration of the client. Clients are asked to imagine a musical orchestra in which each instrument represents a different emotion. The composition they are playing represents the motivational pulls in their lives. Ideally, the composition of the orchestra is harmonious, and the music moves us to take some action in our lives. However, for individuals with chronic anxiety and recurring depression, the "anxiety tuba," the pull toward security, ends up drowning the "reward-piccolo." Clients are encouraged to listen to the orchestral piece in a way wherein each and every part of the orchestra can be heard and discerned for its contribution to the orchestra composition. This metaphor is the departure point for introducing various practices, all aimed at increasing the clients' experience of their emotions with greater granularity and clarity.[1]

Cue Detection and Self-Monitoring

After learning about the tendency for reactive responding (e.g., snowball metaphor), clients are introduced to "catch yourself reacting (CYR)," which is akin to the self-monitoring or chain analysis practices common in many CBT packages. This practice begins as a simple exercise, in which clients attempt to identify the triggers of their emotions, the actual emotions themselves (e.g., fear, anxiety, or disgust), and the intensity of each emotion they listed. This initial CYR also is intended to help clients better differentiate the emotions that arise in their daily lives as opposed to viewing them as a jumble of negative emotions. In later sessions, the amount of information clients monitor and record becomes more complex. The information includes (1) concurrent levels of security and reward motivation pulls as two independent ratings made on 100-point scales; (2) internally

---

[1] ERT therapists are encouraged to use alternative but congruent metaphors if the metaphors presented above are not expected to or do not resonate with the client.

(e.g., worry, self-criticism) and externally (e.g., reassurance seeking, behavioral avoidance) focused responses to the arising of emotions and motivations; and (3) implementation of skills on-the-spot and the impact that those skills had on the situation. Completing CYRs outside of the sessions and reviewing them as part of homework is one of the mainstays throughout ERT. Therapists and clients review CYR entries each week, with an emphasis on reviewing instances where clients recorded successfully implementing their ERT skills to manage a situation, as well as instances where they had difficulty. Here, clients may have neglected to use their skills, or the outcome of the situation may not have been favorable despite the effort put forth by the client. On these occasions, therapists can choose to conduct a "do-over" with the client. This activity resembles both the cognitive rehearsal task, which is described in traditional cognitive therapy of depression (Beck, Rush, Shaw, & Emery, 1979), and evocative unfolding in experiential therapy (Elliott, Watson, Goldman, & Greenberg, 2004; see also Erickson, Newman, McGuire, Chapter 16, this volume). In ERT, imagery of a difficult situation is evoked for clients to help them engage their counteractive skills and obtain a distanced perspective. From this perspective they can then identify any emotions or motivational pulls, and articulate possible actions to be taken. The CYR "do over" essentially represents a therapist-supervised opportunity to shape and solidify the counteractive skills that clients are practicing throughout ERT.

Mindfulness Exercises

Another important facet of ERT is the utilization of mindfulness practices aimed at building skills for becoming more aware of the different constituents of one's experience and using more adaptive regulatory strategies. Most of the mindfulness exercises are first practiced in an off-line version (e.g. at a set time each day), after which clients are encouraged to deploy a briefer, "on-the-spot" version in their daily lives when difficult emotions arise. The mindfulness exercises are first practiced in-session and are then assigned as between-session homework, which clients are asked to practice six times a week. In introducing mindfulness as a concept and its accompanying practices, ERT walks a fine line between cultivating attention skills and inducing distress relief. Distress relief in the here-and-now is not the primary purpose of the practices, but clients are told that the practices are an important part of training their "attention muscle" that may or may not have the by-product of relaxation and relief.

ATTENTION

In ERT, clients learn three mindfulness practices designed to promote single-pointed and flexible attention with a particular emphasis on minimally elaborative and linguistic processing of one's experience. In effect, these practices help to cultivate the skill of attending to one's experience and becoming aware of the constituting emotions and underlying motivations. The first exercise is *mindful belly breathing*, which is a brief diaphragmatic breathing practice aimed at gathering one's attention onto sensations in the body (see Roemer & Orsillo, 2009). This practice can be used both as an offline and an on-the-spot exercise. Next, clients learn a practice adapted from the body scan work common in mindfulness-based stress reduction (MBSR; Kabat-Zinn, 1990) and MBCT (Segal et al., 2002), coupled with an awareness-based progressive muscle relaxation approach, which has been effectively utilized in the treatment of GAD (Borkovec, Newman, Pincus, & Lytle, 2002; Roemer & Orsillo, 2009). The offline practice is referred to as *body and muscle awareness* (BAMA) and includes a guided walk-through of the whole body. An on-the-spot version, *recall BAMA*, can be applied when clients are experiencing unpleasant internal physical states such as muscle tensions. Finally, clients are introduced to an offline practice called *mindfulness of emotions* (adapted from Marra, 2004; Williams, Teasdale, Kabat-Zinn, & Segal, 2007), whereby one brings to mind a situation with conflicting emotions and motivations. Clients are then invited to sit with this experience until they can hold and more clearly delineate the emotions and motivational pulls in the situation.

ALLOWING

Building upon the skill of attending, the implementation of allowing (e.g., Hayes, Strosahl, & Wilson, 2011) in ERT is meant to engender a willingness to be "all in" with one's experience without pushing away or avoiding and to be present with emotions and learn how to determine their functional utility in guiding actions. Clients are informed that allowing is not the same as wanting, but instead is the act of embracing whatever thoughts, feelings, emotions, and bodily sensations arise. Two exercises are introduced with the purpose of developing the skill of allowing. The offline practice is based on the *open presence meditation* (Halifax, 2009; Ricard, 2006), which strives to maintain attention on whatever arises without relying on internal (e.g., one's breath) or external (e.g., sounds) cues as an anchor for the practice. The on-the-spot version of this exercise is called the *3-minute breathing space*, which is drawn from MBCT (Segal et al., 2002). It is first practiced in session, after which the clients are asked to do the practice when they feel the need to gather themselves in a situation where they are pulled toward responding reactively. Much like in MBCT, the breathing space is meant to help clients allow an emotional experience to unfold so that they can notice and glean the emotional and motivational aspects of the experience.

DISTANCING (DECENTERING)

ERT then moves toward a greater focus on healthier elaborative regulatory skills. Distancing involves metacognitive awareness (e.g., Teasdale et al., 2002) and decentering (e.g., Fresco, Moore, et al., 2007; Fresco, Segal, et al., 2007; Safran & Segal, 1990). The client is invited to see his or her emotions and underlying motivational pulls from a healthy distance in order to generate emotional clarity rather than automatically responding. Two offline practices are introduced to promote this skill, each of which concerns a specific perspective: perspective in time and perspective in space.

The first practice, focusing on perspective in time and familiar to practitioners of MBSR, is called the mountain meditation. In this guided practice, clients are invited to internalize a living breathing mountain to provide solidity and permanence to their lives, in contrast to the transient emotion upheavals, which are represented as the weather on the mountain (Kabat-Zinn, 1994). The on-the-spot counterpart to this practice is called *invoking the mountain*, which is a brief version of the mountain meditation. As with the other on-the-spot practices, this one is designed to be utilized in either planned or impromptu moments that pull for "security-first" responses. The other exercise aimed at providing distance is called *finding an observer's distance*, which focuses on mental spatial distance. This practice, which draws in part from the *observer you* exercise in ACT (Hayes et al., 1999), is designed to teach clients to bring situations to mind and then to granulize the constituent parts of the situation by placing them externally on objects in the room. This offline practice is an invitation to create a healthy distance in one's mind's eye, so that these products of the mind are more readily observable, and in turn can inform our deliberate actions from a distance. This practice also has a corresponding on-the-spot skill, called *bringing it with you*, where clients imagine placing products of their mind on objects that they ordinarily carry in their daily lives.

REFRAMING

In ERT, reframing is defined as the ability to change one's evaluation of an event such that the event is altered in its emotional significance (Gross, 2002). Thus, with respect to ERT, reframing is regarded as the most elaborative of the emotion regulation skills and is employed when additional cognitive elaboration is necessary to manage emotions and motivational pulls while providing an alternative to negative self-referential processing (Beck et al., 1979; Mennin & Fresco, 2014). In reframing a situation, clients are first encouraged to adopt a courageous perspective from which they can address the response tendencies associated with their motivational pulls. They are encouraged to articulate alternative statements that reflect their strength in the face of uncertainty and distress. In addition, clients are encouraged to adopt a self-compassionate stance, wherein they can imagine telling a very caring, interested, compassionate individual about their difficult thoughts and feelings and remind themselves of their strengths and coping ability (Gilbert, 2010; Segal et al., 2002). An offline mindfulness practice accompanies teaching the skill of reframing. This practice is called *meditation on courage and compassion*, in which clients are asked to imagine a past difficult emotional situation and then to develop courageous and compassionate responses in order to feel strength in the emotionally intense situation and reduce the likelihood of engaging in reactive responses. Noticing one's self-critical thoughts is encouraged, and "softening" them when they arise is accomplished by invoking alternative, self-validating statements. These courageous and compassionate statements are typically written down on the back of an index or business card and carried with the patient in a pocket, or put on a smartphone, as a recurrent reminder. As the clients increase their ability to employ these new perspectives, they are encouraged to simply tap their pocket or smartphone containing the written statements to quickly regain this sense of perspective.

TAKING ACTION

Building upon the client's sense of how emotions and corresponding motivations have led one to orient his or her life toward security and reactive responding, the concept of opposite action (e.g., Linehan, 1993) is introduced in ERT as a way of restoring motivational balance. Drawing from the work of behavioral activation, ERT clients are encouraged to adopt an outside-in approach (cf. Jacobson et al., 2001; Martell, Addis, & Jacobsen, 2001), meaning that one engages in actions that might be opposite to one's current feelings and motivational pulls. While motivations and emotions guide our actions, the opposite is also the case, that is, an opposite action can ultimately change our motivational pulls and emotions (Linehan, 1993). Clients are introduced to this concept with the practice *envisioning opposite orientation* (adapted from Linehan, 1993; Martell et al., 2001). In this exercise, clients are asked to envision a troublesome situation and then to imagine what it would feel like with a different motivational configuration, thereby possibly changing one or both of the pulls for security and reward.

ERT Part 2: Experiential Exposure to Promote New Contextual Learning

Whereas the first half of ERT represents the movement from being "reactive" to "counteractive" in response to emotional states, the second half invites clients to become "proactive" in the service of broadening one's behavioral repertoires. Thus, taking a proactive stance involves exposure to potentially rewarding but often anxiety-inducing experiences. Exposure exercises are typically understood as a way to *reduce* emotion (especially fear) (cf. Foa & Kozak, 1986). However, recent empirical and theoretical advances have advocated for a broader focus than simple emotion reduction. Indeed, modern learning theory suggests that exposure is effective not because previously associated emotional meanings are unlearned or erased, but because new emotional meanings are strengthened (Bouton, Mineka, & Barlow, 2001; Craske et al., 2008). Thus, a consensus is emerging such that exposure therapies should emphasize emotional processing and the creation of new personal meanings, which may be facilitated through experiential engagement, where new meanings occur from the utilization of emotional information rather than its mere reduction (cf. Greenberg, 2002a; Teasdale, 1999).

ERT echoes these advances and uses a number of modified, classic experiential techniques (i.e., imaginal exposure and experiential dialogue) to prepare clients for real-world exposure. In ERT, exposure to threat–reward contrasts is accomplished by focusing clients on their personal values, which represent a person's highest priorities and most cherished principles (Hayes et al., 1999, 2011; Wilson & Murrell, 2004). Values-based exposure is derived from ACT (e.g., Hayes et al., 1999, 2011) and involves turning a problem on its head; rather than exposing oneself to feared outcomes, one is exposed to the way that he or she would like to be living. As such, values can be considered "top-down" decisions. However, the motivational configuration of the individual at any given point in time may introduce conflicts and pull the individual in a value-incongruent direction. Therefore, ERT expands values-based exposure to address more than just "top-down" decisions related to the person's values. It also concerns "bottom-up" influences of security and reward motivational pulls, as well as their interaction. In this field of "top-down"–"bottom-up" influences, exposure-related fears, disappointments, and judgments may arise. ERT treats such entities as obstacles to being able to live a valued life. Specifically, ERT delineates three main exposure components to promote valued living: (1) imaginal action related to values-informed goals, (2) experiential dialogue tasks to explore perceived internal conflicts related to the client's motivational configuration that may prevent valued actions (Greenberg, 2002a), and (3) planned between-session exercises wherein clients engage valued actions outside of session. Finally, experiential engagement continues into the concluding sessions, where gains are consolidated and the client is preparing for the end of treatment. Clients and therapists discuss how the new skill set can continue to be utilized in service of responding to difficult events that might arise. In doing this, future stressful and painful life circumstances are explored in experiential exposure exercises that center on hypothetical situations related to core themes that may appear in the future.

Proactive Valued Action

ERT draws from ACT (Hayes et al., 1999, 2011) in stressing the importance of *commitment,* or a willingness to act in accordance with one's values despite the presence of strong security motivations and accompanying distress. This willingness may also involve allowing reward motivations to become more salient and to follow these motivations in the service of valued action. In ERT, commitment is considered to be proactive as it involves intentional actions toward goals that are reflective of stated values. However, outcome and goal achievement are not the purpose of engaging values (Hayes et al., 1999, 2011; Wilson & Murrell, 2004). Rather, values are engaged to be more congruent with what matters most to the client and to help the client be open to the opportunities that come with that flexibility.

The client is invited into the values-identification process through the *stranded on a desert island* exercise (Batten, 2011; Hayes et al., 2011). In this exercise, clients are asked to imagine that they survived an airplane crash and are stranded on a desert island. Before being rescued, the family has a memorial service during which they do not merely say positive things about the client, but rather talk about how the client has actually lived his or her life. The client is then asked to reflect on these things and write down his or her thoughts. Based on this exercise, the therapist and client identify cherished values in the domains (e.g., family, friends, relationships, work, and personal care) wherein the client reports discrepancies between the importance he or she places on this value and how consistently the client been living his or her life accordingly (Wilson & Murrell, 2004).

Imaginal Exposure Task

Wilson and Murrell (2004) note that clients often have difficulty engaging in values work. Thus, ERT approaches values action through systematic experiential exploration, given that clients may still struggle with avoidance of emotional experiencing and could potentially employ their newly acquired skills in an avoidant manner. By encouraging active exploration of valued actions therapists can teach clients how to form a better blueprint for how to live by their values and create new meaningful change. Specifically, imaginal exposure tasks that focus on engaging in *specific* valued actions are conducted (1) to provide the client with an experientially rich rehearsal of the steps that might be necessary to live by her or his values and (2) to confront the emotional challenges that are likely to come up as the client imagines engagement of valued action. In this imagery exposure task, therapists help clients imagine each step involved in engaging this value-congruent action, while noticing changes in the motivational configuration and encouraging utilization of skills to address arising difficulties and obstacles.

Exploring Conflict Themes in Obstacles to Valued Living

The second experiential exposure component involves addressing perceived obstacles to taking valued action. Obstacles reflect the client's internal struggle that prevents him or her from engaging in this valued action. In ERT, obstacles are approached via "conflict themes" including primarily (1) a *motivational conflict* (e.g., security motivations are blocking or interrupting reward efforts) and (2) *self-critical reactive responses to emotions* (i.e., judgmental negative beliefs about one's emotional responses and associated motivations). These conflict themes are addressed in session using an experiential dialogue task derived from emotion-focused therapy (i.e., "chair dialogues"; Elliot et al., 2004; Greenberg, 2002a; see also Thoma & Greenberg, Chapter 11, this volume). In ERT, the motivational conflict is addressed by encouraging clients to engage in a dialogue between the parts of themselves that represent the conflict: the part that is strongly motivated to obtain security and the part that is motivated toward a more unified motivational stance conducive to valued action. Resolution comes from both sides being able to hear and acknowledge the needs of the other and coming to an agreement to commit to the valued action, while allowing a place for a softened obstacle voice to be present without total control. This dialogue task is meant to serve several purposes. First, it serves as exposure to conflict themes, which can cultivate a greater sense of emotional tolerance. Second, the task aims at generating new perspectives (i.e., new meaning) on the obstacles that hinder valued action engagement. Clients are invited to use this greater emotional tolerance and these new perspectives to reflect on their stated values and bring about a greater commitment to taking valued actions.

Translating In-Session Experiential Work to Between-Sessions Valued Living

Finally, valued action is promoted through between-session exercises that expand on the work conducted during the experiential exposure practices. Clients are reminded that protection and avoidance will always be a hindrance to living a values-informed life. Instead of eliminating these struggles, clients are asked to bring these struggles with them and to make appropriate choices to engage valued actions. Clients engage both planned (i.e., specific valued actions related to salient values explored in session and committed to in the presence of therapists) and spontaneous (i.e., any other valued actions clients notice themselves engaging in) valued actions outside of session (Hayes et al., 1999, 2011). Furthermore, clients are encouraged to utilize skills both proactively, when they are planning to engage valued actions, and counteractively, when they notice themselves getting unexpectedly anxious and beginning to respond reactively with worry, reassurance seeking, self-criticism, or behavioral avoidance. Finally, external barriers (i.e., obstacles in the environment that are outside the client's control), which might have been deferred during in-session practices, can also be addressed more actively in between-session exercises.

Future Directions

Individuals with chronic anxiety and recurring depression are characterized by temperamental features that reflect heightened emotional experience (Mennin et al., 2007) and sensitivity to underlying motivational systems related to threat/safety and loss/reward (Klenk et al., 2011; Woody & Rachman, 1994). Typical responses include reactive efforts at avoiding or dampening the emotional experience, often via negative self-referential processing. ERT reflects an attempt to improve treatment for these individuals with a greater delineation of the functional role of emotion than has been the case in traditional therapies. As such, the first half of ERT introduces a number of mindfulness-based practices aimed at providing clients with a set of skills with which they can fully engage their emotional experiences, and approach them in a counteractive rather than a reactive fashion. Building on this set of skills, the second half of ERT is centered on experiential exposure, oriented toward proactive living through values-informed actions.

With promising, albeit preliminary, outcome and mechanism data, ERT continues to be developed and tested. Our model is based on current findings in affect and clinical sciences; however, central tenets of the emotion regulation model await further investigation. Nonetheless, preliminary data are supportive of our hypotheses that ERT may exert its therapeutic impact in part through normalization of emotional processes. As such, it may be most effective for individuals with distress disorders in whom this system is most impaired. We argue that efforts to demonstrate the mechanisms by which treatment produces clinical improvement is best tied to *common* target mechanisms. Experiential processing may reflect a common principle underlying different treatment approaches (Mennin, Ellard, Fresco, & Gross, 2013), and it should be further investigated in terms of how and when it leads to clinical improvement. We seek to more formally test how experiential processing is related to different components of our treatment, including the mindfulness practices and experiential exposure. Some particular lines of research that are under way in our laboratories and clinics include experimental studies of motivational responding and regulation both normatively and in patient subgroups of GAD and MDD while monitoring indices in both the central nervous system (i.e., electroencephology/evoked response potentials; functional magnetic resonance imaging assessment of implicit and explicit emotion regulation) and the parasympathetic nervous system (i.e., tonic, phasic, and ambulatory heart rate variability). We also continue to examine the degree to which these biobehavioral markers are associated with acute and enduring treatment change in the course of ERT. Thus, we continue to refine our perspective as a mechanism-targeted intervention focusing on patterns of motivational dysfunction while cultivating regulation skills with varying degrees of verbal elaboration. We are optimistic that this approach will allow us to make a greater contribution to understanding the mechanisms by which CBTs provide their acute and enduring treatment effects.

Further Resources

- For formative and congruent approaches to mindfulness, acceptance, and compassion, see Gilbert (2010); Hayes, Strosahl, and Wilson (2011); Linehan (1993); Roemer and Orsillo (2009); and Segal et al. (2013).
- For formative and congruent approaches to experiential deepening, see Elliot, Watson, Goldman, and Greenberg (2004) and Greenberg (2002a).
- For further information regarding the developing ERT approach, see Fresco et al. (2013) and Mennin and Fresco (2009, 2013), and *www.emotionregulationtherapy.com*.

References

American Psychiatric Association. (2013). *Diagnostic and statistical manual of mental disorders* (5th ed.). Arlington, VA: Author.

Aupperle, R. L., & Paulus, M. P. (2010). Neural systems underlying approach and avoidance in anxiety disorders. *Dialogues in Clinical Neuroscience, 12,* 517–531.

Bar, M. (2009). A cognitive neuroscience hypothesis of mood and depression. *Trends in Cognitive Sciences, 13,* 456–463.

Barlow, D. H. (2002). *Anxiety and its disorders: The nature and treatment of anxiety and panic* (2nd ed.). New York: Guilford Press.

Batten, S. (2011). *Essentials of acceptance and commitment therapy.* London: Sage

Beck, A. T., Rush, A. J., Shaw, B. F., & Emery, G. (1979). *Cognitive therapy of depression.* New York: Guilford Press.

Borkovec, T. D., & Ruscio, A. M. (2001). Psychotherapy for generalized anxiety disorder. *Journal of Clinical Psychiatry, 62*(Suppl. 11), 37–42.

Borkovec, T., & Sharpless, B. (2004). Generalized anxiety disorder: Bringing cognitive-behavioral therapy into the valued present. In S. C. Hayes, V. M. Follette, & M. M. Linehan (Eds.), *Mindfulness and acceptance: Expanding the cognitive-behavioral traditional* (pp. 209–242). New York: Guilford Press.

Bouton, M. E., Mineka, S., & Barlow, D. H. (2001). A modern learning theory perspective on the etiology of panic disorder. *Psychological Review, 108,* 4–32.

Chorpita, B. F., Albano, A. M., & Barlow, D. H. (1998). The structure of negative emotions in a clinical sample of children and adolescents. *Journal of Abnormal Psychology, 107,* 74–85.

Cougle, J.R., Fitch, K.E., Fincham, F.D., Riccardi, C.J., Keough, M.E., & Timpano,

K.R. (2012). Excessive reassurance seeking and anxiety pathology: Tests of incremental associations and directionality. *Journal of Anxiety Disorders, 26*, 117–125.

Craske, M. G., Kircanski, K., Zelikowsky, M., Mystkowski, J., Chowdhury, N., & Baker, A. (2008). Optimizing inhibitory learning during exposure therapy. *Behaviour Research and Therapy, 46*, 5–27.

Cuijpers, P., van Straten, A., Andersson, G., & van Oppen, P. (2008). Psychotherapy for depression in adults: A meta-analysis of comparative outcome studies. *Journal of Consulting and Clinical Psychology, 76*, 909–922.

Elliott, R., Watson, J., Goldman, R. N., & Greenberg, L. S. (2004). *Learning emotion-focused therapy: The process–experiential approach to change*. Washington, DC: American Psychological Association Press.

Etkin, A., Prater, K. E., Hoeft, F., Menon, V., & Schatzberg, A. F. (2010). Failure of anterior cingulate activation and connectivity with the amygdala during implicit regulation of emotional processing in generalized anxiety disorder. *American Journal of Psychiatry, 167*, 545–554.

Etkin, A., & Schatzberg, A. F. (2011). Common abnormalities and disorder-specific compensation during implicit regulation of emotional processing in generalized anxiety and major depressive disorders. *American Journal of Psychiatry, 168*, 968–978.

Farabaugh, A. H., Bitran, S., Witte, J., Alpert, J., Chuzi, S., Clain, A. J., et al. (2010). Anxious depression and early changes in the HAMD-17 anxiety–somatization factor items and antidepressant treatment outcome. *International Clinical Psychopharmacology, 25*, 214–217.

Foa, E. B., & Kozak, M. J. (1986). Emotional processing of fear: Exposure to corrective information. *Psychological Bulletin, 99*, 20–35.

Fresco, D. M., Mennin, D. S., Heimberg, R. G., & Ritter, M. (2013). Emotion regulation therapy for generalized anxiety disorder. *Cognitive and Behavioral Practice, 20*, 282–300.

Fresco, D. M., Moore, M., van Dulmen, M., Segal, Z., Ma, S., Teasdale, J., et al. (2007). Initial psychometric properties of the Experiences Questionnaire: Validation of a self-report measure of decentering. *Behavior Therapy, 38*, 234–246.

Fresco, D. M., Segal, Z. V., Buis, T., & Kennedy, S. (2007). Relationship of posttreatment decentering and cognitive reactivity to relapse in major depression. *Journal of Consulting and Clinical Psychology, 75*, 447–455.

Gilbert, P. (2010). An introduction to compassion focused therapy in cognitive behavior therapy. *International Journal of Cognitive Therapy, 3*, 97–112.

Gohm, C. L., & Clore, G. L. (2002). Four latent traits of emotional experience and their involvement in well-being, coping, and attributional style. *Cognition and Emotion, 16*, 495–518.

Gray, J. A., & McNaughton, N. (2000). *The neuropsychology of anxiety: An enquiry into the functions of the septo-hippocampal system* (2nd ed.). Oxford, UK: Oxford University Press.

Greenberg, L. S. (2002a). *Emotion-focused therapy: Coaching clients to work through their feelings*. Washington, DC: American Psychological Association Press.

Greenberg, L. S. (2002b). Integrating an emotion-focused approach to treatment into psychotherapy integration. *Journal of Psychotherapy Integration, 12*, 154–189.

Gross, J. J. (2002). Emotion regulation: Affective, cognitive, and social consequences. *Psychophysiology, 39*, 281–291.

Gross, J. J., & Thompson, R. A. (2007). Emotion regulation: Conceptual foundations. In J. J. Gross (Ed.), *Handbook of emotion regulation* (pp. 3–24). New York: Guilford Press.

Halifax, J. J. (2009). *Being with dying: Cultivating compassion and fearlessness in the presence of death.* Boston: Shambhala.

Hayes, S. C., Strosahl, K. D., & Wilson, K. G. (1999). *Acceptance and commitment therapy: An experiential approach to behavior change.* New York: Guilford Press.

Hayes, S. C., Strosahl, K. D., & Wilson, K. G. (2011). *Acceptance and commitment therapy: The process and practice of mindful change* (2nd ed.). New York: Guilford Press.

Jacobson, N. S., Martell, C. R., & Dimidjian, S. (2001). Behavioral activation treatment for depression: Returning to contextual roots. *Clinical Psychology Science and Practice, 8*, 255–270.

Joormann, J., Nee, D. E., Berman, M. G., Jonides, J., & Gotlib, I. H. (2010). Interference resolution in major depression. *Cognitive Affective and Behavioral Neuroscience, 10*, 21–33.

Joormann, J., & Tran, T. (2009). Rumination and intentional forgetting of emotional material. *Cognition and Emotion, 23*, 1233–1246.

Kabat-Zinn, J. (1990). *Full catastrophe living: Using the wisdom of your body and mind to face stress, pain, and illness.* New York: Delta Trade.

Kabat-Zinn, J. (1994). *Wherever you go, there you are.* New York: Hyperion Press.

Keltner, D., & Gross, J. J. (1999). Functional accounts of emotion. *Cognition and Emotion, 13*, 467–480.

Keng, S.-L., Robins, C. J., Smoski, M. J., Dagenbach, J., & Leary, M. R. (2013). Reappraisal and mindfulness: A comparison of subjective effects and cognitive costs. *Behaviour Research and Therapy, 51*(12), 899–904.

Klenk, M. M., Strauman, T. J., & Higgins, E. T. (2011). Regulatory focus and anxiety: A self-regulatory model of GAD–depression comorbidity. *Personality and Individual Differences, 50*, 935–943.

Krueger, R. F., & Markon, K. E. (2006). Reinterpreting comorbidity: A model-based approach to understanding and classifying psychopathology. *Annual Review of Clinical Psychology, 2*, 111–133.

Lang, P. J. (1995). The emotion probe: Studies of motivation and attention. *American Psychologist, 50*, 372–385.

Linehan, M. (1993). *Cognitive-behavioral treatment for borderline personality disorder.* New York: Guilford Press.

MacNamara, A., & Hajcak, G. (2010). Distinct electrocortical and behavioral evidence for increased attention to threat in generalized anxiety disorder. *Depression and Anxiety, 27*, 234–243.

Marra, T. (2004). *Depressed and anxious: The dialectical behavior therapy workbook for overcoming depression and anxiety.* Oakland, CA: New Harbinger.

Martell, C. R., Addis, M. E., & Jacobson, N. S. (2001). *Depression in context: Strategies for guided action.* New York: Norton.

Mennin, D. S., Ellard, K. K., Fresco, D. M., & Gross, J. J. (2013). United we stand: Emphasizing commonalities of cognitive-behavioral therapies. *Behavior Therapy, 44*, 234–248.

Mennin, D. S., & Farach, F. J. (2007). Emotion and evolving treatments for adult psychopathology. *Clinical Psychology: Science and Practice, 14*, 329–352.

Mennin, D. S., & Fresco, D. M. (2009). Emotion regulation as an integrative framework for understanding and treating psychopathology. In A. M. Kring & D. S. Sloan (Eds.), *Emotion regulation and psychopathology: A transdiagnostic approach to etiology and treatment* (pp. 356–379). New York: Guilford Press.

Mennin, D. S., & Fresco, D. M. (2011, November). *Emotion regulation therapy for complex and refractory presentations of anxiety and depression.* A spotlight

presentation delivered at the annual meeting of the Association for Behavioral and Cognitive Therapies, Toronto, Ontario.
Mennin, D. S., & Fresco, D. M. (2013). What, me worry and ruminate about DSM-5 and RDoC?: The importance of targeting negative self-referential processing. *Clinical Psychology: Science and Practice, 20,* 259–268.
Mennin, D. S., & Fresco, D. M. (2014). Emotion regulation therapy. In J. J. Gross (Ed.), *Handbook of emotion regulation* (2nd ed., pp. 469–490). New York: Guilford Press.
Mennin, D. S., Fresco, D. M., Heimberg, R. G., & Ciesla, J. (2012, April). Randomized control trial of emotion regulation therapy for generalized anxiety disorder and comorbid depression. In M. Fraire & T. Ollendick (Chairs), *Emotion regulation in anxiety disorders across the lifespan: Comorbidity and treatment.* Symposium presented at the annual meeting of the Anxiety Disorders Association of America, Arlington, VA.
Mennin, D. S., Fresco, D.M., Heimberg, R.G., & Ritter, M. (2014). *An open trial of emotion regulation therapy for generalized anxiety disorder and comorbid depression.* Unpublished manuscript.
Mennin, D. S., Holaway, R. M., Fresco, D. M., Moore, M. T., & Heimberg, R. G. (2007). Delineating components of emotion and its dysregulation in anxiety and mood psychopathology. *Behavior Therapy, 38,* 284–302.
Michelson, S. E., Lee, J. K., Orsillo, S. M., & Roemer, L. (2011). The role of values-consistent behavior in generalized anxiety disorder. *Depression and Anxiety, 28,* 358–366.
Mogg, K., & Bradley, B. P. (2005). Attentional bias in generalized anxiety disorder versus depressive disorder. *Cognitive Therapy and Research, 29,* 29–45.
Muraven, M. R., & Baumeister, R. F. (2000). Self-regulation and depletion of limited resources: Does self-control resemble a muscle? *Psychological Bulletin, 126,* 247–259.
Newman, M. G., & Llera, S. (2011). A novel theory of experiential avoidance in generalized anxiety disorder: A review and synthesis of research supporting a contrast avoidance model of worry. *Clinical Psychology Review, 31,* 371–382.
Newman, M. G., Przeworski, A., Fisher, A. J., & Borkovec, T. D. (2010). Diagnostic comorbidity in adults with generalized anxiety disorder: Impact of comorbidity on psychotherapy outcome and impact of psychotherapy on comorbid diagnoses. *Behavior Therapy, 41,* 59–72.
Porges, S. W. (2001). The polyvagal theory: Phylogenetic substrates of social nervous system. *International Journal of Psychophysiology, 42,* 123–146.
Ricard, M. (2006). *Happiness: A guide to developing life's most important skill.* New York: Little Brown
Roemer, L., & Orsillo, S. M. (2009). *Mindfulness- and acceptance-based behavioral therapies in practice.* New York, NY: Guilford Press.
Roemer, L., Orsillo, S. M., & Salters-Pedneault, K. (2008). Efficacy of an acceptance-based behavior therapy for generalized anxiety disorder: Evaluation in a randomized controlled trial. *Journal of Consulting and Clinical Psychology, 76,* 1083–1089.
Safran, J. D., & Segal, Z. V. (1990). *Interpersonal process in cognitive therapy.* New York: Basic Books.
Salters-Pedneault, K., Roemer, L., Tull, M. T., Rucker, L., & Mennin, D. S. (2006). Evidence of broad deficits in emotion regulation associated with chronic worry and generalized anxiety disorder. *Cognitive Therapy and Research, 30,* 469–480.
Schultz, D., Izard, C. A., Ackerman, B. P., & Youngstrom, E. A. (2001). Emotion knowledge in economically disadvantaged children: Self-regulatory antecedents

and relations to social difficulties and withdrawal. *Development and Psychopathology, 13,* 53–67.
Segal, Z. V., Williams, J. M. G., & Teasdale, J. D. (2002). *Mindfulness-based cognitive therapy for depression: A new approach to preventing relapse.* New York: Guilford Press.
Segal, Z. V., Williams, J. M. G., & Teasdale, J. D. (2013). *Mindfulness-based cognitive therapy for depression* (2nd ed). New York: Guilford Press.
Stein, M. B., & Paulus, M. P. (2009). Imbalance of approach and avoidance: The yin and yang of anxiety disorders. *Biological Psychiatry, 66,* 1072–1074.
Teasdale, J. D. (1999). Emotional processing, three modes of mind and the prevention of relapse in depression. *Behaviour Research and Therapy, 37,* 553–577.
Teasdale, J. D., Moore, R. G., Hayhurst, H., Pope, M., Williams, S., & Segal, Z. V. (2002). Metacognitive awareness and prevention of relapse in depression: Empirical evidence. *Journal of Consulting and Clinical Psychology, 70,* 275–287.
Thayer, J. F., Åhs, F., Fredrikson, M., Sollers, J. J. 3rd, & Wager, T. D. (2012). A meta-analysis of heart rate variability and neuroimaging studies: Implications for heart rate variability as a marker of stress and health. *Neuroscience and Biobehavioral Reviews, 36,* 747–756.
Watson, D. (2005). Rethinking the mood and anxiety disorders: A quantitative hierarchical model for DSM-V. *Journal of Abnormal Psychology, 114,* 522–536.
Williams, J. M. G., Teasdale, J. D., Kabat-Zinn, J., & Segal, Z. V. (2007). *The mindful way through depression: Freeing yourself from chronic unhappiness.* New York: Guilford Press.
Wilson, K. G., & Murrell, A. R. (2004). Values work in acceptance and commitment therapy. In S. C. Hayes, V. M. Follette, & M. M. Linehan (Eds.), *Mindfulness and acceptance: Expanding the cognitive-behavioral tradition* (pp. 120–151). New York: Guilford Press.
Woody, S., & Rachman, S. (1994). Generalized anxiety disorder (GAD) as an unsuccessful search for safety. *Clinical Psychology Review, 14,* 743–747.

PART V

WORKING WITH INTERPERSONAL PROCESS

Using Clients' and Therapists' Emotional Reactions to Each Other as Vehicles for Change

CHAPTER 15

Relational Techniques in a Cognitive-Behavioral Therapy Context

"It's Bigger Than the Both of Us"

Jeremy D. Safran
Jessica Kraus

Although the therapeutic relationship has been the subject of growing interest within contemporary cognitive-behavioral therapy (CBT) and has come under increased scrutiny by both researchers and practitioners as an important aspect of treatment, there is nevertheless a persistent tendency to see the relationship as something that is independent from the active mechanism of change—a precondition for change rather than the agent of change (cf. Castonguay, Constantino, McAleavey, & Goldfried, 2010). Challenging this view, Safran and his colleagues have long maintained that it is the human encounter—the relationship—between the patient and the therapist that is both a mediating variable for and an important mechanism of change (e.g., Safran & Segal, 1996; Safran & Muran, 2000). From this perspective, any technical intervention—creating a thought record, setting the session agenda, identifying and challenging core beliefs—is inherently inseparable from the patient–therapist relational context in which it occurs.

Our approach to treatment—alliance focused training (AFT)—evolved out of an effort to broaden the scope of cognitive behavioral therapy through the integration of more relationally oriented principles. AFT is conceptualized as a set of core principles and intervention strategies that can be taught to cognitive therapists (or therapists of other orientations) as an adjunctive form of training. These principles and strategies have also been manualized and empirically evaluated as a stand-alone form of treatment known as brief relational therapy (BRT; Safran, 2002; Safran & Muran, 2000). From a theoretical standpoint, AFT draws from a wide range of influences, including writings from the interpersonal tradition, notably Harry Stack Sullivan (1956) and Donald Kiesler (1996); seminal thinking on attachment and mother–infant dyads by Bowlby (1969, 1973, 1980), Ed Tronick (1989), and Beatrice Beebe and Frank Lachmann (2002); contemporary relational psychoanalysis, as exemplified in the writings of Stephen Mitchell (1993), Lewis Aron (1996), and Jessica Benjamin (2004); and postmodern constructivist notions found in the writings of theorists such Irwin Hoffman (1998) and Donnel Stern (1997). While these traditions are diverse, they all converge on the centrality of relational factors in human development and change.

Placing the therapeutic relationship at the center of the change process in psychotherapy does not mean, however, that there is neither theory for therapists to learn nor skills for them to acquire. Rather it means that the theory must clarify the process through which relational encounters bring about change, and that the skills must draw on the therapist's ability to cultivate self-awareness and remain affectively attuned to the subtle interpersonal shifts that occur in the course of treatment. In our practice, an AFT-informed approach to CBT keeps in mind the relational dimension of all interventions in order to broaden therapists' conceptualization of the therapeutic process and the range of strategies available to them (e.g., Safran & Segal, 1996; Safran & Muran, 2000).

For over two decades, Safran and colleagues (e.g., Safran, Muran, Samstag, & Stevens, 2002; Safran, Muran, & Eubanks-Carter, 2011) have endeavored to identify and delineate, through close clinical observation and empirical study, the relationally focused intervention principles that that can promote meaningful psychological change. Over the years, our research has focused on the role of the alliance in the therapeutic process; the identification of alliance ruptures or therapeutic impasses (regarded as strains or breakdowns in the therapeutic alliance); and the development of models of resolution, strategies that offer practitioners guidance for working with patients to successfully work through these episodes of strain or deterioration in the alliance. While a breach or a rupture in the therapeutic alliance can be a serious barrier to treatment, it can also provide an indispensible opportunity to foster growth, insight, and change in both patient and therapist.

This chapter is intended to serve as a brief introduction to the underlying theory, empirical evidence, and clinical application of techniques that guide a relationally orientated approach to CBT.

Background and Theoretical Orientation

Interpersonal Theory and Self-Schemas

While working as a CBT practitioner during the 1980s, Safran became intrigued by moments in treatment when the adherent application of cognitive techniques led to deterioration in the quality of patient–therapist relationship and the therapeutic alliance (Safran, 1998). Turning to the interpersonal theory of the influential and iconoclastic American psychotherapist and treatment consultant Harry Stack Sullivan (1956) as a means of addressing what he regarded to be the limitations of cognitive strategies, Safran found that Sullivan's theories were not only congenial to a CBT approach but offered the potential of enriching it (Safran, 1984). Sullivan believed that at a fundamental level all human behavior was driven by the need for human relatedness. Consequently, it was impossible to understand the individual outside of the interactional field or interpersonal context in which interactions with others occurred. Sullivan maintained that this principle extended across all relationships, including the relationship occurring between patient and therapist in the course of treatment (Sullivan, 1956).

Sullivan theorized that people organize information about new acquaintances on the basis of expectations developed through their earliest interactions (Sullivan, 1956). Central to his system is the concept of *personifications*, the self–other cognitive models that inform and direct perception and behavior. Because Sullivan held that an individual's sense of security in the world was predicated on potential relatedness to others, he argued that activation of anxiety played a crucial role in the maintenance and regulation of interpersonal or "me–you patterns," as he termed them. Thus, any interaction inconsistent with one's *self-personification* could potentially evoke intense anxiety.

Consistent with this line of reasoning and based on ethological observations (the scientific study of animal behavior), John Bowlby (1969) hypothesized that infants have an instinctive need to maintain proximity to their primary caregivers or attachment figures in order to maximize survival and maintain a sense of security. When the infant's relationship to his or her caregiver is disrupted, behavioral systems that maintain proximity with the caregiver become activated. Bowlby theorized that infants develop *internal working models* (IWMs) to enable them to anticipate interactions with attachment figures and minimize the potential threat of separation or loss.

Maladaptive Schemas, Cognitive–Interpersonal Cycles, and Metacommunication

Both interpersonal and attachment theories posit that relational schemas or IWMs persist throughout life. Although these play an adaptive role in a developmental context, early experiences with primary caregivers that are maladaptive can lead to the development of interpersonal schemas that are dysfunctional within new situations; the persistence of such schemas within subsequent relationships becomes a maladaptive means of seeking connection (Bowlby, 1969; Safran, 1990a). For example, the individual who as a child had to suppress feelings of vulnerability to maintain interpersonal closeness with early caregivers may come to habitually stifle or disown these "unacceptable" feelings. Within the context of new relationships, this behavior may make him appear remote or emotionally disengaged. Accordingly, the distancing responses that are characteristically evoked in others reinforce the individual's belief that his feelings are indeed unacceptable, confirming the conviction of being fundamentally flawed and unlovable (Safran, 1984; Safran & Segal, 1996). Because relational schemas continue to shape the way that people interact with others, they in turn define and limit the ways in which others relate to them.

Such negative interpersonal patterns that are repeatedly enacted have been referred to as *vicious circles* (Wachtel, 1997) or *cognitive–interpersonal cycles* (e.g., Safran, 1990a). The development and ongoing perpetuation of rigid concepts of self and others is a central source of psychological dysfunction. By unwittingly clinging to these patterns, people blind themselves to the ever-changing nature of experiences and foreclose the possibility of new ways of relating. Sullivan believed one of the most effective means therapists had of assessing and working with patients' dysfunctional interpersonal schemas was to monitor their own emotional reactions in response to patients' "me–you patterns" in the course of treatment. He maintained that the therapist acted as a "participant-observer" in the interaction with the patient, both experiencing the tug of the patient's maladaptive interpersonal schema while also seeking to intervene in a fashion that would elicit new and more adaptive behavior (Safran, 1990b; Safran & Segal, 1996; Sullivan, 1956).

Drawing on the work of Sullivan, Kiesler (1996) described and operationalized the ways in which interpersonal exchanges are governed by *complementarity*. This proposition holds that, within relationships, specific interpersonal behaviors on the part of one individual can "pull for" or evoke particular responses in the other. For instance, by acting in a rigidly dominant fashion, one member of a dyad tends to pull for submission in the other. Similarly hostility tends to pull for counterhostility. Because of the subtlety of nonverbal cues, people are often unaware of what they are responding to when reacting in a complementary fashion.

In terms of the therapeutic relationship, the therapist who experiences the characteristic "tug" or "pull" of the patient's interpersonal pattern must be able to identify, disengage from, and, at an appropriate moment, communicate with the patient about the implicit transaction taking place within the treatment. Both therapist and patient can then collaboratively begin to explore, challenge, and disconfirm the patient's maladaptive expectations regarding interpersonal exchanges. Kiesler termed this technique *metacommunication* (Kiesler, 1996). Within our approach metacommunication has become one of a number of important intervention strategies (Safran & Muran, 2000).

Metacommunication is an attempt to bring ongoing awareness to the emergent patient–therapist interactive process. We conceptualize metacommunication as a type of *mindfulness in action* (see Safran & Muran, 2000, and Safran and Reading, 2008, for elaborations of this point). As much as possible, this metacommunication is grounded in the therapist's immediate experience of some aspect of the therapeutic relationship (either the therapist's own feelings or his or her experience of some aspect of the patient's actions or affect). The objective is to initiate an explicit exploration of something that is being unconsciously enacted, often through the therapist's disclosure of thoughts or impressions, but it can also involve other acts as well (e.g., sharing observations, asking questions, speculating) (Safran & Muran, 2000). Principles related to metacommunications will be addressed at greater length in the "Clinical Applications" section of this chapter.

From One-Person to Two-Person Approaches

Sullivan's position that the therapist assumes the role of participant-observer represented a radical departure from Freud's original view of the therapist as an objective and neutral observer who serves as a blank screen onto which the patient projects his transferences (Safran, 2012). Though influenced by Sullivan's contributions as well as other theorists, contemporary relational psychoanalytic theorists nonetheless depart from the notion that the therapist can ever fully step outside the interpersonal field. The therapist's goal still remains one of ultimately understanding and helping the patient; however, there is an appreciation that this cannot be accomplished without an ongoing process of self-exploration on the therapist's part (Safran, 2012; Safran & Muran, 2000). Within a contemporary relational two-person approach, both the therapist and the patient are regarded as coparticipants in an unfolding experience who engage in a process of mutual influence at both conscious and unconscious levels (Aron, 1996; Mitchell, 1993; Safran & Muran, 2000).

From our perspective, this two-person approach has a number of important implications for psychotherapy. First, it suggests that clinical formulations must always be guided by and revised in light of information gleaned from an ongoing exploration of what is taking place in the therapeutic relationship. Second, it is critical for the therapist to engage in a continuous examination of his or her contributions to the interaction. Third, because the therapist, from a two-person perspective, is always contributing to the dynamic interaction, the extent to which the interaction parallels relational patterns in the patient's daily life must remain an open question (Safran & Muran, 2000).

The Therapeutic Alliance, Ruptures, and Repairs

Numerous psychotherapy research studies have consistently shown that the quality of the therapeutic alliance is one of the better predictors of outcome across a range of different treatment conditions (Horvath, Del Re, Fluckiger, & Symonds, 2011; Martin, Garske, & Davis, 2000). The concept of the therapeutic alliance has had a long and controversial history in the psychoanalytic tradition (for a fuller discussion, see Safran & Muran, 2000, and Safran & Muran, 2006a). In the past three decades, however, the concept has spread to other therapeutic traditions including CBT, in large measure owing to Bordin's (1979) seminal reformulation of the alliance into transtheoretical terms. He proposed that the alliance is a function of the extent to which the patient and the therapist are able to maintain a strong relational bond as they collaborate on the tasks and goals of treatment. Bordin viewed the alliance as an ongoing process of "building and repair" (Bordin, 1983, p. 36). This view influenced our earliest thinking on the topic of negotiating ruptures in the therapeutic relationship and continues to inform our research and practice (Doran, Safran, Waizmann, Bolger, & Muran, 2012; Safran, Crocker, McMain, & Murray, 1990). Bordin's conceptualization of the alliance is at once mutual and dynamic. Thus, this dyadic negotiation both establishes the necessary conditions for change to take place and is an intrinsic part of the change process.

Alliance ruptures are conceptualized as episodes of tension, deterioration, or breakdown in the collaborative process between patient and therapist and can emerge when both patient and therapist are drawn into maladaptive interpersonal cycles (Safran & Muran, 2006a; Safran et al., 2011). Within our research, alliance ruptures are characterized as either *withdrawal* or *confrontation* events, each of which is defined by distinct patterns of patient communication or behavior. In a *withdrawal rupture*, the patient may fall silent, offer minimal responses to questions, or suddenly shift topic to an unrelated matter. In a *confrontation rupture*, the patient may directly express anger, resentment, or dissatisfaction with the therapist or some aspect of the treatment. Whether the behavior manifests as withdrawal or as confrontation, once the therapist becomes aware of the rupture, he or she can begin to disengage from the cycle of enactment. The therapist does this by drawing the patient's attention through metacommunication to what is taking place within the relationship as a means of exploring the patient's habitual interpersonal pattern. We emphasize the need for therapists to cultivate a stance of ongoing awareness of their subjective reactions as a vital source of information that enables them to break the cycle rather than continuing to react in a way that is consistent with the patient's maladaptive beliefs (Safran & Muran, 2000; Safran & Segal, 1996).

When therapist and patient begin to explore a rupture in the alliance, change can occur by way of two parallel processes: *decentering* and *disconfirmation* (Safran & Segal, 1996). *Decentering* involves expanding patients' awareness of both their internal processes and how they interact with others. As patients become more aware of their interpersonal schemas and self-defeating interactional patterns, the therapeutic relationship also provides an opportunity for the *disconfirmation* of these schemas. When the therapist does not respond to the patient in the complementary fashion that the patient has come to expect (e.g., the therapist responds to hostility with compassion rather than counterhostility), he or she is granted a new and affirming experience, one that suggests that there may be other ways of interacting than with the limited relational repertoire in which they habitually engage. The therapist's capacity to understand and tolerate the patient's painful emotions during a rupture can, in turn, help patients discover that neither they nor their relationships will necessarily be destroyed by painful, aggressive feelings. The patient can gradually see the other as potentially available and the self as capable of negotiating relatedness, even in the context of relational strain or tension (Safran & Muran, 2000; Safran & Segal, 1996).

Learning to negotiate the needs of the self versus the needs of others is both a critical developmental task and an ongoing challenge of human existence. Many of the problems that people bring into therapy are thus influenced, at least in part, by difficulties they have in negotiating this tension in a constructive fashion. The development of a relationship with the therapist inevitably involves this type of ongoing negotiation between two different subjectivities at both conscious and unconscious levels (Safran & Muran, 2000). This process can have an important impact on the patient's fundamental sense of the extent to which he or she lives in a potentially negotiable world or needs to compromise his or her own sense of integrity in order to hold onto relationships (Mitchell, 1993).

Empirical Evidence

Beginning in the mid-1980s at the Clarke Institute of Psychiatry of the University of Toronto, and continuing at Beth Israel Medical Center in New York in 1990, Safran and colleagues (most notably Chris Muran) developed and manualized a treatment approach specifically designed for negotiating or resolving ruptures in the therapeutic alliance (Safran & Muran, 2000). As previously noted, this approach can be administered as a stand-alone treatment modality known as brief relational therapy (BRT) or incorporated into the training and supervision of cognitive therapists in the form of alliance-focused training (AFT) in order to enhance their ability to work constructively with alliance ruptures.

Our focus on identifying and addressing alliance ruptures builds on the strong consensus in the research literature that the quality of the alliance is a robust predictor of outcome across a wide range of therapeutic approaches (e.g., see Horvath et al., 2011, and Martin et al., 2000, for meta-analyses). Several studies have found that close attention to alliance ruptures in the session may play an important role in successful treatment (e.g., Foreman & Marmar, 1985; Lansford, 1986; Rhodes, Hill, Thompson, & Elliott, 1994).

Our program of alliance rupture research comprises four iterative stages: model development, model testing, treatment development, and treatment evaluation (Muran, Safran, Samstag, & Winston, 2005; Safran & Muran, 1996; Safran et al., 2002). In the first stage of the research program, we conducted a series of intensive analyses of therapy sessions in which alliance ruptures had reached some degree of resolution (Safran & Muran, 1996). Based on our observations, we developed a stage-process model of rupture resolution in which: (1) the therapist becomes aware of the behavior/communication associated with rupture ("rupture marker"), (2) the therapist initiates collaborative exploration of the rupture experience, (3) the therapist helps patient to overcome avoidance of addressing feelings or response to rupture, and (4) an exploration of the emergence of patient's underlying wish or need is revealed in the course of working through the rupture event. We also conducted a series of analyses to verify the existence of the hypothesized sequences of events within resolution sessions and to demonstrate a difference between resolution and nonresolution sessions (Safran & Muran, 1996). This study confirmed that when therapists addressed alliance ruptures in a manner consistent with our model, this approach facilitated resolution of the rupture. The goal of the model is not to set forth a rigid prescriptive, but rather to help clinicians develop pattern-recognition abilities that can facilitate the intervention process (for a full description of the stage-process model, see Safran & Muran, 2000).

In the treatment development stage of our program, we drew on our findings from the model development and testing stages, and developed a treatment that includes interventions that facilitate rupture resolution (Safran, 2002; Safran & Muran, 2000). The treatment evaluation stage of our research program served to assess the efficacy of the treatment and to provide a verification of the model. We conducted a clinical trial comparing BRT with CBT and a short-term dynamic treatment (STDP) with 128 patients with Cluster C and those with personality disorder not otherwise specified diagnoses (Muran et al., 2005). The majority of the patients in this sample were also comorbid for DSM-IV Axis I diagnoses. The results of this study showed that BRT was as effective as CBT and short-term dynamic psychotherapy and had fewer patient dropouts than the other two treatments. In a related pilot study, Safran, Muran, Samstag, and Winston (2005) found evidence that BRT was more effective for patients with whom it was difficult to establish a therapeutic alliance than either CBT or STDP.

Safran, Muran, and colleagues are currently exploring ways to integrate relational alliance-focused principles into standard cognitive therapy. A study funded by the National Institute of Mental Health is under way to investigate whether integrating rupture resolution training improves therapy process and outcome. Preliminary findings suggest that after therapists receive eight sessions of AFT while treating an ongoing cognitive therapy case, there is less evidence of negative interpersonal process (defined as patient hostility) than there is prior to receiving AFT (Safran et al., 2014). In recent years a number of independent research teams have found evidence regarding the positive impact of augmenting cognitive therapy and other treatment modalities with alliance-focused treatment principles derived from our research program (e.g., Castonguay et al., 2004; Constantino et al., 2008; Crits-Christoph et al., 2006; Harmon et al., 2007; Newman, Castonguay, Borkovec, Fisher, & Nordberg, 2008).

Although the empirical evidence for both the process and the outcome of treatment interventions informed by the principles described in this chapter is promising, there are important limitations. Some of the research is limited by small samples. Other commonly cited findings in the area are based on qualitative research studies that have not yet been validated with quantitative research designs (cf. Safran et al., 2011). Although the number of empirical studies in the area has increased in recent years, there is an important need for more research conducted with large samples of patients with different characteristics by independent investigators. Empirical evidence is also limited by lack of racial/ethnic diversity of both patients and therapists.

Clinical Applications of Relational Methods

In a study we are currently conducting, therapists who have already been trained to conduct CBT and have completed one short-term case while adhering to the CBT protocol, are subsequently introduced to AFT while treating a second CBT case (Safran et al., 2014). Through AFT, therapists are taught to monitor what is taking place in the therapeutic relationship on an ongoing basis and asked to attend to their own feelings as important sources of information about what may be happening within the relationship. In cases in which patients appeared to be benefiting from the use of cognitive-behavioral interventions, therapists are encouraged to continue using these interventions, while at the same time becoming more mindful of distinctive relational patterns or subtle ruptures that might be playing out between them and their patients in sessions. In other cases, in which the use of cognitive interventions appeared to be problematic, therapists are encouraged to modify their approach more dramatically—in some instances actually abandoning the use of cognitive-behavioral interventions in order to focus more intensively on the use of relational interventions (e.g., metacommunication, therapists' exploration of their own contributions to enactments, in-depth exploration of patients' emerging feelings in context of the therapeutic relationship).

Throughout treatment, therapists guided by AFT principles make extensive use of therapeutic metacommunication (i.e., communicating about implicit relational communications) as a means of increasing the patient's awareness of what is transpiring in the session. Below are some basic metacommunication principles (for a fuller elaboration of these principles, see Safran & Muran, 2000).

1. *Explore with skillful tentativeness and emphasize one's own subjectivity.* Therapists should communicate observations in a tentative and exploratory fashion. The message at both explicit and implicit levels should be one of inviting patients to engage in a collaborative attempt to understand what is taking place. It is also crucial to emphasize the subjectivity of one's perceptions since this encourages patients to use the therapist's observations as a stimulus for self-exploration rather than feeling compelled to react to what could seem like either positive or negative authoritative statements. For example, if a patient's response to a suggested homework assignment is muted or he or she exhibits signs of anxiety or tension, the therapist might metacommunicate in the following way: "I noticed that you began to twist your ring when I suggested the assignment and my sense is that perhaps there was something about this that caused you discomfort, or made you feel criticized. I realize I may be off the mark, but I wonder if this at all relates to what you may be feeling right now."

2. *Do not assume a parallel relationship with other relationships.* A therapist should be wary of prematurely attempting to establish a link between the configuration that is being enacted in the therapeutic relationship and other relationships in the patient's life. In addition to being inconsistent with a two-person psychology, interpretations of this type can be experienced by patients as blaming. Instead, the focus should be on exploring patients' internal experiences and actions in a nuanced fashion, as they emerge in the moment.

3. *Accept responsibility.* Ground all formulations in awareness of one's own feelings and accept responsibility for one's own contributions in an open and nondefensive manner. Since each participant is contributing to the interaction in ways of which they are unaware, it is essential to continually attempt to clarify the nature of the contribution. This process can help patients become more aware of feelings that they have but are unable to articulate clearly, in part because they fear the therapist's response. For example, if the therapist becomes aware of sounding critical or blaming, the therapist might say: "I'm aware that I may have sounded harsh or impatient just now. I wonder if that was your experience as well." Such an acknowledgement on the part of the therapist has the potential of freeing patients to express feelings of hurt or resentment; validate their experience of the interaction; and teaching them that they can trust their own judgment.

Increasing patients' confidence in their own judgments may also help to decrease their need for defensiveness, in turn facilitating their exploration and acknowledgment of their own contribution to the interaction.

4. *Start where you are.* Metacommunication should be based on the therapist's feelings and intuitions that emerge in the moment. What was true in one session may not be true in the next, and what was true at the beginning of a session may not be true later in that same session. Therapists should not simply apply supervisors' or colleagues' suggestions; rather, they should seek to become aware of their own experience of patients and to accept and work through their feelings in the moment. For example, the therapist may provide specific feedback related his or her immediate experience of the patient: "Right now, I sense that you seem very wary of me." Or, "As you're speaking, I'm aware of feeling excluded by you now, like you're pushing me away. Do you have any sense of that?" Such metacommunications may facilitate the exploration of thoughts or feelings that the patient regards as unacceptable or frightening.

5. *Focus on the concrete and specific.* Whenever possible, questions, observations, and comments should focus on concrete instances in the moment rather than on generalizations. This promotes experiential awareness rather than abstract, intellectualized speculation. For example, "I am experiencing you as pulling away from me right now. Do you have any awareness of doing this?" When providing therapeutic feedback, rather than saying, "You tend to speak in a very abstract way," the therapist can say, "What you're saying right now seems kind of abstract to me." This type of concreteness and specificity helps patients to cultivate greater self-awareness.

6. *Evaluate and explore patients' responses to interventions.* Therapists should monitor the quality of patients' responsiveness to interventions on an ongoing basis. Does the patient use the therapist's intervention as a stimulus for further exploration? Does he or she respond in a minimal fashion without elaboration? Does he or she not respond? It is important here for the therapist to attend to subtle intuitions about the quality of the patient's responsiveness. If an intervention leads to a decrease in relatedness, then the therapist needs to explore the patient's experience of the intervention. Close attention to patients' responses to interventions can help to clarify their interpersonal schemas. It can also lead to a progressive refinement in therapists' understanding of their own contribution to the interaction.

7. *Establish a sense of collaboration and we-ness.* Patients often feel alone during a rupture. It can be helpful for therapists to frame the impasse as a shared dilemma that patient and therapist will explore collaboratively by acknowledging that "we are stuck together." For instance, a therapist

might say, "It feels like the two of us are playing chess." Or, "It feels like we're both being very tentative right now." Or, "It feels like I'm constantly intruding, and you're trying to politely keep me out. What do you make of that?" In this way, instead of being yet one more in an endless succession of figures who do not understand the patient's struggle, the therapist can become an ally who joins the patient.

8. *Expect resolution attempts to lead to more ruptures, and expect to revisit ruptures.* Even the most thoughtfully and sensitively delivered metacommunication can exacerbate a rupture or lead to a new one. Metacommunication is not an ultimate intervention, but a step in the process of rupture resolution. In addition, therapists often find that the same impasse is revisited many times. Therapists should try to appreciate the ways in which each occurrence is unique, and respond in the immediacy of the moment.

9. *Judiciously disclose and explore your own experience.* Therapists' feelings of being stuck or paralyzed often reflect their difficulty in acknowledging and articulating to themselves what they are currently experiencing. The process of articulating one's feelings to patients can free the therapist to intervene more effectively. It can also clarify the nature of the cognitive–interpersonal cycle in which the patient and the therapist are caught. Another valuable intervention that is related to self-disclosure is inviting patients to suggest ways that the therapist might be contributing to the interaction or to speculate about what the therapist might be experiencing internally. For example, a therapist might ask, "I wonder if you have any thoughts about what may be going on for me right now?" This invitation can help to clarify the patient's experience of the therapist and may lead to further elaboration of the patient's interpersonal schemas. It can also provide new insight into the therapist's contributions to the impasse.

Case Illustration

The following case was first described in Safran and Muran (2000).[1] Ruth contracted to receive 30 sessions of BRT as part of an ongoing psychotherapy research program. She was an attractive, young-looking 52-year-old woman who had been divorced for 16 years. She had one daughter in her 20s, who was no longer living at home. She had ended her marriage of 12 years at the age of 36 because she felt her husband was controlling, emotionally abusive, and generally unable or unwilling to be responsive to her emotional needs. Since her divorce, she had had a series of short-term affairs with men, which typically would end because of her dissatisfaction with her partners. She tended to become involved with men she looked

---

[1] Portions of this case have been adapted from Safran and Muran (2000). Copyright 2000 by The Guilford Press. Adapted by permission.

down on and reported feeling afraid of pursuing men she was more interested in out of fear of being rejected. At the beginning of treatment she admitted that as she grew older she desperately wanted to be in a "real relationship" but felt hopeless about the possibility. A second presenting problem revolved around her feelings of being "disempowered" and not being treated respectfully by colleagues at work.

Although the therapist initially felt very sympathetic toward her, a pattern developed fairly rapidly in which he had difficulty maintaining a sense of emotional engagement with her and found himself biding time until the sessions ended. He became aware of a tendency on her part to tell long stories with considerable obsessional detail, and to do so in an unemotional, droning fashion that left the therapist feeling distant and unengaged. In addition, he found that she seldom paused as if to welcome his input or feedback. Although he would often begin sessions with a renewed intention of taking an interest in her, he typically ended up feeling bored and vaguely irritated.

In an attempt to understand what was being enacted between them, the therapist began to metacommunicate about his emotional disengagement. She seemed responsive to his feedback and indicated that on various occasions she had received feedback of a similar kind from others in her life and that she was eager to come to understand how her own inner struggles and characteristic way of coping with them might be contributing to this dynamic. Over time, Ruth and the therapist's understanding of the configuration's being enacted in the relationship became clearer to some extent. She was able to articulate an underlying fear of abandonment that led her to defend against her vulnerable feelings by controlling her style of presentation. Although the therapist felt encouraged by her openness to exploring what was going on between them, he had an intuition that something did not feel quite right—perhaps an element of compliance in her response or a vague sense of himself beginning to play the sadistic role in a sadomasochistic enactment. At different points the therapist shared with Ruth his sense that she seemed all too ready to work with whatever he presented. At one level, she seemed to take this observation in and work with it, but, at another level, it felt as if even this response had an element of compliance.

During Session 16, after listening to an extended and rather difficult-to-follow monologue about a conflict Ruth was having with her neighbors over the custody of a stray dog, the therapist finally interrupted and metacommunicated to her in the following way:

THERAPIST: I find myself poised to start talking with you about it . . . but sort of waiting for an opening.
RUTH: Oh . . . OK . . .

THERAPIST: I also find myself wondering a little bit about the extent to which you're really wanting or inviting my input.

RUTH: I really do.

THERAPIST: You do?

RUTH: Well . . . I want it to whatever extent you feel comfortable getting involved.

THERAPIST: Yeah?

RUTH: I mean . . . I guess . . . that's why there's a hesitancy . . . I guess there's an assumption on my part . . . that you don't want to be involved . . . that you're throwing it back to me.

THERAPIST: So it sounds like you're reluctant to directly ask me for my help because you assume I won't respond.

RUTH: Yeah.

The therapist's metacommunication about her impact on him (i.e., his feelings of uncertainty about whether she wants his input) seems to facilitate Ruth's capacity to express her desire for help more directly. This led to an extended exploration of Ruth's feelings about asking for and receiving help.

RUTH: Umm . . . (*voice shaky*) I think it's really hard for me to say . . . what I want . . . and it's even harder . . . and why I think it's so hard is it's . . . I can't imagine that I'll get it. You know that, umm . . . and I've really just become aware of how . . . kind of at such a core level, there is this kind of . . . a sense of having been disappointed in getting what I want.

THERAPIST: Uh-huh.

RUTH: So, I mean, I think that's, you know, umm . . . kind of a very big defense I have, like kind of shrouding what I want in a way.

An important shift took place several weeks later during session 19, which Ruth began by telling the therapist about how she had experienced a minor comment of his at the end of the previous session as extremely validating. During the previous session she talked about a situation at work in which she was feeling chastised and infantilized by her superior and felt powerless to change the situation. Since the session was at the end, the therapist had remarked something to the effect of, "This seems like something important to talk about. There are some important issues here."

When the therapist asked Ruth what she had found helpful about his comment, she remarked that it had reassured her that he didn't think she was petty or that she had set up the problem situation at work herself. At the same time, she began to wonder out loud why she had such a lack of confidence that the therapist's minor comment at the end of the session was so important to her. When the therapist responded that he had been wondering about the same thing, she spontaneously connected her response to times in the past when he had commented on his feelings of being disengaged from her, and she had responded by attempting to work with his observation. At this point, she began to shift the topic, and the therapist encouraged her to explore what had occurred internally at the moment prior to the shift. She responded: "What came to mind is, 'Well, that's probably good because I'm a good patient,' and then I just think of saying, 'Well, now I want to be a bad patient. Like now I don't want to be nice.'" Then she went on to tell a story about a friend who had been in therapy and had one day knocked her therapist's books off the shelf in anger. In the rest of the session the therapist and Ruth began to explore the way in which her tendency to comply in an attempt to be a "good girl" was a theme that cut across many situations for her.

In the following session, she began, for the first time, to complain more directly about what she felt she was not getting from the therapist in treatment. Whereas the previous session felt like a preliminary, playing with the possibility of acknowledging her dissatisfaction, in this session, her frustration, anger, and disappointment felt more tangible. She began the session by indicating that she was aware that the treatment was more than halfway through—she asked for the therapist's evaluation of how things were going so far and for a plan for the rest of the treatment. With his encouragement, she was eventually able to tell him that she needed more emotional engagement from him and that she did not want to try to be a more interesting person in order to keep his interest.

In contrast to the previous session, there were times in this session when the therapist felt strongly chastised and pressured to provide her with something that he was not sure he was able to provide. At the same time, her ability to express her need for more emotional engagement helped the therapist to empathize more fully with her experience of not feeling accepted and validated by him. In this and subsequent sessions she was also able to contact sad and painful feelings of being hurt by the therapist's failure to accept and prize her as she wished him to. Witnessing the emergence of these feelings led to a subtle but irrevocable shift in the therapist's perception of her. Although there continued to be periods during which her characteristic, emotionally flat, droning style of speaking continued, the therapist found himself more engaged during these times than he had been in the past. It was as if he were now unable to experience this aspect of her without simultaneously seeing her as a whole person with hopes, dreams, and frustrated yearnings.

The experience of challenging him and seeing that the relationship was able to survive enabled her subsequently to bring her feelings of despair and the underlying vulnerable and dependent feelings into the relationship. She began the following session by saying that, although she had left the previous session "all fired up" and ready to make changes in her life, she found herself sinking back into an apathetic inertia. She then made a passing allusion to feeling that she needed someone to help her out of her inertia. When the therapist asked her if she felt as though she needed help from him right now, she began to cry slightly and to speak about her feelings of disappointment and loss in life in general. The therapist was aware of feeling somewhat touched by her tears, but also somewhat distanced, as if he were not being allowed fully into her experience. The therapist asked if she was aware of her shift to a general focus rather than on the situation unfolding between them in the moment. She acknowledged that she was aware and that she felt that she wanted to push her feelings back inside because she felt she was being self-pitying.

Further exploration led her to articulate a fear of "blubbering and not even being able to talk," her anticipation of consequent embarrassment, and a desire to be by herself. At this point the therapist conveyed to her his sense of being "kept outside," and his remark led to an exploration of the way in which she was pulling away from him in her pain and sadness. This helped her to articulate a fear of being abandoned by him, accompanied by deep and heartfelt sobbing. There followed a tearful exploration of how she had spent so much of her life depriving herself of real contact and support from people because of her difficulty in acknowledging to herself how deeply she wanted to be nurtured and cared for. She then expressed her relief at being able to share her painful feelings and longings with the therapist, mixed with sadness and feelings of loss in the acknowledgment of having spent so many years without receiving the contact and support she needed.

In subsequent sessions together they explored Ruth's fears and sadness about imminent abandonment by him, as well as her anger. Ruth began Session 23 by talking about her fears of abandonment in general.

RUTH: I have this fear of being abandoned and disappointed. And so I guess I just shut down and cut people out of my life.

THERAPIST: In the back of my mind I'm thinking that we only have six or seven more sessions, and so I'm wondering about this whole issue of opening up and being abandoned in this context.

RUTH: Well, it does make me sort of scared when I start thinking about the ending. And I guess that's true of me in general. I guess I'm reluctant to really involve myself deeply in relationships . . . but the desire is still there.

THERAPIST: Uh-huh . . . I have a sense of a real yearning inside of you. (*Ruth begins to cry and then stops herself.*) What's happening for you?

RUTH: Well, it starts to hurt, and then I think, intellectually, "It's so inappropriate for me to be upset about therapy ending."

THERAPIST: It doesn't seem inappropriate to me. We've worked together for a while now and really started to develop a relationship, and my sense is that you're beginning to open up and trust. And we're ending soon . . . and that's got to be painful.

RUTH: Well, and I guess part of it is the finiteness of it. I leave with whatever feelings I have, and for you, it's like, "Good. That was a tough one. That's over." And then you go on with something else.

Ruth and the therapist began to discuss the inequity of the situation and her anger at him. She also spontaneously drew a parallel between the asymmetry of their investment in the relationship and a general tendency for the men she felt deeply about to not reciprocate the depth of her feelings. In the following session, the theme of inequity emerged once again. Ruth returned to the concern that the therapist would be glad when things were over. She then spontaneously told him that she did not want the therapist to tell her whether she was right about his feelings, because, if he denied what she claimed, she might not believe him, and, if he did not she would be upset.

Further exploration helped her to elaborate on her concerns about the therapist's feelings toward her and to articulate her desire that he really care about her. Putting this yearning into words led to more sadness, but also to a feeling of satisfaction about her ability to take the risk of revealing her desires. The session ended with Ruth returning to her feelings of hurt and anger about the fact that the therapist had not volunteered to meet beyond the preestablished termination session. The therapist empathized with her feelings and told her that he believed it was legitimate for her to feel both hurt and angry with him.

She began Session 28 by talking about her difficulty trusting that men are interested in her or care about her, unless they go overboard in their attempts to woo her. When they did do this, however, she said she had a tendency to lose herself. She maintained that given this pattern, she felt good that she was starting to feel OK about her relationship with the therapist, despite his not having actively reassured her. She told a story about a recent encounter with a male friend, in which she had difficulty trusting that he would be there for her, despite evidence to the contrary.

THERAPIST: It sounds as though normally there's a real lack of faith that relationships will work out.

RUTH: Yeah. (*Appears touched by this comment.*) That really captures something important. Normally I tend to devalue relationships when I don't get much active reassurance from people. And I guess there's a risk of my doing that to some extent with our relationship because you're not proposing that we extend our meetings.

THERAPIST: What I'm thinking is that you really need and deserve somebody to be there for you on an ongoing basis, and I'm wondering if you can still find anything of value in our relationship despite the fact that I'm not going to be there for you in the future in the way you deserve.

RUTH: (*beginning to cry slightly*) I'm thinking about it, and I think it's OK. I don't feel abandoned by you. I'm sad, I think, because I'm so aware in this moment of the way my lack of faith in people and fear of abandonment have acted as obstacles to my getting into a good relationship. And I'm thinking about my daughter as well . . . how her lack of faith in relationships gets in the way. I know this is a bit of a digression, but I guess I'm identifying with her. . . . This is an important place to come to. And I thought I wasn't going to cry today (*said with a slightly jocular tone followed by a short period of silence*). I feel like thanking you. And then saying goodbye (*said quickly in a jocular tone*).

THERAPIST: This feels like an awkward moment?

RUTH: Yeah. It feels a little difficult staying with the feeling of contact with you.

THERAPIST: So some of what's going on is that, along with the pain, you feel a sense of connection with me and of gratitude. That's what's uncomfortable.

RUTH: Yeah. Any sort of closeness. It's almost like I have to cut that feeling. I think one time we talked about how I start to feel suffocated when I feel intimate. [During a previous session, Ruth and her theripist had begun to explore such feelings when they emerged during a moment of intimacy between them, and this had led to some associated childhood memories.]

THERAPIST: Can you say anymore about this feeling of suffocation?

RUTH: I guess it's something about the welling up of all these emotions. There's some part of me that always wants to push it down. I don't know what would happen if I didn't. I don't know if it's about being exposed or being out of control. I don't know. But I want to contain it. It's bigger than the both of us (*laughing, then pause*). I don't know what love really is. I think I have it with my daughter . . . but even that . . . it's not direct. The direct expression of feelings is very hard.

THERAPIST: Uh-huh. I was wondering when you said, "It's bigger than the both of us." I know you were laughing, but it sounded interesting.

RUTH: Well, when you ask what am I afraid of . . . I'm afraid that feelings . . . they're consuming. . . . I think I've been in an environment where feelings were so measured . . . It's almost like a family image that comes to me . . . where things aren't stopped, where they're not repressed . . . where they're bountiful. I think my natural exuberance as a child was prohibited. But it's just that letting things tumble out of you in an unrestrained way and letting yourself be doesn't mean that horrible things are going to tumble out.

THERAPIST: But it sounds as if the fear is that it's all consuming and that you don't really know where it's going to lead, in a way.

RUTH: Yes.

THERAPIST: And maybe that's what you mean when you say, "It's bigger than the both of us."

RUTH: Yes.

THERAPIST: Because there's a kind of uncharted territory in a way.

RUTH: Yeah.

THERAPIST: For me as well. I feel a sense of contact with you right now . . . a sense of connection and intimacy, and there's a sense that the feelings are not something I have control of.

RUTH: Yeah. I think that's it. "You've got to keep the reins on." But the idea of it is such a wonderful image for me.

THERAPIST: Well I was struck by your words before, "A family image." "Bountiful." There's a real sense of richness there."

The final two sessions were devoted to summing up and consolidation. Ruth's feeling was that the seed of a new way of being in relationships was beginning to grow in her. She was able to acknowledge her sadness about separating from the therapist and her anxiety about the future, as well as a growing optimism and belief that things could be different in her life. Things had not changed dramatically at work, nor had she gotten into a new relationship with a man. But she felt a subtle sense of beginning to feel more empowered in general and more hopeful about the possibility that things would be different for her in intimate relationships.

Clinical Discussion

There will inevitably be both subtle and not-so-subtle levels at which we, as therapists, fail to accept our patients. Only by becoming aware of and acknowledging the ways in which we are not being fully accepting can we become more so. This process involves an ongoing internal examination of our contributions to the shifting dynamic and an active engagement in ongoing dialogue with the patient, in which the therapist judiciously shares aspects of his or her subjective experience in an attempt to facilitate an exploration of what is being enacted in the relationship.

The therapist's process of metacommunicating about his difficulty staying engaged with Ruth helped him to make explicit that which was already implicit—that is, his difficulty being there for her in a present and attuned fashion on a consistent basis. By acknowledging to himself and Ruth an aspect of his experience that made it difficult for him to be more accepting, a process was initiated that ultimately allowed him to become more present and emotionally available. There were times within their sessions when the therapist felt strongly chastised, pressured, and momentarily at a loss as to how to respond to Ruth's pressure. At the same time, Ruth's ability to express her need for more emotional engagement helped the therapist to empathize more fully with Ruth's experience of not feeling accepted and validated by him.

By encouraging Ruth to tell him about the impact of his metacommunication on her, and by being receptive to her feedback, the therapist was able to develop an affective appreciation of her dilemma, in part, as a result of his increased experiential appreciation of the way he had become a perpetrator in a victim–abuser cycle. The experience of challenging the therapist and seeing that their relationship was able to survive this challenge enabled Ruth subsequently to bring her feelings of despair, as well as her vulnerability and dependency, more fully into the relationship.

A pivotal moment in treatment arrived as Ruth and her therapist collaboratively explored the "uncharted territory" within their relationship, an experience of expansiveness that was at once "bountiful" and frightening: "It's bigger than the both of us." One way of understanding the experience that Ruth is describing here is that the process of working through the alliance rupture, expressing her wishes and needs to the therapist, and collaboratively negotiating a new type of relatedness with the therapist afforded her intimations of a fuller and more "bountiful" sense of a relational encounter. This type of encounter is referred to by Benjamin (2004) as a cocreated intersubjective space in which both partners surrender to a process, rather than actively trying to shape it.

Although various strands in the work were never completely tied together, and certain issues were touched on but not explored in depth, this lack of closure—although particularly heightened by time-limited treatment—is true of all treatment. Learning to live with this type of ambiguity is one of the important lessons for patients and therapists alike. In a sense, termination can be thought of as the ultimate rupture in the alliance. Thus the termination process can provide a valuable opportunity for patients to learn to negotiate the conflicting needs for agency and relatedness in a constructive fashion without disowning either of the two needs.

Future Directions

In this chapter we have emphasized the centrality of the therapeutic relationship in promoting change. We have attempted to present how technical and relational aspects are always inseparable, irrespective of the mode of treatment. As we have proposed, the exploration and resolution of ruptures within the therapeutic relationship can play a critical role in helping patients to overcome self-limiting interpersonal patterns. Moreover, ruptures or breaches are particularly important moments to explore because they are representative of a fundamental dilemma of human existence—the innate desire for interpersonal relatedness and the reality of our separateness. In life, we must negotiate the paradox that by the very nature of our existence we are both alone and yet inescapably in the world with others (Safran, 1993). In this regard, our emphasis on the use of the inevitable ruptures within the therapeutic relationship provides opportunities for patient and therapist to negotiate and explore authentic connection yet allows them to maintain a healthy sense of autonomy. We encourage CBT practitioners to consider how the dynamic patient–therapist relational principles we have presented can be used as a framework for setting the course of treatment and guiding technique.

Further Resources

Books

- For a comprehensive guide to negotiating ruptures in the therapeutic alliance that synthesizes theory, empirical research, training, and clinical experience, see Safran and Muran (2000).
- For a fuller investigation of the integration of cognitive with interpersonal traditions illustrated with clinical vignettes, see Safran and Segal (1996).
- See Safran (1998) for a collection of key papers on broadening the theoretical and technical scope of CBT.
- For an informative and concise primer on the evolution of psychoanalysis and psychodynamic therapies, see Safran (2012).

DVDs

- See Safran (2008 & 2010) and Safran & Muran (2006b) for a series of training videos that demonstrate basic principles of therapeutic metacommunication in negotiating and repairing ruptures in the patient–therapist alliance.

References

Aron, L. (1996). *A meeting of minds: Mutuality in psychoanalysis.* Hillsdale, NJ: Analytic Press.
Beebe, B., & Lachmann, F. M. (2002). *Infant research and adult treatment.* Hillsdale, NJ: Analytic Press.
Benjamin, J. (2004). Beyond doer and done to: An intersubjective view of thirdness. *Psychoanalytic Quarterly, 73,* 5–46.
Bordin, E. (1979). The generalizability of the psychoanalytic concept of the working alliance. *Psychotherapy: Theory, Research, and Practice, 16,* 252–260.

Bordin, E. S. (1983). A working alliance based model of supervision. *Counseling Psychologist, 11,* 35–42.
Bowlby, J. (1969). *Attachment and loss: Vol. 1. Attachment.* New York: Basic Books.
Bowlby, J. (1973). *Attachment and loss: Vol. 2. Separation, anxiety and anger.* New York: Basic Books.
Bowlby, J. (1980). *Attachment and loss: Vol. 3. Sadness and depression.* New York: Basic Books.
Castonguay, L. G., Constantino, M. J., McAleavey, A. A., & Goldfried, M. R. (2010). The therapeutic alliance in cognitive-behavioral therapy. In J. C. Muran & J. P. Barber (Eds.), *The therapeutic alliance: An evidence-based guide to practice* (pp. 150–171). New York: Guilford Press.
Castonguay, L. G., Schut, A. J., Aikins, D. E., Constantino, M. J., Laurenceau, J. P., Bologh, L., et al. (2004). Integrative cognitive therapy for depression: A preliminary investigation. *Journal of Psychotherapy Integration, 14,* 4–20.
Constantino, M. J., Marnell, M. E., Haile, A. J., Kanther-Sista, S. N., Wolman, K., Zappert, L., et al. (2008). Integrative cognitive therapy for depression: A randomized pilot comparison. *Psychotherapy: Theory, Research, Practice, Training, 45,* 122–134.
Crits-Christoph, P., Gibbons, M. B., Crits-Christoph, K., Narducci, J., Schramberger, M., & Gallop, R. (2006). Can therapists be trained to improve their alliances?: A preliminary study of alliance-fostering psychotherapy. *Psychotherapy Research, 16,* 268–281.
Doran, J. M., Safran, J. D., Waizmann, V., Bolger, K., & Muran, J. C. (2012). The Alliance Negotiation Scale: Psychometric construction and preliminary reliability and validity analysis. *Psychotherapy Research, 22,* 710–719.
Foreman, S. A., & Marmar, C. R. (1985). Alliances in psychotherapy. *American Journal of Psychiatry, 142,* 922–926.
Harmon, S. C., Lambert, M. J., Smart, D. M., Hawkins, E., Nielsen, S. L., Slade, K., et al. (2007). Enhancing outcome for potential treatment failures: Therapist–client feedback and clinical support tools. *Psychotherapy Research, 17,* 379–392.
Hoffman, I. Z. (1998). *Ritual and spontaneity in the psychoanalytic process: A dialectical–constructivist view.* Hillsdale, NJ: Analytic Press.
Horvath, A. O., Del Re, A. C., Flückiger, C., & Symonds, D. (2011). Alliance in individual psychotherapy. *Psychotherapy: Theory, Research, Practice, Training, 48,* 9–16.
Kiesler, D. J. (1996). *Contemporary interpersonal theory and research: Personality, psychopathology, and psychotherapy.* New York: Wiley.
Lansford, E. (1986). Weakenings and repairs of the working alliance in short-term psychotherapy. *Professional Psychology: Research and Practice, 17,* 364–366.
Martin, D. J., Garske, J. P., & Davis, M. K. (2000). Relation of the therapeutic alliance with outcome and other variables: A meta-analytic review. *Journal of Consulting and Clinical Psychology, 68,* 438–450.
Mitchell, S. A. (1993). *Hope and dread in psychoanalysis.* New York: Basic Books.
Muran, J. C., Safran, J. D., Samstag, L. W., & Winston, A. (2005). Evaluating an alliance-focused treatment for personality disorders. *Psychotherapy: Theory, Research, Practice, Training, 42,* 532–545.
Newman, M. G., Castonguay, L. G., Borkovec, T. D., Fisher, A. J., & Nordberg, S. S. (2008). An open trial of integrative therapy for generalized anxiety disorder. *Psychotherapy Theory, Research, Practice, Training, 45,* 135–147.
Rhodes, R. H., Hill, C. E., Thompson, B. J., & Elliott, R. (1994). Client retrospective recall of resolved and unresolved misunderstanding events. *Journal of Counseling Psychology, 41,* 473–473.
Safran, J. D. (1984). Assessing the cognitive-interpersonal cycle. *Cognitive Therapy and Research, 8,* 333–347.

Safran, J. D. (1990a). Towards a refinement of cognitive therapy in light of interpersonal theory: I. Theory. *Clinical Psychology Review, 10,* 87–105.
Safran, J. D. (1990b). Towards a refinement of cognitive therapy in light of interpersonal theory: II. Practice. *Clinical Psychology Review, 10,* 107–121.
Safran, J. D. (1998). *Widening the scope of cognitive therapy: The therapeutic relationship, emotion, and the process of change.* Northvale, NJ: Aronson.
Safran, J. D. (2002). Brief relational psychoanalytic treatment. *Psychoanalytic Dialogues, 12,* 171–195.
Safran, J. D. (2008). *Relational psychotherapy.* Washington, DC: American Psychological Association Press.
Safran, J. D. (2010). *Psychoanalytic therapy over time.* Washington, DC: American Psychological Association Press.
Safran, J. D. (2012). *Psychoanalysis and psychoanalytic therapies.* Washington, DC: American Psychological Association Press.
Safran, J. D., Crocker, P., McMain, S., & Murray, P. (1990). Therapeutic alliance rupture as a therapy event for empirical investigation. *Psychotherapy: Theory, Research, Practice, Training, 27,* 154–165.
Safran, J. D., & Muran, J. C. (1996). The resolution of ruptures in the therapeutic alliance. *Journal of Consulting and Clinical Psychology, 64,* 447–458.
Safran, J. D., & Muran, J. C. (2000). *Negotiating the therapeutic alliance: A relational treatment guide.* New York: Guilford Press.
Safran, J. D., & Muran, J. C. (2006a). Has the concept of the therapeutic alliance outlived its usefulness? *Psychotherapy: Theory, Research, Practice, Training, 43,* 286–291.
Safran, J. D., & Muran, J. C. (2006b). *Resolving therapeutic impasses.* Santa Cruz, CA: Customflix.
Safran, J. D., Muran, J. C., Demaria, A., Boutwell, C., Eubanks-Carter, C., & Winston, A. (2014). Investigating the impact of alliance-focused training on interpersonal process and therapists' capacity for experiential reflection. *Psychotherapy Research, 24,* 269–285.
Safran, J. D., Muran, J. C., & Eubanks-Carter, C. (2011). Repairing alliance ruptures. In J. C. Norcross (Ed.), *Psychotherapy relationships that work* (2nd ed., pp. 224–238). New York: Oxford University Press.
Safran, J. D., Muran, J. C., Samstag, L. W., & Stevens, C. (2002). Repairing alliance ruptures. In J. C. Norcross (Ed.), *Psychotherapy relationships that work: Therapist contributions and responsiveness to patients* (pp. 235–254). New York: Oxford University Press.
Safran, J. D., Muran, J. C., Samstag, L. W., & Winston, A. (2005). Evaluating an alliance-focused treatment for potential treatment failures. *Psychotherapy, 42,* 512–532.
Safran, J. D., & Reading, R. (2008). Mindfulness, metacommunication, and affect regulation in psychoanalytic treatment. In S. Hick & T. Bien (Eds.), *Mindfulness and the therapeutic relationship* (pp. 122–140). New York: Guilford Press.
Safran, J. D., & Segal, Z. V. (1996). *Interpersonal process in cognitive therapy.* New York: Basic Books.
Stern, D. B. (1997). *Unformulated experience.* Hillsdale, NJ: Analytic Press.
Sullivan, H. S. (1956). *Clinical studies in psychiatry.* New York: Norton.
Tronick, E. Z. (1989). Emotions and emotional communication in infants. *American Psychologist, 44,* 112–119.
Wachtel, P. L. (1997). *Psychoanalysis, behavior therapy, and the relational world.* Washington, DC: American Psychological Association Press.

CHAPTER 16

Adding an Interpersonal–Experiential Focus to Cognitive-Behavioral Therapy for Generalized Anxiety Disorder

Thane M. Erickson
Michelle G. Newman
Adam McGuire

Interpersonal and emotional processing therapy (I/EP) is an integrative psychotherapy that was developed and tested to complement standard cognitive-behavioral therapy (CBT) in the treatment of clients suffering from generalized anxiety disorder (GAD). This approach draws on experiential and interpersonal principles in order to target core dysfunctions not adequately addressed in traditional CBT. The present chapter provides the background and theory of I/EP, preliminary evidence of efficacy, detailed elaboration of the treatment strategies, and discussion of limitations and future directions.

Background and Theory

CBT for GAD

GAD is defined by the cardinal symptom of uncontrollable worry about multiple topics not circumscribed to other DSM-5 disorders, and at least three symptoms among restlessness, fatigue, concentration problems, irritability, muscle tension, and sleep disturbance (American Psychiatric Association, 2013). These symptoms persist for most days over 6 months or more and cause significant impairment (American Psychiatric Association, 2013), as consistent with evidence of impact of GAD on quality of life, employment, finances, and health (e.g., Kessler, Greenberg, Mickelson, Meneades, & Wang, 2001; Massion, Warshaw, & Keller, 1993). CBT has demonstrated efficacy as the "gold standard" treatment of GAD, surpassing effects of receiving no treatment, pill placebo, and nondirective and psychoanalytic therapy (Borkovec & Ruscio, 2001; Durham, Chambers, MacDonald, Power, & Major, 2003). This treatment typically incorporates self-monitoring, progressive muscle relaxation, identification and cognitive restructuring of worries, and self-control desensitization. Nonetheless, CBT is less efficacious for GAD than for other anxiety disorders (Brown, Barlow, & Liebowitz, 1994), with approximately 50% of clients reaching high end-state functioning after treatment, at best (Newman, Castonguay, Borkovec, & Molnar, 2004); thus, there exists much room for improvement.

Problems Not Targeted in Traditional CBT for GAD

Although CBT alleviates some of the core GAD symptoms, it fails to fully address factors theorized to contribute to or maintain GAD—namely, avoidance of emotional processing (Borkovec, Alcaine, & Behar, 2004) and problematic interpersonal behaviors in significant relationships and the therapeutic relationship (Newman et al., 2004). First, excessive worry in GAD has been conceptualized as a way to avoid experiential awareness or emotional processing of fears. Individuals with subclinical or clinical GAD seem particularly sensitive to specific emotions (Turk, Heimberg, Luterek, Mennin, & Fresco, 2005), emotional disclosure (Erickson & Newman, 2007), or, in our most recent formulation, shifts from positive to negatively valenced emotions (Newman & Llera, 2011). Worry may prohibit full experiential engagement with other, deeper emotional concerns (Borkovec et al., 2004). Exposure therapy is one traditional CBT technique that has been used to therapeutically increase clients' affective arousal. However, the approach still tends to emphasize control over emotions (Wiser & Goldfried, 1993) rather than deepening of experience to increase clients' awareness of emotional needs (Greenberg, Rice, & Elliott, 1996), many of which pertain to significant relationships.

Research has demonstrated robust links between interpersonal factors and GAD or worry (see Newman & Erickson, 2010). First, GAD clients report troubled childhood relationships with their parents (e.g., Cougle et al., 2010) and disrupted attachment (Cassidy, Lichtenstein-Phelps, Sibrava, Thomas, & Borkovec, 2009). Second, chronic worry and GAD status predict negative social-cognitive processes such as worries about relationships (Roemer, Molina, & Borkovec, 1997), self-reported interpersonal sensitivity (Hoehn-Saric, Hazlett, & McLeod, 1993), and biased attention to threatening faces (Mogg, Millar, & Bradley, 2000). Third, GAD is linked to problematic social behavior, as suggested by self-reported interpersonal problems (e.g., Przeworski et al., 2011), lack of close friends (Whisman, Sheldon, & Goering, 2010), and increased likelihood of divorce or separation (Whisman, 2007) or low marital satisfaction (Whisman et al., 2000). In addition, interpersonal problems (Borkovec, Newman, Pincus, & Lytle, 2002; Crits-Christoph, Gibbons, Narducci, Schamberger, & Gallop. 2005), marital tension (Durham, Allan, & Hackett, 1997), partner hostility (Zinbarg, Lee, & Yoon, 2007), and personality disorders (Ansell et al., 2011) predict lower GAD remission or response to CBT, implying that interpersonal processes may maintain GAD symptoms. Additionally, experiential avoidance is theorized to contribute to interpersonal problems (Newman et al., 2004). However, conventional CBT fails to address such processes.

Given evidence of problems in significant relationships, individuals with GAD may also engage in problematic processes in the therapeutic relationship. Analogue GAD participants in social interaction tasks have shown relatively poor awareness (over- or underestimation) of their interpersonal impact on confederates (Erickson & Newman, 2007). Similarly, worry uniquely (controlling social anxiety and depressive symptoms) predicted significant others' ratings of hostile interpersonal impact, in contrast to self-reported interpersonal styles (Erickson, Newman, & Abelson, 2010). Studies have not yet examined the therapy relationship in GAD treatment, but the foregoing findings are consistent with clinical observations of low awareness of impact on therapists in GAD clients (Newman et al., 2004). Additionally, findings that CBT therapists using manualized treatments may overlook the therapeutic alliance (Castonguay, Hayes, Goldfried, & DeRubeis, 1995) provide impetus for increased attentiveness to this relationship, beyond traditional CBT foci.

Overview of I/EP

Because of the limitations of conventional CBT for GAD, Newman et al. (2004) developed the I/EP therapy to target avoidance of emotional processing and interpersonal processes with significant others and in the therapeutic relationship. I/EP was designed to augment, rather than to replace, CBT. Like CBT, I/EP strives to identify and replace maladaptive behaviors, but the two approaches differ in the behaviors targeted and the strategies employed (Newman et al., 2004). Whereas CBT teaches skills consistent with GAD clients' existing strengths in the cognitive domain (e.g., analyzing situations and using thoughts to manage emotions), I/EP focuses on experiential engagement with avoided emotional, often interpersonal, content—a skill deficit seemingly common in persons with GAD. Such a goal requires disclosure and vulnerability with others, experiencing feared emotions, and receptivity to feedback about one's impact on others, as well as tolerance for discussing the therapy relationship. Although these strategies are more common in experiential and psychodynamic therapies, we conceptualize them in terms of general CBT principles applied integratively: detailed examination of clients' cognitive and interpersonal strategies to avoid emotional processing (functional analysis), experiential deepening of particular emotional states (exposure), therapist disclosure of emotional and interpersonal reactions to clients (modeling), and learning new ways to manage emotions (skills training).

I/EP was developed as a sequential module to complement traditional CBT. The two therapies have been "packaged" sequentially into 2-hour sessions for 14 weeks. Each session consists of 55 minutes of CBT, followed by 55 minutes of I/EP (Newman et al., 2004). This division of components within each session derives from both scientific and practical rationales. The scientific reasoning for distinct modules is that an additive design permits empirical "dismantling" of incremental effects of I/EP beyond traditional CBT. From a practical perspective, separate modules ensure dedication of time to both skill sets. We have observed that clients with GAD often naturally favor in-session work on cognitive strategies to regulate emotion (e.g., CBT)—strategies consistent with their tendencies toward cognitive analysis—and prefer to avoid working on experiential awareness of emotion and its impact on others. Scheduling time to work separately on both distinct domains prevents such avoidance.

Evidence

Several elements integrated into I/EP have demonstrated therapeutic effects in psychotherapy process and outcome studies with non-GAD samples. For instance, meta-analyses show that alliance rupture repair is robustly associated with enhanced treatment outcomes (Safran, Muran, & Eubanks-Carter, 2011), and strategies designed to enhance emotional awareness (e.g., empty-chair and two-chair techniques) do indeed predict deeper emotional experiencing (Greenberg, Elliott, & Lietaer, 1994). However, the overall package has also been tested in several preliminary psychotherapy treatment outcome studies examining the effects of CBT plus I/EP for GAD.

The initial open trial ($N = 21$) tested the efficacy of 14 sessions of this treatment package (Newman, Castonguay, Borkovec, Fisher, & Nordberg, 2008). First, the results showed clinically significant changes in anxiety and interpersonal problems. Using a 20% improvement in at least four of six anxiety outcome measures as a marker for clinically significant changes in anxiety, 83.3% of participants demonstrated clinically significant change at posttreatment, 58.8% at a 6-month follow-up, and 76.5% at a 1-year follow-up. Similarly, 95% of participants were classified as low functioning interpersonally at pretest, whereas this percentage reduced to 55.6% by posttreatment. Combined CBT + I/EP demonstrated a larger pre–post effect size for anxiety symptoms when compared to the average effect size in a meta-analysis of CBT (Borkovec & Ruscio, 2001).

Subsequent to these promising results, Newman et al. (2011) conducted a randomized controlled trial testing the CBT + I/EP treatment ($N = 43$) versus CBT plus supportive listening (CBT + SL; $N = 40$). SL encouraged self-reflection in a supportive context without direct advice. Both conditions adopted the sequential format. This additive design permitted a rigorous test of the incremental effect of I/EP, controlling for the amount of time clients spent with therapists. The treatments did not differ in attrition, credibility, or client expectancy for success, and both led to pre–post improvements with large effect sizes for GAD symptom severity, depression, and interpersonal problems, along with the maintenance of benefits from posttreatment to a 2-year follow-up. Additionally, medium effect sizes in the direction of higher clinically significant change for CBT + I/EP on end-state functioning at 6 and 24 months emerged. Because the sample size was only powered to detect large effects, the advantages of CBT + I/EP did not reach statistical significance. However, the findings do suggest that a larger sample size with increased statistical power may have more robustly shown the incremental benefits of I/EP. Thus, the extant trials establish that CBT + I/EP for GAD is feasible, well-tolerated, and as efficacious or trending toward higher efficacy relative to standard CBT, as demonstrated in an extremely conservative study design. In future publications we plan to examine treatment moderators, mediators, and process measures.

Application

Exploration of Current Interpersonal Patterns

The foundation for I/EP is a thorough (one to two sessions) inventory of a client's interpersonal relationships. The inventory examines current problematic interpersonal patterns and past, developmentally important relationships (e.g., those from clients' families of origin). However, once a broad assessment of these relationships is conducted, I/EP emphasizes exploration of present relationships with immediate emotional primacy.

Subsequent to the inventory, exploration of current problematic relational patterns comprises the first main task of I/EP. Several principles govern this process. First, consistent with core experiential/Gestalt sensibilities, a *present-moment focus* permeates the exploration of relationships where possible. Individuals with GAD often use worry to avoid more pressing or emotionally evocative issues (Borkovec & Roemer, 1995); they may perseverate on past experiences or discuss abstractions of their problems in a way that halts emotional immediacy. The therapist must attentively monitor such behaviors and their functions, gently discouraging them, and inviting elaboration about "here-and-now," emotionally alive situations from daily life.

Second, the I/EP therapist emphasizes *specificity* in the exploration of interpersonal patterns. The client is invited to discuss concrete, "blow-by-blow" descriptions of interpersonal transactions with other people, in contrast to the topographically "flat" descriptions that are common in worriers. Therapists help clients identify particular recent problematic interactions, with in-session changes in affect as a marker for material that warrants exploration. Consistent with functional analysis of behaviors in CBT, I/EP entails an *interpersonal* functional analysis in which the therapist and client closely examine concrete interactions, clarifying the client's behaviors, their intended function (interpersonal goals), concomitant emotions, impact of these behaviors on the other person, and whether the behaviors met the desired outcome or goal.

Third, exploration of current relationships requires therapist and client attentiveness to *emotionally evocative content and needs* during examination of particular interactions. As clients are encouraged to concretely examine or relive such interactions, they may experience emotions that they originally experienced *in situ*. Clients are challenged to permit themselves to fully experience the emotion evoked, prior to higher-order cognitive analysis. Typically, a salient interpersonal need (e.g., desire for intimacy) or fear (e.g., fear of rejection) is present in such interactions. After promoting experiential deepening around these needs or fears, therapists help clients to identify cognitive, behavioral, or interpersonal strategies they used to dampen awareness of these emotions in the situation (e.g., their function in terms of negative reinforcement). Additionally, they are encouraged to examine not only the *intrapersonal* goal behind such strategies, but also the *interpersonal* consequences for their and others' emotions. Avoidance strategies may elicit undesirable responses from others, or even those very responses that are most feared.

As in CBT, the style of Socratic questioning is present. "Open questions" by the therapist serve as the main technique for orienting clients to the concrete particulars of social interactions. The following open "process" questions are used (therapeutic purpose in parentheses):

"What happened between you and the other person?" (Orients client to specific interaction.)
"What emotions did you feel?" (Invites client to attend to emotional experience.)
"What did you need or hope to get from this person?" (Clarifies goals for the interaction.)

"What did you fear from the other person?" (Clarifies problematic interpersonal schemas.)

"What did you do?" (Encourages client to link interpersonal behaviors to goals or fears.)

"How did he or she respond? What happened next between you and the other person?" (Encourages client to notice impact of behavior on partner, and whether the strategy accomplished desired goal.)

The therapist can cycle back through questions as needed.

Here is an illustrative therapist–client exchange:

CLIENT: I'm so annoyed and stressed over my boss. He doesn't get that I don't want to work overtime. And my daughter obviously doesn't respect me, given that she won't do her chores even when I ask repeatedly. I got so irritated from nagging her that I eventually had to just let her do what she wanted because I couldn't handle the conflict. And my husband is driving me crazy. He's so busy with his hobbies that I don't know how I'll get him to make family time . . .

THERAPIST: As I hear you listing off the stressful situations in your life right now, it's clear that you have a lot on your plate. I wonder if you are aware of jumping from one stressful topic to the next, without fully attending to any of these important issues.

CLIENT: I guess that talking about one stressful situation just blurs into the next for me sometimes.

THERAPIST: If you could check in with yourself, especially your shoulders and neck . . . which of these situations feels the most intense?

CLIENT: Hmmm. When I think about my daughter and power struggles with her, my chest and neck feel tight. I don't like it.

THERAPIST: This situation seems important for you, . . . and important for us to examine closely. What did you want to happen when you were interacting with your daughter?

CLIENT: I really wanted for her to just dump the trash and clean out the cat litter without my nagging. I wish I could help her to see herself as a contributing member of the family and to take pride in the little things like that. I worry that she won't ever learn that.

THERAPIST: So what did you do, in order to pursue these goals?

CLIENT: Well, I just felt helpless and got more irritated, so I guess I just started barking at her.

THERAPIST: How did that work?

CLIENT: (*wry smile*) It didn't. I just felt . . . guilty.

THERAPIST: What was that like?

CLIENT: It was a big knot in my stomach. I just wanted to hide.

THERAPIST: You felt strong anger and guilt. How did you deal with those feelings?

CLIENT: I felt bad so I just backed off and dropped the conversation.

THERAPIST: How did that impact her? What message do you think she walked away with?

CLIENT: Well, she looked fearful when I was badgering her, and then was quiet when I left the room. I guess she probably didn't know what to make of it.

THERAPIST: You felt understandably upset, but nagging only led to guilt, which led to leaving the situation. Unfortunately, rather than your daughter learning to feel pride over participating in family chores, she was left confused. I wonder if there might be other, more effective strategies that you could experiment with in this situation.

In this vignette, the therapist helped the client notice her process of worrying out loud" while recounting emotion-evoking events from the week, shifting attention to current emotions as a marker to guide exploration of a specific, evocative social interaction. One situation was dissected with greater concreteness and specificity in terms of relevant emotions, goals, and behaviors, laying the groundwork for consideration of alternative social strategies.

Exploration of Past Relationships

Although I/EP therapists encourage clients to first process current or recent emotionally salient social interactions, this focus does not preclude examination of past relationships. I/EP assumes that clients' social needs and fears, as well as their problematic interpersonal strategies for dealing with them, have likely been learned in formative relationships in earlier developmental epochs. One feature that makes I/EP "integrative" is its explicit examination of developmental experiences in detail. Akin to psychodynamic/analytic therapies promoting "insight," I/EP helps clients to understand links between current interpersonal strategies and the developmental matrices out of which they arise. Whereas traditional cognitive therapies permit brief examination of these experiences as explanations for current beliefs and schemas, I/EP encourages vivid, extended recall of emotionally laden childhood experiences. Exploring past relational experiences helps clients conceptualize their maladaptive interpersonal strategies as understandable efforts to meet developmental needs, promoting emotional acceptance rather than self-judgment. Ultimately, though, as in CBT, such explorations culminate in renewed focus on current social interactions and functional analysis thereof.

Additionally, the impact of clients' consideration of past–present links is most pronounced when clients, not therapists, make the links. Open-ended questions that invite clients to explore are again central, welcoming active engagement instead of passive receptivity. The therapist may invite the client to recall a particularly evocative relational memory, providing emotional and physiological details. Alternatively, following experiential processing of current situations, the therapist may ask whether the needs, fears, or interpersonal strategies discussed in session played a role in earlier relationships (transitions from both present to past and vice versa are acceptable, provided that discussion facilitates emotional salience rather than abstract reflection). Once the client selects a past particular memory, he or she is encouraged to concretely examine the sequence of interpersonal transactions and emotions as they unfolded, using the same open questions (above) as described for current interactions. After experiential processing of current and relevant past interactions, clients are asked for perceived links between childhood experiences, resultant needs and fears, and adult interpersonal strategies they use to manage them (albeit not successfully).

For instance, in the following vignette, the client explores an emotionally evocative memory encapsulating her interpersonal wish, and the therapist helps her to recognize links to a current situation and her behavior therein:

THERAPIST: In discussing your hopes for your relationship with your daughter, you used the word "pride" several times, and hinted at your own childhood experiences. What does pride mean to you, in this situation?

CLIENT: I have this vivid memory of having dinner with my best friend's family when I was maybe 10. She put a ton of care into setting the table, and her brother cleaned up afterward; they both seemed so proud to contribute to their family by doing chores, and to share this with me. They just beamed. It was just so different from my family, where none of us were expected to do much, and there was no sense of teamwork. Back then, I felt jealous of my friend's family. I wished we felt more like a family, like we were working toward something.

THERAPIST: So "pride" for you is a sense of working together, of feeling like a close-knit family. You saw it in another family, and wanted to feel that in your own family, where it was absent. How does that emotion connect back to the events of this week?

CLIENT: Um . . . now that I have kids, I'm afraid it's going to be just like my childhood. I'm worried that we can't do any better, that the type of family I want isn't possible for me.

THERAPIST: So you worry that you won't find it. And that leads to the irritability and nagging your daughter, which you mentioned hasn't brought you any closer to meeting this need.

CLIENT: Exactly. It's weird to admit it, but I guess that this desire to have a close family . . . and fear that it won't happen . . . are in the back of my mind a lot of the time.

Attending to the Therapeutic Relationship

In addition to exploring past and present relationships with significant others, the therapeutic relationship itself constitutes a means for clients to learn experientially about their typical strategies and more effective alternatives. The I/EP therapist must attend closely to the therapist–client relationship. Informed by psychodynamic and interpersonal therapies, I/EP assumes that clients commonly enact their characteristic interpersonal strategies with the therapist, often without metacognitive awareness. Thus, attending to this relationship is a means of managing the risk of interpersonal processes interfering with therapy, as well as providing another emotionally alive context for learning. Several steps comprise the process of learning from instances of clients acting out problematic interpersonal behaviors in session.

First, therapists must be willing to permit themselves to be temporarily "hooked" into the client's typical interaction pattern (Safran & Segal, 1990). On the basis of the principle of interpersonal complementarity, one person's social behavior probabilistically constrains the behavior of an interaction partner. For example, the client's yielding behavior invites dominant therapist behavior and vice versa; the client's cold or warm behavior invites similar behavior by the therapist (Kiesler, 1996). As "participant-observers" (Sullivan, 1953) in social interactions, therapists cannot always avoid falling into predictable responses elicited by clients. Initially, the therapist may be unwittingly drawn into behaviors that confirm the client's interpersonal schemas or expectations, reinforcing interpersonal or emotional avoidance. This process is normal but may derail therapy if therapists remain stuck in collusion. However, when managed well, the process forms an important basis for subsequent learning.

While attending to the interpersonal processes in therapy sessions, and in particular to the therapist's own internal emotional experience, the therapist becomes aware of having been "hooked." Rather than mounting a direct challenge to the client or premature encouragement of behavior change, the therapist first conducts a brief self-assessment, monitoring his or her own emotional reactions and (often unintentional) contributions to the problematic client-therapist interaction pattern. For instance, the therapist may experience a sense of impasse or shared helplessness in the therapy, feelings of low attachment to the client, or even irritability. Additionally, therapists may become aware of colluding by avoiding clients' emotionally evocative material. Common examples include excessive joking, prematurely comforting clients (vs. gentle encouragement toward experiential contact with emotions), or passively permitting clients to engage in tangential, worry-like, or abstract accounts of problems. The latter can be a common, persistent, problem in working with GAD clients.

Allowing oneself to temporarily recapitulate client patterns in session prevents premature challenges to clients and provides an experiential window into client behaviors that may generalize to other relationships; however, the therapist must "unhook" from such patterns to prevent undue confirmation of client schemas. After examining the transactional pattern and his or her own contributions to it, the therapist invites the client to shift attention to the "here-and-now" interpersonal process. This further heightens clients' awareness of interpersonal expectations, needs, and strategies for dealing with them. Metacommunication about therapist–client interaction patterns is a relatively neutral, noncomplementary interpersonal response to client's behavior (Kiesler, 1996), providing an opportunity for new learning.

Such metacommunication may be conducted by first inviting the client to examine the current social interaction, reminding the client of this core feature of I/EP. Adopting a communication style of curiosity and avoiding blame or defensiveness, the therapist models owning his or her own perception of specific client behaviors and associated emotional responses (e.g., "I felt _____ when you _____"). The therapist then seeks client feedback in a way to encourage attention to emotions (e.g., "How are you feeling about what I just said?"), monitoring the client's reaction for open disclosure versus defensiveness. The therapist should empathically reflect and validate the client's emotional reactions, asking additional open questions to further process associated feelings, goals, and the function of in-session social behavior. Finally, the therapist elicits discussion of how particular in-session behaviors function in other social interactions in daily life. Consistent with I/EP principles previously discussed, emotionally evocative reactions to concrete particulars are processed prior to higher-order formulation.

In the following example, the therapist models metacommunication to the client:

THERAPIST: I'd like for us to check in about our own interaction here today. As we discussed, being able to do this is one of the helpful things about this kind of therapy.

CLIENT: Um . . . OK. What's up?

THERAPIST: Just now, when we started to examine the stressful interaction with your daughter this week, you shifted into rapidly listing all your worries about your spouse, the bills, parenting, your work. . . . I started to feel a bit less clear about where you were at emotionally. It almost felt like, for a few minutes, you took upon yourself both of our jobs . . . and you were too busy to need my help. But this is just my experience of it; what was yours?

CLIENT: Wow. I guess I just went into "autopilot" and started listing off all my worries. I didn't really notice it happening . . . and I really didn't think about how you would perceive it.

THERAPIST: Can you tune into the moment when you went there? What was happening for you?

CLIENT: I started thinking about my daughter, and got afraid I wouldn't improve my relationship with her, and my body got tense. It scares me to hope that things could be better, because it would be worse to expect it to get better and then fail. That freaks me out. I think I just felt the need to run through all my worries so that I would be ready for the worst.

THERAPIST: That's really interesting. You very much want to connect with your daughter, but it feels risky to hope for it . . . even triggering physical tension. So to deal with it, you shifted into worrying so that . . . at least you wouldn't be caught off guard if things don't work out.

CLIENT: Yeah . . . I do that all the time! And it's also a way for me to express how scared I feel.

THERAPIST: So listing off worries is comfortable for you, as it protects you from being "blindsided" when you let yourself feel a positive emotion in a vulnerable way. So it works for you in some ways. However, during the worry listing, it felt like a one-sided conversation; I actually felt a bit further away from you rather than more understanding of your struggles.

CLIENT: Really? I'm sorry. I wasn't really aware of that. It's sort of a habit.

THERAPIST: It's a habit. Have you noticed this habit in other relationships?

CLIENT: . . . Well, I do it a lot. Sometimes it turns into nagging my daughter and my husband. And we've talked about how that usually turns out.

THERAPIST: Right. You're frustrated that they seem to tune you out rather than being more attentive. A bit like how I felt less engaged with you when you listed off worries. This seems like an important pattern for us to watch in here. How about if we keep watch for it, and check in if you start to slip into listing off worries during session?

CLIENT: That's a good idea. Let me know, because I probably won't realize I'm doing it.

THERAPIST: My guess is that you'll get better at catching it earlier. We can also talk about your fear of being vulnerable and different ways to pursue your goals in these family relationships.

The foregoing discussion focuses on the impact of the client on the therapist, but we have found that therapists must actively monitor the therapeutic relationship for signs that clients experience negative interpersonal impacts by the therapist as well. Accordingly, we have incorporated strategies for managing ruptures of the therapeutic alliance based on the work of Safran and colleagues (Safran, Crocker, McMain, & Murray, 1990). Because Safran and Kraus (in Chapter 15, this volume) address these procedures in detail, we note them only briefly here. First, the therapist identifies ruptures as evidenced by markers such as client passivity, defensiveness, or disagreement about therapy tasks. Next, the therapist communicates awareness of such behaviors and invites the client to disclose any negative reactions to therapist behavior. Next, the therapist reflects and affirms the client's emotional experience. Last, resisting urges toward defensiveness or passive appeasement, the therapist acknowledges his or her own contribution to the client's experience, seeking to identify understandable concerns.

Developing New Interpersonal Strategies to Meet One's Needs

Unlike classical psychoanalysis, the I/EP model does not assume that "insight" into current struggles and their developmental origins will ameliorate clients' difficulties. Furthermore, experiencing one's emotions and relational needs/fears is assumed to be helpful given the penchant for cognitive avoidance in worriers, but not therapeutically sufficient in itself. Rather, both processes ultimately lead back to the client's current problems, providing conceptual and experiential awareness as a springboard for learning new interpersonal strategies to meet needs. In this regard, I/EP is a behavioral treatment focused on social skill building.

Once the client gains experiential awareness of his or her underlying interpersonal motives and needs and views previous interpersonal strategies as no longer productive, the therapist helps the client brainstorm alternative behaviors. Clients are encouraged to learn by behavioral engagement and experimentation, practicing previously avoided or underused strategies. For instance, GAD clients' "all-or-none" thinking often translates into similarly binary interpersonal strategies such as avoiding disclosure of emotion versus being intrusive, passive sulking versus hostility, or submissive appeasement versus domineering. Clients are invited to consider flexible alternatives to these dichotomous options. For example, many GAD clients benefit from learning to practice warm, yet assertive interpersonal skills (i.e., communicating that the needs of both the self and others are important) rather than hostile assertiveness or warm, but appeasing behavior.

In-session role plays provide an experiential means for learning new interpersonal strategies for meeting one's needs and how to attend to interpersonal impact on others. Typically, the client first plays the role of him- or herself acting in relation to the therapist in the role of a significant other. This clarifies concrete interpersonal strategies currently used in specific situations, increasing awareness of verbal and nonverbal behaviors. It also permits the therapist to observe such behaviors in preparation for switching roles:

THERAPIST: If you could role-play yourself in that recent frustrating interaction with your daughter, that would help me get a more vivid sense of what it was like. Imagine that you're back in that moment, and you're upset with her for not doing her chores. I'll play her role. What are you saying and doing in this situation?

CLIENT: OK. . . . If I've told you once, I've told you a thousand times: Do your chores without asking! It's not like you have more important things to be doing. You're 8 years old. The least you could do is to clean out the kitty litter, you know? But maybe I'm just expecting too much of you, your dad, and everyone else. . . . Why do I even bother?

THERAPIST: Good! This can feel awkward at first, but is seems like you really got into the role.

CLIENT: Yeah. It definitely put me back there.

THERAPIST: What's that like for you?

CLIENT: I can feel my stomach tightening a little bit.

THERAPIST: I believe it. I could see your face tighten up—especially your eyebrows. You looked really irritated.

Next, the therapist adopts the role of the client, emulating his or her social behaviors and asking the client to attend to what it feels like to experience the interaction from the perspective of the significant other. This process cultivates clients' empathy and awareness of their own interpersonal impact on others, an important skill that seems to be lacking in many worriers (Erickson & Newman, 2007). Thus, role plays target experiential awareness, as well as skill building, in the interpersonal domain:

THERAPIST: Now that we have a clear picture of how you spoke with your daughter, let's switch roles so that you can get a sense of how you might have come across to your daughter. OK?

CLIENT: All right.

THERAPIST: (*leaning forward, with furrowed brow and lower jaw protruding*) I've told you a thousand times to do your chores! It's the least you could do! What else do you need to do? You're only 8! I don't know why I even try with you and this family! I guess it's too much to ask! . . . (*now out of role*) What was it like being on the receiving end? What did you notice?

CLIENT: Did I really look that angry?

THERAPIST: Yes. Angry eyebrows, jaw, posture. . . . That surprises you?

CLIENT: Yeah. I guess I came across as more grumpy than I thought.

THERAPIST: What was it like to receive that anger? What did you think I wanted?

CLIENT: I felt like . . . shrinking back or avoiding you. That sorta got in the way of hearing anything else.

THERAPIST: So you can see now how your anger in the situation was very real, but kept you from paying full attention to your deeper desire for connection, and pushed your daughter away rather than helping her see that desire.

CLIENT: Yeah. It's not surprising that she tends to tune me out.

Subsequent to new awareness of interpersonal impact and shortcomings of clients' existing interpersonal strategies, traditional social skills-training role plays may be practiced. Clients experiment with alternative interpersonal strategies for need satisfaction, factoring in a fresh sense of what they want and how particular strategies have been ineffective. Then clients practice the strategy in session, receiving therapists' reinforcement and shaping. For example:

THERAPIST: You're describing how listing off all your worries about your relationship to your daughter is understandable, but it comes off as nagging to her. And it doesn't seem to move you any closer to the relationship you want with her.

CLIENT: Yeah. I wear her out and wear myself out! Then it's easier to just back off and give up.

THERAPIST: So we don't yet know what strategies might work better, but we know that these strategies really aren't working for you. Let's brainstorm some other options to experiment with. You said that you strongly desire to feel closer to your daughter, and you also want to help her participate in family chores. What are alternatives to worrying, nagging, and withdrawing?

CLIENT: I don't know. I could first try to limit nagging. Remind myself of the reality that it never works. I think it would be nice to have a nag-free zone or something like that.

THERAPIST: A great idea! How will that serve your goal?

CLIENT: I don't want her to remember me for nagging. If I can knock that off and just be with her for 20 minutes after she comes home in the afternoon, maybe that will be a start. She loves to do puzzles after school. I could join in and try to limit myself to listening to her.

THERAPIST: Sounds like a great thing to try out this week. What about the issue of chores?

CLIENT: Well, if the goal is to reduce nagging . . . maybe I need to find more fun ways to get her involved or get her motivated, or at least be more consistent about my expectations.

THERAPIST: Good, but it would be worth figuring out *how* you would want to let her know you will be trying some new approaches, while trying to stay connected to your gut sense of what you want with her. I'll take on her role. I just got home from school. "Hi mom. The bus just dropped me off. I'm going to play with my toys . . . "

CLIENT: Um . . . (*out of role*) I need to think . . .

THERAPIST: Take your time, but please give it a try. "Mom, I feel like playing and skipping chores today."

CLIENT: OK. "Hi honey. I want to check in with you. You know how Mom has been nagging you a lot lately about chores?"

THERAPIST: "Yeah, you've been nagging a lot. Makes me annoyed." (*out of role*) Use the emotion here to keep you focused . . .

CLIENT: "I am sad about nagging you. I do think we should check in about chores, but I'm sorry for nagging. What I really want is to feel closer to you and our family. Tell you what . . . Mom will set aside 20 minutes of time after school to play with you on whatever you want, and we can wait on chores until after that."

THERAPIST: (*out of role*) Wow. You came across as really meaning it, and both loving and firm, without either nagging or withdrawing. If you're open to it, I'd be happy to share some tips, based on research, on strategies for setting up play time and consequence systems. Of course, we will need to tailor them to your situation, and treat them as an experiment.

CLIENT: Sounds good . . . I think I could talk to her this week.

Client role plays of new interpersonal strategies typically require repetition, with the therapist shaping" and reinforcing successive approximations. For instance, in the above-mentioned example, the therapist might help the client first inhibit nagging behaviors, then attend to emotional needs when communicating, then develop increasingly adaptive (i.e., balancing emotional disclosure and assertiveness) communications informed by therapist feedback about their interpersonal impact.

After in-session role plays facilitate rehearsal of the interpersonal skills that the client and therapist collaboratively agree to be more adaptive, the therapist assigns homework targeting real-life practice. Consistent with a focus on specificity and lived experience, clients are encouraged to select specific interaction goals and relational contexts in which to experiment with new social skills. Additionally, the therapist sets client expectations to debrief these experiments in the subsequent session, permitting therapist reinforcement and affirmation of successful attempts or further problem solving and shaping as needed.

Emotional Processing

As should be clear by now, processing and deepening emotions is integral to I/EP. Emotional processing is not necessarily a separate target from examination of interpersonal issues, given that strong emotion is often tied to interpersonal needs, goals, and fears. When engaging the aforementioned tasks of examining problematic interpersonal patterns in one's current close relationships, family of origin, or therapeutic relationship, I/EP therapists must help clients attend to avoided, often unpleasant, emotions. Regardless of context, the following considerations are important when clients discuss emotionally evocative material. First, the therapist must track markers of intense emotional experience on the part of the client. For instance, the quality of client vocalization, such as fluctuation in pitch or increased/decreased pace of verbalization, may change. Other markers include affect appropriate to content (e.g., tears when discussing loss) or affect inconsistent with content (e.g., smiling when discussing painful experiences). The therapist should gently encourage the client to stay with here-and-now experiencing of such emotions, acknowledging the often scary nature of this process and conveying acceptance of whatever emotions clients share. When clients are observed in attempts to suppress or dampen present emotions (e.g., through intellectual abstraction, changing the subject, or postural changes such as "curling into a ball"), the therapist continues to encourage contact with uncomfortable affects. Moreover, given that clients with GAD are sometimes prone to experience anger more easily than more vulnerable states, the therapist elicits client attention to "primary emotions," such as feeling weak, vulnerable, or sad, which may underlie secondary anger. For instance, in the aforementioned vignette, the client found it easier to express irritability than to experience the risky vulnerability of wanting and hoping for family intimacy.

In addition to an experiential focus interwoven into all I/EP discussions of interpersonal and emotional issues, I/EP integrates existing experiential techniques. Namely, therapists attend to clients' *problematic reactions*, *internal conflicts*, and *unfinished business*, each of which are emotional-processing problems that arise in session and correspond to specific interventions developed and studied in the context of emotion-focused therapy (EFT; see Elliott, Watson, Goldman, & Greenberg, 2004; Greenberg et al., 1996). We briefly describe these foci here, but refer readers to Thoma and

Greenberg (Chapter 11, this volume) for further details, particularly for the latter two "chair-work" interventions.

Some clients experience "problematic reactions," or confused reactions to emotions. Such reactions are identified via markers such as client surprise in response to an emotion (Elliott et al., 2004; Greenberg et al., 1996). Some clients are surprised by tearful reactions when clarifying their previously unacknowledged interpersonal needs, almost as if these were the needs of someone else. In "systematic evocative unfolding" (or simply "unfolding") clients close their eyes and imagine the evocative situation, making first-person, sensory descriptions in vivid detail. They describe associated bodily senses and emotions, which may serve as exposure to interoceptive cues and avoided emotions, as well as opportunities to connect with the needs/action tendencies suggested by the emotions. This process amplifies emotions to help clients differentiate aspects of a situation and their emotional reaction to it, clarifying underlying "emotion schemes" (the network of situational appraisals, bodily and expressive features, needs and action tendencies, and symbolic-conceptual understandings associated with an emotion). Once therapists (1) identify markers such as clients' perplexity about an emotion, the subsequent steps include (2) inviting them to re-evoke the memory of the situation that evoked the emotion, slowly examining concrete features of the memory as if it making a movie; (3) tracking the "two sides" of perception of the external situation and internal reactions; (4) finding a "meaning bridge" or link that makes sense of how the situation generated their unique emotional reaction; (5) helping clients explore how the same process occurs in other situations; and finally (6) considering how the new understanding can empower personal change. The following brief vignette encapsulates this process:

CLIENT: Given that [my daughter] has been doing so much better with her chores, I was caught off guard by how upset I was with her yesterday. I really lost it. It makes no sense to me.

THERAPIST: So it's hard for you to understand why you had such a strong reaction to this situation. Would it be helpful to spend some time working through the situation to make sense of what you felt?

CLIENT: Yeah. I feel like I shouldn't be this upset. It bugs me that I didn't expect this reaction.

THERAPIST: And we know that feeling caught off guard is particularly frustrating for you.

CLIENT: Every time!

THERAPIST: OK. Starting with how things were going before the upsetting situation, can you walk me through the situation in slow motion, almost like a movie?

CLIENT: All right. I was having a pretty good day. I was off work. Sunday morning. Got to sleep in a little. We had a slow morning.

THERAPIST: How was your mood?

CLIENT: Not bad. Just coasting along.

THERAPIST: So you wake up in a decent mood. You feel rested. You're enjoying a low-key Sunday morning. Then what happens?

CLIENT: I'm sitting, drinking my coffee, and I notice my daughter cleaning out the cat litter.

THERAPIST: What happens for you at that moment?

CLIENT: Well, I guess my first reaction was just feeling happy. Maybe even a little grateful. I'm watching her doing her chores, and thinking of how good it feels that she is doing better with . . . doing her part in the family.

THERAPIST: Sounds like a pleasant moment. You didn't even have to nag her, and she's taking care of the cat. Then what?

CLIENT: . . . Somewhere around that time . . . she walks up to me and asks to be paid for doing her chores . . . and something just hits me.

THERAPIST: What was going on for you then?

CLIENT: It was like getting the wind knocked out of me.

THERAPIST: Something important there—that moment when she asks to be paid—that hit you hard.

CLIENT: Definitely, yeah. It was like . . . even though I knew we had agreed to give an allowance for chores . . . I was upset that she ruined the moment by asking then.

THERAPIST: You were enjoying this sense of her doing her part, but her asking to be paid right then meant that . . .

CLIENT: That maybe she was just doing her chores only because we would pay her. That she wasn't really interested in the sort of family I want to have.

THERAPIST: . . . You first thought her taking care of the cat meant she was joining your picture of a happy family, but maybe it was purely motivated by money. Maybe it really means you'll never have the family you want!

CLIENT: Exactly!

THERAPIST: So we're starting to understand why you had such a strong reaction to what initially seemed like no big deal. We're again finding this powerful desire for a type of family connection that you never had, and real anger associated with a sense of your daughter stopping you from having it. Does this sound familiar?

CLIENT: *(smiling)* Yeah. This is my problem . . . .I need to figure out to how to work toward a close family without making her carry the whole thing.

In other instances, clients present "internal conflicts" between parts of themselves. Therapists track markers for such conflicts by noting when clients seem to be "of two minds" about a concern or when one part of the self criticizes or blocks the expression of another part of the self. The "two-chair exercise" provides an experiential means for clients to enact different sides of the conflict, experiencing emotions from each side and attaching labels to them (Elliott et al., 2004; Greenberg et al., 1996). Many clients with GAD, for example, experience conflicts between wishes and fears. They often listen to a part of themselves that prefers to defensively expect the worst rather than be disappointed, ignoring another part of the self that optimistically hopes for desired outcomes. The therapist may invite the client to fully own and enact the role of the part of the self that embodies the wish or something they are hopeful will happen, differentiating and articulating what that part is experiencing. Clients are then encouraged to shift into speaking from the "afraid self" to the wishful part of themselves (with actual shifting between chairs encouraged). Continued deepening of this split and contact between parts of the self lead to softening of the part of the self that badgers the other via worry, and ultimately a new self-experience integrates both sides while finding more adaptive ways to deal with primary emotions.

Last, clients may bring up unresolved feelings about a relationship, or "unfinished business." Again, therapists track markers of unfinished business such as complicated, prolonged grief or emotional reactivity to reminders of painful memories. In the "empty chair" exercise, clients imagine that the person in question is sitting present in a chair; they talk directly to this empty chair, imagining, enacting, and communicating what they feel or wish the other person could understand (Elliott et al., 2004; Greenberg et al., 1996). This first-person, verbal-motoric process often evokes and deepens strong emotions, which can then be explored to help clients determine important needs or wishes.

Future Directions

I/EP possesses numerous strengths, including a strong conceptual rationale based on previous theory and research germane to GAD, integration of a variety of therapy strategies, and preliminary evidence of efficacy. However, its limitations warrant mention. First, some might question the format of adding the I/EP module to the CBT module rather than truly integrating them within single sessions. Nonetheless, in the initial trial (Newman et al.,

2011), clients and therapists informally suggested that they found focusing on one set of skills at a time (e.g., cognitive restructuring, then emotional deepening) to be helpful, not problematic. One way to adapt the modular approach to clinical practice (given constraints of time and reimbursement by insurance companies) would be to retain the format, but simply shorten the time devoted to each module (e.g., half of a 60-minute session devoted to CBT, and the second half devoted to I/EP). Alternatively, recent data show that clients with more chronic GAD may respond better to single component therapies (e.g., cognitive therapy) than to comprehensive CBT packages (Newman & Fisher, 2013), so therapists might provide a full dose (e.g., 14 sessions) of CBT as a first-line treatment and then offer I/EP to clients who have not yet responded adequately.

Second, the existing data establish general efficacy for CBT + I/EP, but leave some questions unaddressed. Specifically, although this treatment trended toward greater efficacy than CBT plus supportive listening, its treatment specificity remains undetermined. Adherence and quality checks attested to treatment fidelity (Newman et al., 2011), but therapy process research must investigate whether I/EP clients differentially engaged in emotional processing in an interpersonally immediate manner, relative to CBT + SL clients, and whether such processes mediate treatment outcomes. If not, ways to facilitate client engagement in tasks that target theorized mechanisms of GAD would require reexamination. Moreover, our clinical experience and theoretical formulation suggest that not all GAD clients may require the I/EP module in addition to standard CBT; clients' whose functional analyses reveal systematic avoidance of particular emotional experiences and specific interpersonal strategies (e.g., avoidance of setting boundaries, avoidance of softening boundaries to allow intimacy) may derive greater benefit from this module. In contrast, clients with GAD endorsing excessive worry and tension without the associated avoidance of emotional processing may fare well in CBT without I/EP. Future studies will probe aptitude by treatment interactions to test these predictions, as well as testing differential response based on particular clusters of interpersonal problems.

Alternatively, ongoing research may reveal that I/EP successfully engaged clients in theoretically important emotional and interpersonal processes without leading to associated incremental treatment efficacy beyond standard CBT. If so, this would merit reconsideration of the precise nature of the emotional/interpersonal mechanisms that maintain GAD. In fact, since the time of the original rationale and study design for testing I/EP, a new model of emotional mechanisms for GAD has developed: the contrast avoidance model of worry (Newman & Llera, 2011). This model proposes that individuals with GAD possess hypersensitivity to shifts from relatively neutral or positive mood states to negative moods. People with GAD seem so exquisitely reactive to strong emotional shifts that they may prefer to worry to remain in a negative affective state, in order to prevent "negative emotional contrasts" or unprepared-for impacts of negative events (i.e., "If I expect the worst, then I can never be surprised by it!"). A recent literature review showed that, contrary to the notion that worry is reinforced by facilitating avoidance of negative emotion, worry fails to suppress or limit negative emotionality and physiological arousal; in fact, worry promotes and prolongs negative emotions and physiological activation (Newman, Llera, Erickson, Przeworski, & Castonguay, 2013). Individuals with GAD reported higher distress than nonanxious controls following shifts from euthymic to negative states and actually report finding worrying before emotional video exposures *more helpful* than neutral or relaxation inductions, a preference opposite to those of nonanxious controls (Llera & Newman, 2011). As a result, individuals with GAD are theorized to employ worry and interpersonal strategies to avoid negative emotional contrast experiences, with such processes negatively reinforced by perceived reduction of these experiences.

The general justification for I/EP remains strong, given the extant research linking worry and GAD to interpersonal dysfunction and avoidance of emotional processing. However, it remains possible that research on the contrast avoidance model may lead to further enhancements or adaptations of I/EP. An I/EP that incorporates insights from the contrast avoidance model would employ all of the same treatment techniques, but would attend to the role of negative emotional contrasts. For instance, functional analysis of worry and interpersonal behaviors would delineate ways in which these processes prevent emotional contrasts in daily life and social contexts. Examination of interpersonal transactions with significant others or the therapist would scrutinize similar themes. Furthermore, experiential deepening strategies would target emotional shifts, for instance, by exposing clients to negative emotional stimuli immediately following euthymic mood inductions by relaxation exercises. Ongoing research will investigate these possibilities.

In conclusion, I/EP stands as an integrative psychotherapy incorporating experiential and interpersonal therapy strategies to complement standard CBT techniques. Such integration is guided by basic research into mechanisms that may maintain GAD. Individuals with GAD demonstrate emotional sensitivities and employ worry as a maladaptive compensatory strategy. Facilitating their capacity for emotional deepening to reduce such sensitivities and enhance awareness of their own needs and values is an important therapeutic goal. Allowing and embracing the reality of emotional shifts may uncover previously neglected perspectives and opportunities for learning. We hope that continued research into mechanisms and moderators of I/EP, as well as mechanisms that maintain GAD, will lead to enhanced well-being for individuals with GAD in their emotional and interpersonal lives.

Further Reading

Articles

- For the initial open trial of CBT + I/EP, see Newman, Castonguay, Borkovec, Fisher, and Nordberg (2008).
- For the randomized controlled trial of CBT + I/EP versus CBT + supportive listening, see Newman et al. (2011).

Books

- See Newman, Castonguay, Borkovec, and Molnar (2004) for an earlier review of I/EP strategies.
- See Elliott, Watson, Goldman, and Greenberg (2004) for detailed examples of techniques drawn from emotion-focused therapy.
- See Safran and Segal (1990) for elaboration on ways to examine in-session interpersonal processes.

References

American Psychiatric Association. (2013). *Diagnostic and statistical manual of mental disorders* (5th ed.). Arlington, VA: Author.

Ansell, E. B., Pinto, A., Edelen, M. O., Markowitz, J. C., Sanislow, C. A., Yen, S., et al. (2011). The association of personality disorders with the prospective 7-year course of anxiety disorders. *Psychological Medicine, 41*, 1019–1028.

Borkovec, T. D., Alcaine, O. M., & Behar, E. S. (2004). Avoidance theory of worry. In R. Heimberg, D. Mennin, & C. Turk (Eds.), *Generalized anxiety disorder: Advances in research and practice* (pp. 77–108). New York: Guilford Press.

Borkovec, T. D., Newman, M. G., Pincus, A. L., & Lytle, R. (2002). A component analysis of cognitive-behavioral therapy for generalized anxiety disorder and the role of interpersonal problems. *Journal of Consulting and Clinical Psychology, 70*, 288–298.

Borkovec, T. D., & Roemer, L. (1995). Perceived functions of worry among generalized anxiety disorder subjects: Distraction from more emotionally distressing topics? *Journal of Behavior Therapy and Experimental Psychiatry, 26*, 25–30.

Borkovec, T. D., & Ruscio, A. M. (2001). Psychotherapy for generalized anxiety disorder. *Journal of Clinical Psychiatry, 62*, 37–45.

Brown, T. A., Barlow, D. H., & Liebowitz, M. R. (1994). The empirical basis of generalized anxiety disorder. *American Journal of Psychiatry, 151*, 1272–1280.

Cassidy, J., Lichtenstein-Phelps, J., Sibrava, N. J., Thomas, C. L., & Borkovec, T. D. (2009). Generalized anxiety disorder: Connections with self-reported attachment. *Behavior Therapy, 40*, 23–28.

Castonguay, L. G., Hayes, A. M., Goldfried, M. R., & DeRubeis, R. J. (1995). The focus of therapist interventions in cognitive therapy for depression. *Cognitive Therapy and Research, 19*, 487–505.

Cougle, J. R., Timpano, K. R., Sachs-Ericsson, N., Keough, M. E., & Riccardi, C. J. (2010). Examining the unique relationships between anxiety disorders and childhood physical and sexual abuse in the National Comorbidity Survey—Replication. *Psychiatry Research, 177*, 150–155.

Crits-Christoph, P., Gibbons, M. B. C., Narducci, J., Schamberger, M., & Gallop, R. (2005). Interpersonal problems and the outcome of interpersonally oriented psychodynamic treatment of GAD. *Psychotherapy: Theory, Research, Practice, Training, 42,* 211–224.

Durham, R. C., Allan, T., & Hackett, C. A. (1997). On predicting improvement and relapse in generalized anxiety disorder following psychotherapy. *British Journal of Clinical Psychology, 36,* 101–119.

Durham, R. C., Chambers, J. A., MacDonald, R. R., Power, K. G., & Major, K. (2003). Does cognitive-behavioural therapy influence the long-term outcome of generalized anxiety disorder?: An 8–14 year follow-up of two clinical trials. *Psychological Medicine, 33,* 499–509.

Elliott, R., Watson, J. C., Goldman, R. N., & Greenberg, L. S. (2004). *Learning emotion-focused therapy: The process–experiential approach to change.* Washington, DC: American Psychological Association Press.

Erickson, T. M., & Newman, M. G. (2007). Interpersonal and emotional processes in generalized anxiety disorder analogues during social interaction tasks. *Behavior Therapy, 38,* 364–377.

Erickson, T. M., Newman, M. G., & Abelson, J. L. (2010, November). *Discrepant perspectives on the interpersonal characteristics of worriers based upon self versus peer assessment.* Paper presented at 44th annual meeting of the Association for Behavior and Cognitive Therapies, San Francisco, CA.

Greenberg, L. S., Elliott. R., & Lietaer, G. (1994). Research on experiential therapies. In A. Bergin & S. Garfield (Eds.), *Handbook of psychotherapy and behavior change* (pp. 509–539). New York: Wiley.

Greenberg, L. S., Rice, L. N., & Elliott, R. K. (1996). *Facilitating emotional change: The moment-by-moment process.* New York: Guilford Press.

Hoehn-Saric, R., Hazlett, R. L., & McLeod, D. R. (1993). Generalized anxiety disorder with early and late onset of anxiety symptoms. *Comprehensive Psychiatry, 34,* 291–298.

Kessler, R. C., Greenberg, P. E., Mickelson, K. D., Meneades, L. M., & Wang, P. S. (2001). The effects of chronic medical conditions on work loss and work cutback. *Journal of Occupational and Environmental Medicine, 43,* 218–225.

Kiesler, D. J. (1996). *Contemporary interpersonal theory and research: Personality, psychopathology, and psychotherapy.* New York: Wiley.

Llera, S. J., & Newman, M. G. (2011, November). *An experimental examination of emotional avoidance in generalized anxiety disorder: Data supporting a new theory of emotional contrast avoidance.* Paper presented at 119th annual convention of the American Psychological Association, Washington, DC.

Massion, A. O., Warshaw, M. G., & Keller, M. B. (1993). Quality of life and psychiatric morbidity in panic disorder and generalized anxiety disorder. *American Journal of Psychiatry, 150,* 600–607.

Mogg, K., Millar, N., & Bradley, B. P. (2000). Biases in eye movements to threatening facial expressions in generalized anxiety disorder and depressive disorder. *Journal of Abnormal Psychology, 109,* 695–704.

Newman, M. G., Castonguay, L. G., Borkovec, T. D., Fisher, A. J., Boswell, J. F., Szkodny, L. E., et al. (2011). A randomized controlled trial of cognitive-behavioral therapy for generalized anxiety disorder with integrated techniques from emotion-focused and interpersonal therapies. *Journal of Consulting and Clinical Psychology, 79,* 171–181.

Newman, M. G., Castonguay, L. G., Borkovec, T. D., Fisher, A. J., & Nordberg, S. S. (2008). An open trial of integrative therapy for generalized anxiety disorder. *Psychotherapy: Theory, Research, Practice, Training, 45,* 135–147.

Newman, M. G., Castonguay, L. G., Borkovec, T. D., & Molnar, C. (2004). Integrative psychotherapy. In R. G. Heimberg, C. L. Turk, & D. S. Mennin (Eds.), *Generalized anxiety disorder: Advances in research and practice* (pp. 320–350). New York: Guilford Press.

Newman, M. G., & Erickson, T. M. (2010). Generalized anxiety disorder. In J. G. Beck (Ed.), *Interpersonal processes in the anxiety disorders: Implications for understanding psychopathology and treatment* (pp. 235–259). Washington, DC: American Psychological Association Press.

Newman, M. G., & Fisher, A. J. (2013). Mediated moderation in combined cognitive behavioral therapy versus component treatments for generalized anxiety disorder. *Journal of Consulting and Clinical Psychology, 81,* 405–414.

Newman, M. G., & Llera, S. J. (2011). A novel theory of experiential avoidance in generalized anxiety disorder: A review and synthesis of research supporting a contrast avoidance model of worry. *Clinical Psychology Review, 31,* 371–382.

Newman, M. G., Llera, S. J., Erickson, T. M., Przeworski, A., & Castonguay, L. G. (2013). Worry and generalized anxiety disorder: A review and theoretical synthesis of evidence on nature, etiology, mechanisms, and treatment. *Annual Review of Clinical Psychology, 9,* 275–297.

Przeworski, A., Newman, M. G., Pincus, A. L., Kasoff, M. B., Yamasaki, A. S., Castonguay, L. G., et al. (2011). Interpersonal pathoplasticity in individuals with generalized anxiety disorder. *Journal of Abnormal Psychology, 120,* 286–298.

Roemer, L., Molina, S., & Borkovec, T. D. (1997). An investigation of worry content among generally anxious individuals. *Journal of Nervous and Mental Disease, 185,* 314–319.

Safran, J. D., Crocker, P., McMain, S., & Murray, P. (1990). Therapeutic alliance rupture as a therapy event for empirical investigation. *Psychotherapy: Theory, Research, Practice, Training, 27,* 154–165.

Safran, J. D., Muran, J. C., & Eubanks-Carter, C. (2011). Repairing alliance ruptures. *Psychotherapy, 48,* 80–87.

Safran, J. D., & Segal, Z. V. (1990). *Interpersonal process in cognitive therapy.* New York: Basic Books.

Sullivan, H. S. (1953). *The interpersonal theory of psychiatry.* New York: Norton.

Turk, C. L., Heimberg, R. G., Luterek, J. A., Mennin, D. S., & Fresco, D. M. (2005). Emotion dysregulation in generalized anxiety disorder: A comparison with social anxiety disorder. *Cognitive Therapy and Research, 5,* 89–106.

Whisman, M. A. (2007). Marital distress and DSM-IV psychiatric disorders in a population-based national survey. *Journal of Abnormal Psychology, 116,* 638–643.

Whisman, M. A., Sheldon, C. T., & Goering, P. (2000). Psychiatric disorder and dissatisfaction with social relationships: Does type of relationship matter? *Journal of Abnormal Psychology, 109,* 803–808.

Wiser, S., & Goldfried, M. R. (1993). Comparative study of emotional experiencing in psychodynamic-interpersonal and cognitive-behavioral therapies. *Journal of Consulting and Clinical Psychology, 61,* 892–895.

Zinbarg, R. E., Lee, J. E., & Yoon, K. L. (2007). Dyadic predictors of outcome in a cognitive-behavioral program for patients with generalized anxiety disorder in committed relationships: A "spoonful of sugar" and a dose of non-hostile criticism may help. *Behaviour Research and Therapy, 45,* 699–713.

CHAPTER 17

Functional Analytic Psychotherapy

Using Awareness, Courage, Love, and Behaviorism to Promote Change

Mavis Tsai
Andrew P. Fleming
Rick A. Cruz
Julia E. Hitch
Robert J. Kohlenberg

Functional analytic psychotherapy (FAP) uses behavioral principles to create a therapeutic environment that nurtures awareness, courage, and therapeutic love and views the therapeutic relationship as the primary vehicle for client healing and transformation. The essential clinical interventions center on the therapist noticing, evoking, and responding effectively to client problems and improved behaviors as they occur during the session. Thus, FAP uses what happens in session between therapist and client to create more authentic and effective ways for clients to connect with others, ultimately bringing about closer, more intimate relationships in their daily lives.

Using a highly individualized intervention that requires a thorough assessment and case conceptualization of each client, FAP therapists identify clinically relevant behaviors occurring in the therapy room that are related to the client's daily life issues (Kohlenberg & Tsai, 1991; Tsai et al., 2009). Such clinically relevant behaviors (CRBs) are defined as functional classes based on similar antecedents and consequences and the purpose they serve, with specific form or appearance varying from client to client (Tsai, Callaghan, & Kohlenberg, 2013; Tsai, Kohlenberg, Kanter, Holman, & Plummer Loudon, 2012). A common misunderstanding of behaviorism is that behavior is defined in terms of how it appears. In fact, the appearance of a behavior is of little interest to a behaviorist without understanding the context in which it occurs. For example, in order to understand the typical CRB of avoiding genuine intimate expression (that, in turn, interferes with forming close relationships in daily life), we try to understand the contexts that trigger this behavior and the consequences that follow. Essentially, the client avoids expressing closeness when faced with the opportunity to do so, thus avoiding feared negative consequences (e.g., rejection). This avoidance may appear very different from one client to the next, possibly taking the form of missing sessions, making jokes, or expressing anger. All of these behaviors in this example, however, even though their appearance is markedly different, would be considered to be in the same functional class.

In this chapter, we briefly describe research evidence for the efficacy of FAP and then focus on the essence of FAP by discussing its five rules and illustrating how they are applied clinically. Our goal is to point to phenomena and interventions that could be useful to all clinicians, regardless of their orientation. Finally, we consider limitations, precautions, and future directions.

Evidence for Outcome and Mechanism of Change

In essence, FAP's focus on the therapeutic relationship involves watching for, noticing, and responding to CRBs. We contend that adding such a focus may improve the intensity and power of psychotherapy, broadly defined. Some strong supportive evidence is provided by Kohlenberg, Kanter, Bolling, Parker, and Tsai (2002) in a nonrandomized controlled study for depression that involved a comparison between cognitive therapy and FAP-enhanced cognitive therapy (FECT). Results indicated that clients receiving FECT showed a more favorable reaction to the FAP rationale, and significantly improved on the GAF (Global Assessment of Functioning), interpersonal functioning as measured by the SSQ (Social Support Questionnaire), with trends found on the HRSD (Hamilton Rating Scale for Depression) and SCL-90 (Symptom Check List–90). The incremental effectiveness of adding FAP to CBT also has been demonstrated via single-subject design studies (Gaynor & Lawrence, 2002; Kanter et al., 2006).

In addition, a variety of process–outcome studies support FAP's basic principles (see Baruch et al., 2009) as well as some FAP-specific research that focuses on measuring therapist and client behavior during session and exploring the relationship between in-session therapist behavior and indicators of client outcomes.

Recent research on FAP has defined its mechanism to be *therapist-contingent responding with natural reinforcement to CRBs*. Thus such research aims to isolate and identify FAP's purported mechanism of action and demonstrate the effects of this mechanism on the behavior of individual clients.

With this research goal in mind, the Functional Analytic Psychotherapy Rating Scale (FAPRS) was developed to measure turn-by-turn client and therapist behavior and thus to allow for reliable identification of in-session problems (CRB1s), improvements (CRB2s), and contingent therapist responses (Callaghan, Summers, & Weidman, 2003; Callaghan, Follette, Ruckstuhl, & Linnerooth, 2008). Not only were CRBs identified (supporting the belief in FAP that general interpersonal problems may present themselves in the therapeutic context), but therapist contingent responding to CRB was identified as well. Overall research using the FAPRS has provided support for the mechanism of change (contingent responding) and indicates that CRB1s decreased and CRB2s increased over the course of FAP (Kanter et al., 2006; Busch et al., 2009).

In order to assess whether a therapist's attending to the therapy relationship (termed an "*in-vivo* hit") had beneficial effects on session-by-session indicators of outcome, Kanter, Schildcrout, and Kohlenberg (2005) evaluated the relationship between the number of *in-vivo* hits in a session and both overall progress and relationship-specific improvements reported by the client for the week following the session. Results indicated a statistically significant relationship between *in-vivo* hit rates per session and whether or not clients reported that the session was helpful in making progress with their problems. The turn-at-speech analysis found that for every five *in-vivo* hits that are added by therapists in a session, there is an incremental improvement in outcome. Our explanation for this finding is that an increased number of *in-vivo* hits are consistent with a therapist following FAP Rule 1 (observing CRB). The relationship between the number of *in-vivo* hits and positive outcome is likely to be curvilinear depending on the individual client or session; the average optimal number of *in-vivo* hits has not yet been empirically established.

In the only randomized-controlled study incorporating FAP, Gifford and colleagues (2011) randomly assigned 303 smokers from a community sample to bupropion, a widely used smoking cessation medication or bupropion plus a combination of FAP and ACT (acceptance and commitment therapy; see Germer & Chan, Chapter 1, this volume) in a smoking cessation trial. There were no differences between conditions at posttreatment; however, participants in the FAP and ACT condition experienced significantly better outcomes at 1-year follow-up.

This research focusing on CRBs is still in its infancy. Nevertheless, taken together, there is accumulating support for the specific mechanism of action in the therapy relationship according to FAP.

Clinical Application of FAP

Given that therapy is a complex interactional process, our suggestions for technique are not intended to be complete or to exclude the use of procedures not described here. Instead, other therapy methods can be complemented and augmented by taking advantage of therapeutic opportunities that may otherwise go unnoticed. Our procedures are given in the form of "rules" not in a rigid sense, but more as suggestions that are expected to produce greater therapeutic effects. What follows is a description of the five FAP rules, or guidelines, specifying ways for therapists to notice, evoke, and naturally reinforce clinically relevant behaviors so that positive changes that take place in session can generalize to clients' daily lives. Initially, therapists who follow these rules are engaging in rule-governed behavior, but as they gain experience, therapist behavior comes under direct control of the contingencies, for example, successful outcomes. When this process occurs, therapist behavior is less under conscious control and is then referred to as "contingency-shaped behavior."

Rule 1. Watch for CRBs (Be Aware)

This rule forms the core of FAP. In order to use Rule 1, therapists continually attend to the question: "How do the client's daily life problems show up in this therapeutic relationship?" When clients' problem behaviors or corresponding improvements appear in session, they are termed "clinically relevant behaviors" (CRBs), which we divide into CRB1s and CRB2s. CRB1s are client problem behaviors that occur in session. For example, common CRB1s include avoidance of expressing emotions or avoidance of asserting needs with the therapist. These CRB1s may correspond to daily life problems such as stifling emotional expression or avoiding assertion of needs with loved ones, friends, and others. CRB2s are client improvements that occur in session. Continuing the previous example, for a client who avoids expressing emotion (CRB1), any in-session behavioral step toward greater emotional expression would be a CRB2. It is important to note that in contrast to a traditional psychodynamic approach, a specific behavior can be a CRB1 or a CRB2 depending on the nature of the client's daily life problems. For example, a client who has obsessive–compulsive disorder and comes late to or misses a session might actually be engaging in a CRB2 and thus should be reinforced by the therapist.

A therapist's personal reactions to the client are a valuable guide for identifying CRBs. Useful questions can include:

> "What are the ways your client has a negative impact on you?"
> "Does your attention wander because you experience him as droning on and on?"
> "Does she avoid responding to your questions?"

"Does he frustrate you because he procrastinates on his homework assignments?"
"Does she say one thing then do another?"
"Is he mean or unreasonable with you?"
"Is she late with her payments?"
"Is he critical of your every intervention?"
"Does she shut down when you are warm?"
"Does he pull away when the two of you have had a close interaction?"
"Does she seem to have no interest or curiosity about you as a person?"

In order to use personal reactions as an effective guide, FAP therapists strive to notice when their own responses are idiosyncratic and related to their own learning histories versus broadly representative of how others might generally react to the client. When a therapist reacts similarly to how others in the client's life might react, these therapist reactions provide an accurate measure of the client's CRBs. It is important, therefore, when using one's own reactions as a guide, to have some understanding of how important people in the client's life might respond. Overtly, this may include asking, "I am having X reaction to you right now—how would your significant other [or boss, co-worker, family member, friend] react?" This approach, however, requires a continued effort over time to truly understand the consequences that have shaped and maintained the client's behavior in the outside world.

It also is imperative that therapists continually engage in self-awareness practice, striving to notice how their reactions to clients are influenced by their own personal learning history. This prevents the potentially iatrogenic effect of shaping the client to act in such a way that is likely to be reinforced by the therapist but unlikely to be reinforced by those in the client's life. To this end, we recommend ongoing peer consultation to assist in evaluating the degree to which positive and negative reactions toward clients are representative of how others in the clients' daily lives might respond. When therapists succeed in tuning into their own broadly representative reactions to the client, implementing Rule 1 becomes more natural, effortless, and powerful.

Rule 2. Evoke CRBs (Be Courageous)

From an FAP standpoint, the ideal client–therapist relationship is one that evokes CRB1s; these CRB1s then become the precursors for developing and nurturing CRB2s. Because CRBs are idiographic and arise from the unique circumstances and life histories of individual clients, the ideal therapeutic relationship evokes behaviors relevant to the specific daily life problems of a particular client. For example, if a client has difficulty committing to a course of action in life, the therapeutic relationship and the process of therapy may similarly evoke problems in decision making and making commitments (e.g., selecting goals during the initial phase of therapy, committing to a particular change or to a period of therapy). Problems in developing and maintaining meaningful close interpersonal relationships, also referred to as "intimacy," play a role in most disorders (Wetterneck & Hart, 2012).

Many clients report that they struggle with the essential relationship skills and behaviors that foster intimacy, such as the ability to deeply trust others, take interpersonal risks, act authentically, and give and receive love. Thus, in FAP, the therapeutic relationship provides a unique opportunity for clients to develop their behavioral and emotional repertoire in ways that will enhance the client's experience of and satisfaction with relationships in daily life. FAP calls upon therapists to be emotionally present and to structure their therapy in an emotionally evocative manner in order to foster therapeutic relationships grounded in intimacy, authenticity, trust, and interpersonal connection.

Creating an evocative therapeutic relationship also requires therapists to take interpersonal risks and to push their own intimacy boundaries. For example, when a client misses a session without cancelling ahead of time, or shows up late to multiple sessions (possible CRB1s), FAP principles may encourage the therapist to discuss the impact of the client's behavior (e.g., "When you are late, I feel that our sessions are unimportant to you," or "I sense myself feeling frustrated when you miss a session without cancelling ahead of time"), as well as asking how this behavior comes up in client's life and how it impacts his or her other relationships. These evocative statements may open the door for the client to engage in a CRB2, which can then be naturally reinforced by the therapist. When therapists are doing FAP well, they are most likely stretching their limits and venturing beyond their comfort zone to harness the therapy relationship not simply as an analogue for interpersonal relationships, but as a real relationship with real interpersonal consequences. The therapist's willingness to take risks in the therapeutic relationship will set the tone for the therapy and help the client to feel that the therapy relationship is transactional and authentic.

Therapists can evoke CRBs in three major ways, recognizing that all interactions in the context of the therapeutic relationship may be indicative of clinically relevant material.

Structure a Therapeutic Environment That Evokes CRBs

At the very first contact, FAP therapists provide a rationale to gain informed consent and buy-in for the treatment approach, as well as to prepare clients for an intense and evocative therapy that focuses on *in-vivo* interactions. For example, one might say to a depressed client:

"I understand that you are seeking treatment for depression. One reason why people may get depressed is that they find it hard to express how they feel and what they need in their relationships, and find it difficult to assert those needs to important people in their life. Do you find that this is true for you? [The answer is usually "Yes."] Well, one focus of our therapy will be on how you can become a more powerful person by developing ways for you to express your true feelings with conviction and compassion and go after what you want in your relationships and in life. [The response is typically "That sounds good."] The most effective and efficient way for you to develop the skills to become a more expressive person is to start right here, right now, with me, and to discuss with me what you are thinking, feeling, and needing, even if it feels scary or risky. If you can bring forth your best self with me, then you can transfer these behaviors to other people in your life. How does that sound?"

The format and structure of the therapy process often naturally evoke CRBs. Aspects of therapy that may evoke CRBs include scheduling and canceling sessions, paying session fees, and time constraints. The therapist should watch for potential CRBs (Rule 1) and seek to understand how the client's behavior in these situations parallels his or her behavior in daily life. In the example of the client who is consistently late to session, the FAP therapist would approach this problem behavior (CRB1) using functional analysis to (1) help the client understand barriers to arriving on time and (2) discuss the effect of lateness not only on the therapist, but on the client's relationships in daily life. (Note that since FAP therapists pay close attention to the function and not just the form of a behavior, occasionally lateness may constitute an improvement or CRB2 in the case of someone who is compulsively punctual).

In addition, the beginning of therapy naturally calls for clients to share both historical and current details about their lives. FAP often employs a written life history exercise in which clients are asked:

"Reflect on your life from birth to the present in terms of the highlights, challenges, celebrations, relationships, enduring circumstances, turning points, accomplishments, losses, adventures, and the peaks and valleys that have shaped who you are as a person. You can do this in chart form or narrative form."

Based on the client's response, the therapist can begin to get a sense not only of the content of the client's life history, but also of the client's interpersonal style, and approach or avoidance of emotionally charged material.

Use Evocative Therapeutic Methods

FAP is an integrative therapy and calls for varied approaches depending on what will evoke client CRBs and what will naturally reinforce client progress. What is important is not the theoretical origin of a specific method, but rather its function with the client. To the extent that a procedure—any procedure—functions to evoke CRBs, it is potentially useful to FAP. Methods such as free association, writing exercises (i.e., Chapter 6), empty-chair work (see Thoma & Greenberg, Chapter 11, this volume), mindfulness (see Germer & Chan, Chapter 1, this volume), cognitive restructuring (see Daflos, Lunt, & Whittal, Chapter 5, and Leahy, Chapter 13, this volume), evoking emotion by focusing on bodily sensations, and hypnotherapy have all been used in FAP (Kanter, Tsai, & Kohlenberg, 2010; Tsai et al., 2009). The FAP therapist has tremendous flexibility in selecting procedures, given that the key is the function (e.g., evoking, reinforcing), not the form. Often, effective evocative techniques help clients contact and express feelings and thoughts that they typically avoid.

During the course of therapy, a therapist may decide to enlist mindfulness meditation at the beginning of each therapy session as a "grounding" and connecting activity for client and therapist to complete together. A session bridging form is also given to clients after every session (see Tsai et al., 2009, Appendix D) where they are asked to share their candid responses in order to maximize the effectiveness of the therapy. Questions include:

"What stands out to you about our last session? Thoughts, feelings, insights?"
"What would have made the session a more helpful experience?"
"Anything you are reluctant to say or ask for?"
"What issues came up for you in the session with your therapist that are similar to your daily life problems?"
"What risks did you take in session/with your therapist or what progress did you make that can translate into your outside life?"

Structured exercises to evoke CRB may be linked to specific issues that the client is working on. Telling others about one's innermost thoughts and feelings is central to establishing intimacy and reducing emotional avoidance. For clients, these thoughts and feelings may be about the therapeutic relationship or may involve emotionally laden expressions that are not necessarily about the therapist, but the presence of the therapist evokes avoidance. An example of an evocative exercise done in session is the "nondominant handwriting task," which tends to bring forth more potent, less ordinary responses because there has been less historical opportunity to develop avoidance repertoires while writing with the nondominant hand. Stem sentences include: "I feel . . . I need . . . I long for . . . I'm scared . . . I'm struggling with . . . I dream of . . . I pretend that . . . It's hard for me to talk about/tell you . . . If I had the money, I would . . . If I had the courage, I would . . . " The stem sentences are read aloud to clients in session, and they are told that they only have to disclose the responses they feel comfortable sharing. Emotional expressions in the presence of the therapist are potential CRB2s of greater intimacy and openness, but for others, setting a privacy limit until they feel comfortable sharing may be a CRB2 as well.

Use Oneself as an Instrument of Change

To the extent that therapists can allow themselves to be who they really are in the service of client growth, a more powerful and transformative therapeutic relationship can be created. Considering the following questions may help you as a therapist to increase your potency as an agent of change:

1. *What unique qualities make you distinctive as a person and as a therapist? How can you use your distinctiveness to your clients' advantage?* For example, whether you have a great sense of humor, a terrific memory for details, or if you get tearful easily because you are so compassionate, you can assess on an individual basis how each of these qualities can be used to increase connection with particular clients.

2. *Do any of your client's interests match yours?* Consider disclosing this commonality. Similarly, do you have comparable life experiences, such as growing up Catholic, birth order, moving around a lot as a child, being a member of a minority group? A major factor to take into account in making a decision to disclose is whether such disclosure will facilitate clients having greater contact with their issues, or whether it will take them away from their own focus. Other considerations include whether the disclosure will engender more closeness from the client and whether the disclosure is problem behavior or a target behavior for the therapist. That is to say, it is important that therapists carefully consider the function and possible behavioral consequences of self-disclosure.

3. *What is your experience of your client? What do you see as really special about this person, how does he or she positively impact you, and how evocative would it be for you to mirror back what is most special about him or her?* Clients are often only in touch with their flaws and shortcomings; for you to consistently tell them how you experience their positive characteristics is an experience they may not have had before, creating a turning point in self-perception (e.g., "You light a room with warmth when you walk in; the people in your life are really lucky to be in your sphere of caring").

4. *What are the ways you care about your client?* Anyone can say the words "I care about you," but it is far more impactful to describe your behaviors that indicate caring. For example, you can talk about the ways they affect you outside of the therapy hour, such as, "I had a dream about you," "I was thinking the other day about what you said to me," or "I saw a movie and thought at the time, 'I've got to tell you about this movie because you would really like it,'" or "I went to a workshop on art therapy with you in mind because I thought the techniques would be really helpful in our work together." Statements such as these are likely to be both evocative (Rule 2) and naturally reinforcing (Rule 3).

5. *How can you take risks to deepen your therapeutic relationship in ways that serve the client's best interests* (e.g., share a poem that reminds you of the client)? *Are there topics you avoid addressing with your clients* (e.g., her behaviors that push you away, wanting him to say what he is feeling underneath his facade, your caring for her) *because you would feel discomfort? Are there ways you can ask your clients to be more present and open with you* (e.g., When you are more open and vulnerable with me, I feel more connected to you. On a scale of 1–10 with 1 being very shallow and 10 being very deep, where are you right now in terms of how you're talking with me? Are you willing to go a little deeper to increase your sense of connection with yourself and between us) ?

These questions facilitate exploration of how one can become a more compassionate and transparent change agent through disclosing one's own thoughts, reactions and personal experiences. Such disclosures can enhance the therapeutic relationship, normalize clients' experiences, model adaptive and intimacy-building behavior, demonstrate genuineness and positive regard for clients, and equalize power in the therapeutic relationship. From an FAP perspective, these therapist behaviors may serve the client by evoking CRBs, blocking CRB1s, and encouraging and nurturing (reinforcing) CRB2s. Thus, disclosure should be undertaken strategically, with awareness for how the disclosure may evoke, reinforce, or punish CRBs for a particular client (Vandenberghe, Coppede, & Kohlenberg, 2006; Tsai, Plummer, Kanter, Newring, & Kohlenberg, 2010).

In addition to the above strategies, using oneself as a therapeutic agent of change is also exemplified through the FAP "End of Therapy Letter," an important component of the parting process. The letter may include a description of the client's progress and strengths, what the therapist will remember about the client, what the therapist wants the client to take away, hopes and wishes for the client, and parting advice. Each letter is unique to the client–therapist relationship and serves as a tangible reminder of the client's progress and of the relationship itself. The letter is a chance to model how a relationship can end positively, with meaning and feeling. Clients should have a clear sense of the ways in which they are special, and clarity about what they have to contribute to their relationships, their communities, and perhaps even the world.

Rule 3. Naturally Reinforce CRBs (Be Therapeutically Loving)

A fundamental premise of FAP is that the closer in time and place client behavior is to the therapist's intervention (i.e., contingent reinforcement), the stronger the effect of the intervention. Thousands of studies have used immediate reinforcement to establish and maintain behavior in mammals ranging from rats to humans (Catania, 1998). The delay effect—that reinforcement becomes less effective as the delay between a response and reinforcement increases—is most clearly demonstrated in humans with complex tasks (Hockman & Lipsitt, 1961) and when intervening behavior occurs between a response and reinforcement (Atkinson, 1969).

Thus, a therapist can maximize the power of intervention by observing (Rule 1) and evoking (Rule 2) clients' relevant interpersonal behaviors within the session, and then immediately reinforcing behavioral progress (Rule 3) as it occurs. In order to achieve this, one must be skilled in delivering effective reinforcement. In other words, a therapist must respond to client's behavioral progress (e.g., more effective assertion of needs) in such a way that the client is likely to repeat and continue that growth.

Rule 3 presents one of the greatest challenges in using this therapeutic approach. FAP is based on the assertion that therapist reinforcement is the primary mechanism of change, yet deliberate efforts to reinforce run the risk of producing contrived or arbitrary, rather than natural, reinforcement. A contrived or inauthentic response is more likely to punish rather than reinforce client progress. Therefore, inauthentic responses, even if delivered with skillful timing, are unlikely to strengthen client's progress and do not generalize to the client's daily life. For example, if a client exhibits a CRB2 of expressing anger, and the therapist exuberantly says, "It's fantastic you're being angry at me!" but does not seriously address the client's unmet need that led to the anger, such a response does not represent what the client is likely to encounter in daily life, On the other hand, natural but poorly timed responses may fail to contingently reinforce progress, and may even reinforce problem behaviors (CRB1s). Thus, it is essential that the therapist align natural, genuine responding with effective, skillful responding. Natural and contingent therapist responses improve client functioning in a way that promotes generalization and client adaptability.

In order to respond genuinely, FAP therapists must draw on their own private reactions to their clients (thoughts, emotions, physiological responses) and naturally respond to each CRB accordingly. Thus when clients engage in improved behavior (CRB2s)—particularly behavior that breaks the rules they typically adhere to—FAP therapists convey the interpersonal effect of clients' behavior by revealing their reactions to clients in the moment. For example:

CLIENT: Last week's session ended kind of abruptly and that was difficult for me. Can we take more time to wrap up this week?
THERAPIST: I feel a greater sense of trust between us just knowing that you'll ask for what you want with me. Yes, we can do that.

In this example, the therapist shares a natural response that is both genuine and likely to reinforce the client's improved behavior. (Note that the therapist cannot assume that a particular response has had a reinforcing effect on the client; Rule 4 emphasizes the importance of checking for this effect.)

Relevant to this discussion of natural reinforcement are recommendations from the child treatment literature that advocate the importance of therapists working from a "coping model" rather than a "mastery model" (Kendall & Braswell, 1982). A mastery model simply displays success without acknowledging struggle, whereas a coping model demonstrates the initial difficulties, a strategy to effectively manage or overcome the problem, and then success. A therapist's ability to model coping with a challenge, such as anxiety, rather than simply displaying mastery, helps to normalize a client's experience, and emphasizes that coping with one's struggles is a skill to be learned (Podell et al., 2010). From an FAP perspective, a therapist's vulnerability in sharing his or her own struggles that are relevant to the client's may be an evocative risk (Rule 2), but such vulnerability also can be very naturally reinforcing of a client's CRB2s. In this case transcript (edited for clarity), the therapist uses coping modeling as both an evocative risk and as natural reinforcement after she and her 8-year-old client with OCD both touch a public toilet with their bare hands:

THERAPIST: Like you, I can't help feeling a little anxious after we just touched that toilet—I can almost feel the germs on my hands.

CLIENT: I can't believe we just touched a toilet. Yuck! I just want to wash my hands. Are you sure we aren't going to get sick?

THERAPIST: I totally understand being worried because there is no way to be certain that we won't get sick. I know if we wash our hands right now the worry about germs will only get worse and worse over time. Instead I'm going to purposely think about all the germs that might make me sick even though it makes me nervous, not wash my hands, and then do something fun like play a game. Want to try my trick with me?

CLIENT: OK, I guess.

THERAPIST: Great! It will make it so much better to do it with you instead of by myself. I love being a team fighting OCD with you. Ok, now let's imagine every possible gross germ we can crawling all over our skin.

CLIENT: That was so gross but it got easier as the time passed. I still don't like it though.

THERAPIST: I was watching you as you were imagining and you looked so focused and powerful. It's like I could literally see you doing battle with OCD this very moment and winning. Look at all you did today— you touched a toilet, imagined all the things you hate thinking about, and didn't wash your hands!

CLIENT: Yeah, it feels pretty good! . . . Can we play the game now?

THERAPIST: Of course.

To highlight the importance of responding both authentically *and* effectively (contingent on CRB1/CRB2s), we emphasize that naturally reinforcing behaviors are therapeutically loving. Therapeutic love is ethical, is always in the client's best interests, and is genuine. Loving clients does not necessarily mean using the word "love" with them, but it does mean fostering an exquisite sensitivity and benevolent concern for the needs and feelings of clients and caring deeply about them. In behavioral terms, this means that clients' well-being and therapeutic progress are powerfully rewarding and reinforcing *to the therapist*. In order to create and maintain this therapeutically loving stance toward clients, we recommend these therapist practices:

1. *Establish a clear case conceptualization for each individual client, specifically linking in-session behavioral improvements toward their larger life goals.* This enhances therapist awareness of how even small in-session improvements (CRB2s) serve the client's best interests. It is essential to match one's expectations with clients' current repertoires in order to be tuned into successive approximations or nuances of improvement, and thus prevent becoming frustrated or even subtly rejecting of the client.

2. *Practice metta meditation (i.e., loving-kindness meditation), both generally and toward clients in particular.* For example, "May all beings be free of fear and harm; May we all be happy just as we are; May we all be at peace with whatever comes; And may we all rest gently in the softness of our own hearts." (Salzberg, 1995, p. 124–125). This practice of "wishing others well" strengthens compassion and positive emotions toward others (Frederickson, Cohn, Coffey, Pek, & Finkel, 2008), increasing the likelihood a client's progress will naturally evoke a reinforcing response from the therapist.

3. *Practice awareness of the ways in which one's own learning history informs responses to client behavior (i.e., "countertransference"), striving to distinguish idiosyncratic responses from typical responses.* Cultivating this awareness allows the therapist to provide the client with feedback that more strongly generalizes to other relationships in the client's life.

4. *Expand one's own behavioral repertoire to include clients' goal behaviors.* This allows a therapist to genuinely model and reinforce behavioral progress. A therapist who is accepting of intimacy will more naturally display and easily reinforce clients' steps toward intimacy, whereas a therapist who is avoidant of intimacy will be less effective in facilitating intimacy-building behaviors in clients.

5. *Develop poetic and metaphorical language.* A therapist can enhance the strength of verbal responses by developing fluency with powerful language and metaphors, and by expanding vocabulary for

capturing emotion. Because authenticity is essential, it is recommended that therapists cultivate their own "poetic style" that is both powerful and genuine. Further, a range of styles may be required for a range of clients. One recommendation is reading poetry or practicing writing poetry (Fox, 1997).

Rule 4. Notice Your Impact

When therapists respond to clients' CRBs, it is imperative that they pay attention to client reactions and consider the question: "Am I having the desired effect on my client?" By definition, the client has experienced therapeutic reinforcement only if his or her target behavior is strengthened. Therefore, therapists must assess the degree to which their behaviors that were intended to reinforce actually functioned as reinforcers. By continuing to pay close attention to the function of one's own behavior, the therapist can adjust his or her responding as necessary to maximize the potential for reinforcement. It also is important for therapists to focus on the role of therapist in-session problem behaviors (T1s) and therapist in-session target behaviors (T2s) because an increased awareness of oneself goes hand-in-hand with an increased awareness of one's impact on clients. We recommend that therapists set aside time to explore questions such as the following:

> "What do you tend to avoid addressing with your clients?"
> "How does this avoidance impact the work that you do with these clients?"
> "What do you tend to avoid dealing with in your own life (e.g., tasks, people, memories, needs, feelings)?"
> "How do your daily life avoidances impact the work that you do with your clients?"
> "What are the specific T2s you want to develop with each client based on the case conceptualization?"

Rule 5. Provide Functional Interpretations of Behavior (Interpret and Generalize)

A functional analytically informed interpretation includes a history that accounts for how client behavior was adaptive at some point in his or her past, and how to generalize progress in therapy to daily life. Implementing Rule 5 emphasizes "out-to-in parallels" when daily life events correspond to in-session situations and "in-to-out parallels" when in-session events correspond to daily life events (Tsai, Kohlenberg, Kanter, & Waltz, 2009). Both are important, and a good FAP session may involve considerable weaving between daily-life and in-session content through multiple in-to-out and out-to-in parallels. One example involves a client pulling away from her therapist expressing caring (out-to-in parallel) and relaxing into this caring and allowing it to happen in her daily life (in-to-out parallel). Thus, out-to-in parallels typically consist of maladaptive behaviors that manifest in session, and in-to-out parallels consist of newly learned adaptive behaviors in session that are then implemented in daily life.

Provision of homework is also important to Rule 5; the best homework assignments are those in which a client has engaged in a CRB2 and the assignment is for the client to then take the improved behavior "on the road" and test it with significant others (e.g.,"You took the risk of letting yourself be vulnerable by sharing some deep feelings with me, and we felt more connected as a result. Would you be willing to practice taking little steps outside of your comfort zone this next week and keep a log of your interpersonal risks?").

In summary, when these five FAP rules are applied well, we believe that it leads to an increased and meaningful focus on the therapeutic relationship entailing awareness, appropriate risk taking by both clients and therapists, natural reinforcement of positive change, and the generalization of in-session progress to daily life, thus maximizing therapeutic outcome.

Precautions

FAP seeks to create a deep and profound therapeutic experience; the degree of thoughtfulness, care, and caution that FAP therapists bring to their work must be equally deep and profound (Tsai et al., 2012). Thus, these are areas of potential ethical concern:

1. *Avoid exploitation.* The intensity and emotional intimacy that are typically present in FAP relationships may increase the likelihood of situations that may be harmful to clients: an unhealthy dependence on the therapist, sexual involvement, or interminable treatments where both parties are gratified by a relationship that is more like friendship than therapy. In order to minimize the likelihood of exploiting or harming clients, it is important to constantly keep in mind the question, "What is best for my client at the moment and in the long run?"
2. *Titrate the treatment according to the client's tolerance level.* It is important to know what evocative therapist behaviors will encourage growth at a level the client is ready for versus what will lead to undue stress or disengagement, and to titrate the *in-vivo* focus in a way that the client can tolerate.
3. *Be controlled by reinforcers that benefit clients.* Therapists must recognize when they are controlled by reinforcers that are not helpful to the client (e.g., the therapist is reinforced by praise and gratitude, but this behavior is a CRB1 for the client).

FAP-informed treatment does not help all clients, particularly ones who do not agree with the rationale that it is important to focus on in-session behavior and the therapeutic relationship. At times, a client's decision not to continue treatment may be a CRB2—a behavior that should be reinforced.

Future Directions

FAP uses basic learning principles to explain how the focus on the therapeutic relationship leads to change. FAP proposes that the therapist–client relationship lies at the very heart of the change process and offers specific, behaviorally defined therapist guidelines to help clients establish intimacy skills that are transferred to their daily lives. Our behavioral approach takes into account the client's unique history, and, as called for by the American Psychological Association Division 29 Task Force on Empirically Supported Relationships (Norcross, 2001), tailors both discrete methods and relationship stances on a patient-by-patient or moment-to-moment basis. Although it is an approach that will benefit from further empirical evidence, we hope that FAP offers an inspiring and conceptually clear framework that crosses theoretical boundaries and provides additional ways to focus on the therapeutic relationship as a means to facilitate meaningful client change.

Further Resources

Articles

- For a cogent description of how FAP can be integrated with any treatment, see Kohlenberg and Tsai (1994).
- For a review of how intimacy is a transdiagnostic problem for cognitive-behavioral therapy, see Wetterneck and Hart (2012).

Books

- For a theory and clinical practice overview of FAP, see Kohlenberg and Tsai (1991).
- For a guide to FAP methods and how they relate to awareness, courage, and love, see Tsai, Kohlenberg, Kanter, Kohlenberg, et al. (2009).
- For a primer on distinctive features of FAP, see Tsai, Kohlenberg, Kanter, Holman, and Plummer Loudon (2012).

Website

- For handouts, articles, and training information, go to *www.faptherapy.com*.

References

Atkinson, R. C. (1969). Information delay in human learning. *Journal of Verbal Learning and Verbal Behavior, 8,* 507–511.
Baruch, D., Kanter, J., Busch, A., Plummer, M., Tsai, M., Rusch, L., et al.. (2009). Lines of evidence in support of FAP. In M. Tsai, R. Kohlenberg, J. Kanter, B. Kohlenberg, W. Follette, & G. Callaghan (Eds.), *A guide to functional analytic psychotherapy: Awareness, courage, love and behaviorism* (pp. 21–36). New York: Springer.
Busch, A., Kanter, J., Callaghan, G., Baruch, D., Weeks, C., & Berlin, K. (2009). A microprocess analysis of functional analytic psychotherapy's mechanism of change. *Behavior Therapy, 40,* 280–290.
Callaghan, G., Follette, W., Ruckstuhl, L., & Linnerooth, P. (2008). The Functional Analytic Psychotherapy Rating Scale: A behavioral psychotherapy coding system. *Behavior Analyst Today, 9,* 98–116.
Callaghan, G., Summers, C., & Weidman, M. (2003). The treatment of histrionic and narcissistic personality disorder behaviors: A single-subject demonstration of clinical effectiveness using functional analytic psychotherapy. *Journal of Contemporary Psychotherapy, 33,* 321–339.
Catania, C. (1998). *Learning.* Englewood Cliffs, NJ: Prentice-Hall.
Fox, J. (1997). *Poetic medicine: The healing art of poem-making.* New York: Putnam.
Fredrickson, B., Cohn, M., Coffey, K., Pek, J., & Finkel, S. (2008). Open hearts build lives: Positive emotions, induced through loving-kindness meditation, build consequential personal resources. *Journal of Personality and Social Psychology, 95*(5), 1045–1062.
Gaynor, S., & Lawrence, P. (2002). Complementing CBT for depressed adolescents with Learning through In Vivo Experience (LIVE): Conceptual analysis, treatment description, and feasibility study. *Behavioural and Cognitive Psychotherapy,* 79–101.
Gifford, E., Kohlenberg, B., Hayes, S., Pierson, H., Piasecki, M., Antonuccio, D., et al. (2011). Does acceptance and relationship focused behavior therapy contribute to bupropion outcomes?: A randomized controlled trial of functional analytic psychotherapy and acceptance and commitment therapy for smoking cessation. *Behavior Therapy, 42*(4), 700–715.
Hockman, C. H., & Lipsitt, L. P. (1961). Delay-of-reward gradients in discrimination learning with children for two levels of difficulty. *Journal of Comparative and Physiological Psychology, 54,* 24–27.
Kanter, J., Landes, S., Busch, A., Rusch, L., Brown, K., Baruch, D., et al. (2006). The effect of contingent reinforcement on target variables in outpatient psychotherapy for depression: A successful and unsuccessful case using functional analytic psychotherapy. *Journal of Applied Behavior Analysis, 39,* 463–467.
Kanter, J., Schildcrout, J., & Kohlenberg, R. (2005). *In vivo* processes in cognitive therapy for depression: Frequency and benefits. *Psychotherapy Research, 15*(4), 366–373.
Kanter, J., Tsai, M., & Kohlenberg, R. (Eds.). (2010). *The practice of functional analytic psychotherapy.* New York: Springer.
Kendall, P. C., & Braswell, L. (1982). Cognitive-behavioral self-control therapy for children: A components analysis. *Journal of Consulting and Clinical Psychology, 50,* 672–689.
Kohlenberg, R. J., Kanter, J., Bolling, M., Parker, C., &. Tsai, M. (2002). Enhancing cognitive therapy for depression with functional analytic psychotherapy: Treatment guidelines and empirical findings. *Cognitive and Behavioral Practice, 9,* 213–229.

Kohlenberg, R., & Tsai, M. (1991). *Functional analytic psychotherapy: Creating intense and curative therapeutic relationships.* New York: Plenum Press.

Kohlenberg, R. J., & Tsai, M. (1994). Functional analytic psychotherapy: A behavioral approach to treatment and integration. *Journal of Psychotherapy Integration, 4,* 175–201.

Norcross, J. D. (Ed.). (2001). Empirically supported therapy relationships: Summary report of the Division 29 Task Force. *Psychotherapy, 38*(4).

Podell, J. L., Mychailyszyn, M., Edmunds, J., Puleo, C. M., & Kendall, P. C. (2010). The Coping Cat Program for anxious youth: The FEAR plan comes to life. Cognitive and Behavioral Practice, 17(2), 132–141.

Salzberg, S. (1995). *Loving-kindness: The revolutionary art of happiness.* Boston: Shambhala Classics.

Tsai, M., Callaghan, G., & Kohlenberg, R. J. (2013). The use of awareness, courage, therapeutic love, and behavioral interpretation in functional analytic psychotherapy. *Psychotherapy, 50*(3), 366–370.

Tsai, M., Kohlenberg, R., Kanter, J., Holman, G., & Plummer Loudon, M. (2012). *Functional analytic therapy: Distinctive features.* London: Routledge.

Tsai, M., Kohlenberg, R., Kanter, J., Kohlenberg, B., Follette, W., & Callaghan, G. (Eds.). (2009). *A guide to functional analytic psychotherapy: Awareness, courage, love, and behaviorism.* New York: Springer.

Tsai, M., Kohlenberg, R. J., Kanter, J. W., & Waltz, J. (2009). Therapeutic technique: The five rules. In M. Tsai, R. J. Kohlenberg, J. W. Kanter, B. Kohlenberg, W. C. Follette, & G. M. Callaghan (Eds.), *A guide to functional analytic psychotherapy: Awareness, courage, love, and behaviorism* (pp. 61–102). New York: Springer.

Tsai, M., Plummer, M., Kanter, J., Newring, R., & Kohlenberg, R. (2010). Therapist grief and functional analytic psychotherapy: Strategic self-disclosure of personal loss. *Journal of Contemporary Psychotherapy, 40,* 1–10.

Vandenberghe, L., Coppede, A. M., & Kohlenberg, R. J. (2006). Client curiosity about the therapist's private life: Hindrance or therapeutic aid? *Behavior Therapist, 29*(3), 41–46.

Wetterneck, C. T., & Hart, J. M. (2012). Intimacy is a transdiagnostic problem for cognitive behavior therapy: Functional analytical psychotherapy is a solution. *International Journal of Behavioral Consultation and Therapy, 7*(2–3), 167–178.

Conclusion

Experiential Methods, Cognitive-Behavioral Therapy, and Next Steps in Emotional Engagement in Treatment

Dean McKay
Nathan C. Thoma

> Talking to a therapist, I thought, was like taking your clothes off and then taking your skin off, and then having the other person say, "Would you mind opening up your rib cage so that we can start?"
>
> —Julie Schumacher (2008, p. 58)

The degree to which therapy is an intense interpersonal experience can sometimes be lost on therapists, particularly when they are focusing on treatment as a scientific enterprise. Some clinicians approach therapy as empirical, with clearly measured goals, behavioral outcomes, emotional adjustments, and clinically significant change (i.e., a reduction in specific symptoms) as the only meaningful outcomes to be gleaned from the therapeutic endeavor (see Salekin, Jarrett, & Adams, 2013, for a discussion of measurement in therapy). Clearly these are important goals. At the other extreme, some clinicians eschew any hint of data, decamping to the position that the human experience is beyond quantification and that attempts to measure change cheapen the therapeutic relationship (see Bornstein, 2005, for a lament concerning this position among psychodynamic researchers).

Clinicians generally wear multiple hats. They consider data as well as the interpersonal experience of their clients. Most of us in the field share a tacit understanding that while much can (and should) be measured to assess baseline functioning and to assess progress, there are additional components of therapy that are difficult to quantify. Unfortunately, it is the reliance on the difficult-to-quantify side of the therapy experience that leads to approaches that are questionable, unscientific, or pseudoscientic (Garb & Boyle, 2003).

The topic this book attempted to tackle involves one of these difficult-to-quantify aspects of therapy, the experiential feature. This topic should be highly compatible with the work of therapists, both full-time clinicians and those who also work as researchers. Yet there is surprising little experimental work that directly discusses experiential features that impact a client's functioning and response to treatment. At the time of this writing (December 24, 2013), a search of the PubMed and PsycLit databases using the terms "experiential" and "experiment" resulted in 311 peer-reviewed articles; of these, only 24 related directly to therapy. And yet, therapists have been discussing experiential features of therapy for decades, and some have highlighted the challenges facing psychologists who wear the hats of both clinician and researcher. Kohut (1977) described this conflict well: "If we initially have the courage to acknowledge the fact that scientific objectivity in the sciences of man must always include the objective assessment of the observer—the influence of the observed on the observer and, especially, the influence of the observer on the field that he observes—then we can clarify our methodology" (p. 40). Kohut was describing several conflicts that scientifically minded therapists face. First, we are necessarily blinded by our own biases when we begin to engage in assessment. Second, we do well to attend to these biases in order that we can be more objective. But third, we can never completely escape our biases and must therefore calibrate our approaches to account for the inherently subjective nature of our work.

Cognitive-Behavioral Therapy and Emergent Therapy Trends

When cognitive-behavioral therapy (CBT) began to be investigated in earnest (primarily referred to as "behavior therapy" at the time), the scientific approach focused on avoiding the inherent biases that cloud the judgment of scientists in testing their own hypotheses. Most of the research of the early behavior therapists focused on observable and measurable behaviors, with limited attention to cognitions (Kazdin, 1978). This seemed a natural stance, as the early behavior therapists were reacting to what they viewed as excessive "mentalism" in the profession. The desire among behavior therapists to distinguish themselves from therapists concerned with inner processes led in some instances to divisive commentary (for a history of the contentious relation between behavior therapy and other therapeutic approaches, see Staats & Eifert, 1990). However, the early behavior analysts were also keenly aware of learning history (i.e., experience) as a factor critically involved in later learning (see Salzinger, 1996). Salzinger (1996) cites classic, basic behavioral research that showed how prior reinforcement led to specific differential responses under new conditions of reinforcement. These laboratory learning experiences in turn suggest that the experience of individuals is a crucial variable for understanding and treating clients.

The attention paid to behavior over other psychological processes soon gave way to an emphasis on cognitions and associated inner processes as critical components of therapy, leading to the cognitive revolution. There are a number of reasonable sources that can be ascribed significance in this movement, such as the focus on distorted beliefs as functionally important in depression (Beck, 1976), the identification of irrational beliefs as central in neuroses generally (Ellis, 1962), and the general idea that human experiences can lead to distorted thinking as well as behavior (Mahoney, 1979). These cognitive approaches inherently included emotional processes as a marker of improvement, with early research concentrating largely on subjective (i.e., client) report of improvement as indicative of treatment efficacy.

Interestingly, in the course of the CBT movement there have been other efforts to integrate approaches that explicitly include experiential features into treatment. These usually came by way of attempts to integrate aspects of CBT with other prevailing psychotherapeutic methods. For example, Stampfl and Levis (1967) developed a method of exposure therapy that included imagery based on interpretations made by the clinician. Cognitive therapy approaches included methods that required clinicians to creatively develop specific exercises that tied to the client's personal experience in order to activate beliefs. These "behavioral experiments" have come to be viewed as potent methods for changing behaviors and emotional reactions (e.g., in the context of obsessive–compulsive disorder; Abramowitz, Taylor, & McKay, 2005). In short, CBT-oriented therapists have in fact been concerned with experiential features of client functioning for many years now, even if they do not expressly endorse the term.

Modern CBT: Protocols, Dissemination, and Scientific Practice

Cognitive-behavioral therapists typically endorse the empirically supported approach to practice. At the most basic level, this implies that research findings (i.e., randomized controlled trials) guide their decisions about treatment. Indeed, scientific approaches are considered the cornerstone of the discipline. To illustrate, in lists of empirically supported treatments for psychological conditions, the vast majority of protocols are cognitive-behavioral in nature (i.e., Chambless & Ollendick, 2001). Since the time criteria were established for declaring support for different psychological interventions, the support for CBT methods has grown substantially, as evidenced from the online listing of scientifically supported interventions maintained by Division 12 (Clinical) of the American Psychological Association. There are also scientifically supported approaches that are based in other theoretical domains (e.g., interpersonal psychotherapy for depression and other psychological conditions; see *www.psychologicaltreatments.org*).

The fact that so many treatments that are scientifically supported happen to also derive from CBT does not tell the entire story. Indeed, whereas the science is firmly in favor of CBT for most psychological conditions, few practitioners employ these approaches. The reasons for this disparity are well beyond the scope of this chapter,[1] but there are two important points worth raising here that are germane to our discussion of experiential methods. First, there are persistent problems in disseminating empirically supported methods. McHugh and Barlow (2010) discuss the many successful training programs for different presenting problems whereby clinicians can be trained to be effective in administering scientifically based approaches, but when the training protocol ends, so too does the application of scientifically based methods. Others have construed this problem as one that must be addressed at the point of education (Klepac et al., 2012) if there is to be any meaningful reform in the way practitioners understand the relation between science and practice. Efforts toward reform now extend to how clinical scientists are trained, with proposals calling for experiential approaches to foster the ability of nascent clinicians to develop interventions from a scientific base (Shoham et al., 2014).

Second, there is a large gap between the findings from randomized controlled trials and implementation of treatment in everyday clinical settings. This gap has long been acknowledged, but some have pressed simply for clinicians to adopt the manuals into practice with minor deviations from protocol in order to individualize therapy (Wilson, 2007). Alternatively, Gallo, Comer, and Barlow (2013) argue that single-case designs afford a heretofore untapped opportunity to refine protocols by evaluating specific mechanisms as each step of treatment development, allowing for inclusion of therapeutic procedures that may be overlooked in other approaches to protocols. As an illustration of this approach, research from this same group (Satir et al., 2011) demonstrated the importance of the

---

[1] Lilienfeld, Ritschel, Lynn, Cautin, and Latzman (2013) discuss in detail the reasons for resistance among clinicians for adopting scientific approaches to therapy. The authors, echoing a mandate many clinicians are given during training, argue that when clients present with resistance it is the job of the therapist to identify the root causes.

therapeutic alliance in the treatment of anorexia nervosa using a single-case design.

This leads to the unresolved question facing clinicians, namely: What constitutes scientific practice? Empirically derived clinical practice guidelines have been formulated as a means to begin to answer this question (Hollon et al., 2014). What is notable in the newly formulated practice guidelines are provisions for identifying treatments that clinicians are advised against using. Under the existing empirically supported treatment guidelines, treatments can gather empirical support, but null findings or findings that suggest that interventions are detrimental effectively "don't count" in determining whether to recommend an approach.

Experiential Methods and CBT

As this book makes plain, and as the above discussion highlights, experiential approaches are firmly in the purview of CBT. However, until recently, most of the experiential approaches have been implied, not explicit, in the conduct of CBT. By making the conduct of experiential approaches explicit, we hope these can then become mainstream in the everyday practice of clinicians and also receive empirical scrutiny (such that clinical practice guidelines may develop around these procedures). At present, it may be inferred that CBT-oriented therapists rely on a range of other therapeutic methods when the protocols or other empirically supported approaches lack guidance for the presenting problems of our clients, or when clinicians rely on prior experience, personally experienced emotions, or idiographic clinical judgment (i.e., Waller, Stringer, & Meyer, 2012).

References

Abramowitz, J. S., Taylor, S., & McKay, D. (2005). Potentials and limitations in cognitive-behavior therapy for obsessive–compulsive disorder. *Cognitive Behaviour Therapy, 34,* 140–147.

Beck, A. T. (1976). *Cognitive therapy and the emotional disorders.* New York: International Universities Press.

Bornstein, R. A. (2005). Reconnecting psychoanalysis to mainstream psychology: Challenges and opportunities. *Psychoanalytic Psychology, 22,* 323–340.

Chambless, D. L., & Ollendick, T. H. (2001). Empirically supported psychological interventions: Controversies and evidence. *Annual Review of Psychology, 52,* 685–716.

Ellis, A. (1962). *Reason and emotion in psychotherapy.* Secaucus, NJ: Lyle Stewart.

Gallo, K. P., Comer, J. S., & Barlow, D. H. (2013). Single-case experimental designs and small pilot trial designs. In J. S. Comer & P. C. Kendall (Eds.), *The Oxford handbook of research strategies for clinical psychology* (pp. 24–39). New York: Oxford University Press.

Garb, H. N., & Boyle, P. A. (2003). Understanding why some clinicians use pseudoscientific methods. Findings from research on clinical judgment. In S. O. Lilienfeld, S. J. Lynn, & J. M. Lohr (Eds.), *Science and pseudoscience in clinical psychology: Findings from research on clinical judgment* (pp. 17–38). New York: Guilford Press.

Hollon, S. D., Areán, P. A., Craske, M. G., Crawford, K. A., Kivlahan, D. R., Magnavita, J. J., et al. (2014). Development of clinical practice guidelines (CPGs). *Annual Review of Clinical Psychology, 10*, 213–241.

Kazdin, A. E. (1978). *History of behavior modification: Experimental foundations of contemporary research.* Ann Arbor: University of Michigan Press.

Klepac, R. K., Ronan, G. F., Andrasik, F., Arnold, K. D., Belar, C. D., Berry, S. L., et al. (2012). Guidelines for cognitive-behavioral training within doctoral psychology programs in the United States: Report of the Inter-Organizational Task Force on Cognitive and Behavioral Psychology Doctoral Education. *Behavior Therapy, 43*, 687–697.

Kohut, H. (1977). *How does analysis cure?* Chicago: University of Chicago Press.

Lilienfeld, S. O., Ritschel, L. A., Lynn, S. J., Cautin, R. L., & Latzman, R. D. (2013). Why many clinical psychologists are resistant to evidence-based practice: Root causes and constructive remedies. *Clinical Psychology Review, 33*, 883–900.

Mahoney, M. J. (1979). *Self-change: Strategies for solving personal problems.* Oxford, UK: Norton.

McHugh, R. K., & Barlow, D. H. (2010). The dissemination and implementation of evidence-based psychological treatments: A review of current efforts. *American Psychologist, 65*, 73–84.

Salekin, R. T., Jarrett, M. A., & Adams, E. W. (2013). Assessment and measurement of change considerations in psychotherapy research. In J. S. Comer & P. C. Kendall (Eds.), *The Oxford handbook of research strategies for clinical psychology* (pp. 103–119). New York: Oxford University Press.

Salzinger, K. (1996). Reinforcement history: A concept underutilized in behavior analysis. *Journal of Behavior Therapy and Experimental Psychiatry, 27*, 199–207.

Satir, D. A., Goodman, D. M., Shingleton, R. M., Porcerelli, J. H., Gorman, B. S., Pratt, E. M., et al. (2011). Alliance-focused therapy for anorexia nervosa: Integrative relational and behavioral change treatments in a single-case experimental design. *Psychotherapy, 48*, 401–420.

Schumacher, J. (2008). *Black box.* New York: Simon & Schuster.

Shoham, V., Rohrbaugh, M. J., Onken, L. S., Cuthbert, B. N., Beveridge, R. M., & Fowles, T. R. (2014). Redefining clinical science training: Purpose and products of the Delaware Project. *Clinical Psychological Science, 2*, 8–21.

Staats, A. W., & Eifert, G. H. (1990). The paradigmatic behaviorism theory of emotions. *Clinical Psychology Review, 10*, 539–566.

Stampfl, T. G., & Levis, D. J. (1967). Essentials of implosive therapy: A learning-theory-based psychodynamic behavioral therapy. *Journal of Abnormal Psychology, 72*, 496–503.

Waller, G., Stringer, H., & Meyer, C. (2012). What cognitive behavioral techniques do therapists report using when delivering cognitive behavioral therapy for the eating disorders? *Journal of Consulting and Clinical Psychology, 80*, 171–175.

Wilson, G. T. (2007). Manual-based treatment: Evolution and evaluation. In T. A. Treat, R. R. Bootzin, & T. B. Baker (Eds.), *Psychological clinical science: Papers in honor of Richard M. McFall* (pp. 105–132). New York: Taylor & Francis.

Index

Page numbers followed by f indicate figures.

Acceptance, mindfulness and, 14–15
Acceptance and commitment therapy (ACT), 5, 16, 32–58, 91
  and assumptions about client, 42
  client potential for learning and, 42
  client strength as focus in, 44–45
  clinical application of, 38–54
  clinical formulation for guiding, 44–53
  and cognitive fusion in the moment, 45–47
  compassion-focused therapy and, 60
  contextual behavioral science and, 33–34
  debriefing exercises/metaphors in, 53–54
  emotion regulation therapy and, 323
  evidence basis of, 36–37, 55
  experiential work in, 34–35, 39–40
  exposure therapy and, 94–95
  future directions for, 55
  and overly directive therapist, 43–44
  and parallel processes for therapist, 43
  "Passengers on the Bus" in, 40, 43–44
  promoting experiential awareness and acceptance in, 48–53
  questions used in, 38–40
  relational frame theory and, 32, 35–36
  resources for, 56
  stepped approach to, 41
  theory of, 32–36, 33f, 34f
  therapeutic relationship in, 41–44
  timing of experiential work in, 41
  and use of client's metaphors, 47–48
  values in, 47–48
Acceptance-based coping skills, in depression, 128

Acquisition, emotions and, 65
Action, committed, ACT and, 34f
Adaptive beliefs, constructing and testing, 111–112
Adaptive emotions, avoidance of, 146–147; *see also* Affect phobia therapy (APT)
Adult mode, healthy, 270
Affect
  activating *versus* inhibitory, 148
  APT categories of, 147–148
  motivational function of, 147
Affect bridge, 183–184, 279
Affect exposure, 150
Affect forecasting, 299–302
  processes in, 289–290
Affect matching, 70
Affect phobia, defined, 147
Affect phobia therapy (APT), 5, 146–151, 149f, 150f
  adaptive use of affect in, 160–161
  evidence supporting, 155–157
  future directions in, 167–168
  as integrative model, 147
  practical introduction to, 157–167
  psychodynamic approach in, 153
  resources for, 168
  sense of self in, 150–151
  sessions in, 151–153
  theoretical framework of, 146–151, 149f, 150f
  transferrability of, 168
Affect regulation, in compassion-focused therapy, 64–66
Alleviation/prevention, psychology of, 66, 67f

405

Index

Alliance rupture, research on, 338–341, 359–360
Alliance-focused training (AFT)
  empirical evidence for, 339–341
  metacommunication principles in, 341–344
  principles and strategies of, 333–334
Allowing practice, in ERT, 319
Anger, adaptive *versus* maladaptive, 148
Angry Child mode, 267
  empty-chair exercise and, 280–283
  therapist response to, 283
Anxiety; *see also* Generalized anxiety disorder (GAD)
  attentional rigidity in, 313
  cognitive model of, 107
  contextual learning mechanisms in, 313–314
  death, 90–91
  emotion regulation therapy and, 310–311 (*see also* Emotion regulation therapy (ERT))
  resistance and, 11–12
  safety and reward motivations in, 312–313
Anxiety disorders
  acceptance and commitment therapy and, 36
  exposure-based cognitive therapy and, 125
  exposure and emotional processing for, 122–123
  exposure therapy and, 88–89
  and exposure *versus* behavioral experiments, 108–109
  extinction principle and, 84
  processes that maintain, 123
Aristotle, 146–147
Assumptions, identifying, with behavioral experiments, 115–117
Attachment theory, 65–66
Attention
  focused (*see also* Mindfulness)
    in mindfulness practice, 13
  self-focused, 218
Attention training
  in emotion regulation therapy, 318–319
  mindfulness and, 17
  therapist-directed, 223–224
Attentional bias, depressive, 124
Attentional rigidity, in anxiety and depression, 313
Avoidance
  ACT and, 33f
  affect motivating, 148
  depression and, 123–124
  emotion regulation and, 123–124
Avoidance-intrusion-rumination cycle, 122, 128, 139, 141

B

Bayda, Ezra, 11
Beck, Aaron, 240
Becker, Ernest, 90
Behavior
  functional interpretations of, 394–395
  interrelatedness with emotion and thought, 1–2
  safety-seeking, 107
Behavioral activation therapy, 124–125
Behavioral experiments, 5, 105–120
  anxiety and, 107–108
  client selection for, 118
  in clinical practice, 110–118
    case formulation and, 110
    for constructing/testing new adaptive beliefs, 111–112
    difficulties implementing, 117–118
    example of, 115–117
    experiment setup, 112–114
    for identifying beliefs and assumptions, 115–117
    for testing negative cognitions, 110–111
  cognitive mediation and, 109–110
  in cognitive therapy for social anxiety, 224–225
  cognitive *versus* extinction rationales for, 108–109
  evidence supporting, 108–110
  versus exposure, 106–107
  future directions for, 118
  hypothesis testing and, 107–108
  purpose of, 105
  resources for, 118
  strategies in, 106
  for testing maladaptive cognitions, 105–106
Behaviorism, misunderstanding of, 382
Beliefs
  adaptive, constructing and testing, 111–112
  encapsulated, in CT for social anxiety, 228–229
  identifying, with behavioral experiments, 115–117
  maladaptive (*see* Maladaptive beliefs)
Biases, depressive attentional, 122
Body and muscle awareness, in emotion regulation therapy, 319

Body awareness, mindfulness and, 17, 18–19, 21
Borderline personality disorder (BPD)
  imagery rescripting and, 179
  mode work and, 265, 268, 271–272
Bowlby, John, 335
Brain function
  meditation and, 13, 26
  and old-brain psychology, 61–63, 62f
  and real *versus* imagined experiences, 176–177
Breathing
  mindful belly, in ERT, 319
  soothing rhythm, website for, 72
Brief relational therapy (BRT), 334, 339
Bully/Attack Mode, 268

C

Calming/soothing, emotions and, 65
Care, receiving, in imagery rescripting, 177
"Catch yourself reacting (CYR)," in ERT, 317–318
Chairwork, 279
  applications of, 282–283
  in schema therapy, 274–276
  for unfinished business, 282
Change
  in childhood meanings, 177–178 (*see also* Imagery rescripting for personality disorders)
  exposure-based cognitive therapy and, 126–127
  promoting with functional analytic psychotherapy, 381–398 (*see also* Functional analytic psychotherapy [FAP])
  therapist as instrument of, 389–390
  through affect phobia therapy (*see* Affect phobia therapy (APT))
Chesterton, Lord, 289
Child abuse/neglect
  in complex PTSD, 210
  empty-chair exercise and, 254–255
  imagery rescripting and (*see* Imagery rescripting for personality disorders)
Child modes, 266–267
Childhood memories; *see also* Imagery rescripting for personality disorders
  accuracy of, 191, 278
  age of child in, 190–191
  difficulty retrieving, 195–196
  imagery rescripting and, 177–179, 182–195
  reprocessing, 177–178
Chronic pain, ACT and, 37

Churchill, Winston, 216
Clark and Wells model of cognitive therapy, 216–221, 219f
Claustrophobic fears, cognitive mediation and, 109–110
Client-centered therapy (CCT), 4
Clinically relevant behaviors (CRBs)
  defined, 381–382
  evoking, 385–390
  examples of, 384
  interpreting, 394–395
  reinforcing, 390–394
  watching for, 384–385, 394
Cognition(s)
  and detachment from experience, 35–36
  emotion and, 2–3
  evolution of, 61–62
  exposure therapy and, 87
  maladaptive, identifying, 106
  negative, testing with behavioral experiments, 110–111
Cognitive fusion, 60
  ACT and, 33f, 45–47
  clinical significance of, 63–64
  cost of, 47
  defined, 45
Cognitive mediation, 109–110
Cognitive restructuring, during imagery rescripting for social anxiety, 231–232
Cognitive science, embodied mind perspective in, 2
Cognitive theory, event interpretation in, 105–106
Cognitive therapy
  Clark and Wells model of, 216–220, 219f
  contributions of, 3
  limitations of, 14
  schema therapy and, 263–264
  for social anxiety disorder, 216–220, 219f
    behavioral experiments in, 224–225
    decatastrophizing experiments in, 225
    empirical evidence for, 220–221
    experiential past-focused techniques in, 226–229
    experiential present-focused techniques in, 222–226
    future directions for, 233–234
    imagery rescripting session in, 230–233
    resources for, 234
    surveys in, 225–226
    therapist-directed attention training in, 223–224
    video feedback in, 222–223

Cognitive-behavioral therapy (CBT)
  behavior emphasis in, 400–401
  emergent therapy trends in, 400–401
  empirically supported protocols for, 1
  experiential techniques and, 403
  for GAD, 356–358
  and integration with other methods, 401
  key principles of, 311
  modern versions of, 401–403
  neglect of emotion in, 1
  personality disorders and, 175
Cognitive-interpersonal cycles, in relational techniques, 335–337
Compassion
  defined, 66
  mindfulness and, 14–15
  nature of, 66
Compassion flowing in exercise, 73–75
Compassion meditation; *see also* Loving-kindness meditation
  in mindfulness practice, 13
Compassionate Mind Foundation, 76–77
Compassionate Self exercise, 71–73
Compassion-focused therapy (CFT), 59–79
  affect regulation processes in, 64–66
  clinical application of, 69–75
    compassionate flowing in practice in, 73–75
    compassionate self exercise in, 71–73
    reality check in, 69–71
  clinical example of, 62–63
  and contextualizing of mental events, 60–61
  empirical evidence for, 66–69
  evolution, cognition, behavior and, 63–64
  evolutionary context and, 60–61
  future directions in, 75–76
  Internet-based training for, 76
  and nature of compassion, 66, 67f
  old- and new-brain psychology and, 61–63, 62f
  randomized controlled trials of, 76
  resources for, 76–77
Compliant Surrenderer Mode, 268
Conceptualized self, ACT and, 33f
Conflict triangle, 148–151, 149f
  case example of, 155–167
Confrontation, empathic, 269, 274, 276–277
Contextual behavioral science (CBS), ACT and, 33–34
Contextual learning mechanisms
  in anxiety and depression, 313–314
  in emotion regulation therapy, 321–325

Coping modes, 268–269
  maladaptive, 268–269
  overcoming and bypassing, 276–278
Coping strategies
  acceptance-based, in depression, 128
  alternative, 297
  costs *versus* benefits of, 297
  versus defenses, 148
  problematic, identifying with EST, 295–297, 296f
Corrective emotional experience, 1–2
  approaches for creating, 4–5
Couples therapy, emotion-focused therapy in, 245–246
Courage and compassion, meditation on, in emotion-focused therapy, 321
Crying, changing views of, 289
Cue detection, in ERT, 317–318

D

Death anxiety, 90–91
  terror management therapy and, 92
Death instinct, Freud's concept of, 90
Decatastrophizing experiments, in cognitive therapy for social anxiety, 225
Decentering
  in emotion-focused therapy, 320
  in therapeutic alliance ruptures, 338–339
Decision making, emotion in, 2
Defenses, *versus* coping strategies, 148
Defusion, ACT and, 34f
Demanding Parent mode, in two-chair dialogue, 275
Depression, 121–145
  ACT and, 37
  attentional rigidity in, 313
  as avoidance disorder, 123–124
  contextual learning mechanisms in, 313–314
  exposure-based cognitive therapy and, 123–126, 245
    application process in, 127–142
    emotion regulation therapy and, 310–311 (*see also* Emotion regulation therapy (ERT))
    maintenance factors in, 128
    medication *versus*, 121
    mindfulness-based intervention for, 19–23
    Phase I (stress management), 128–129
    Phase II (exposure and processing), 129–138
    Phase III (positive growth), 138–141
    processes that maintain, 123
    resources for, 142

risk factors for, 121–122
safety and reward motivations in, 312–313
future directions for, 141–142
Depressive attentional bias, 122, 124
Depressive network
activation of, 131–136
and activation of positive self, 139–140
EBCT and, 127, 130
emotional engagement and, 130–131
emotional processing and, 131
identifying, 129, 131–132
Detached Protector Mode, 268–269
Dialectical behavior therapy (DBT), 16
Disconfirmation, in therapeutic alliance ruptures, 338–339
Dissociation
during imagery rescripting for personality disorders, 196
during imagery rescripting for PTSD, 211
Distancing practice, in ERT, 320
Distress disorders; *see also* Anxiety; Depression
CBT and, 310–311
Drive systems, 65

E

Elias, Norbert, 289
Embodied mind perspective, 2
EMDR; *see* Eye movement desensitization and reprocessing (EMDR)
Emotion(s); *see also* Affect
acceptance of, 5
versus actions, 305–306
adaptive (*see* Adaptive emotions)
avoidance of, 268
beliefs about duration of, 299–302
challenging self-critical thoughts about, 305
connecting exposure with, 93–96
in decision making, 2
difficult, meditation and, 22
in distress disorders, 311
dysregulation of, 3
EFT concept of, 239
encapsulated beliefs and, 229
functions of, 311–312
guilt and shame and, 305–306
during imagery rescripting for social anxiety, 230–232
incomprehensibility of, 302–303
in-session conceptualization of, 241–244, 242f
instrumental, 241

interrelatedness with thought and behavior, 1–2
linking to higher values, 306–307
linking to rumination and worry, 303–304
linking to thoughts and events, 303
making sense of, 304
maladaptive, examples of, 148
maladaptive use of, 146
nonverbal, assessing, 298–299
normalizing, 305
positive, dismissal of, 128–129
primary, 242, 242f
primary maladaptive, 242–243, 242f, 247f
productive, 246–247
secondary, 241–242, 242f, 247f
self-monitoring of, 300
social construction of, 288–290
as somatic markers, 2
stress-appraisal theory and, 290–293
theories of, 240–241
Emotion differentiation, mindfulness and, 17
Emotion regulation
avoidant styles of, 123–124
mindfulness and, 17
Emotion regulation therapy (ERT), 310–330
application of, 315–325, 316f
experiential exposure in, 321–325
skills building in, 316–321
background and theory, 311–314
between-sessions experiential work in, 324–325
for chronic anxiety and recurring depression, 311
client values and, 322–325
contextual learning mechanisms in, 313–314
future directions in, 325–326
motivational mechanisms in, 312–313
preliminary evidence for, 314–315
regulatory mechanisms in, 313
resources for, 326
target mechanisms in, 312–315, 316f
therapies influencing, 312
Emotion schemes, in emotion-focused therapy, 240–244, 247–248, 250–251, 253–254, 257–258
Emotional anchoring, 299
Emotional arousal, positive outcomes and, 3–4
Emotional engagement, in EBCT, 130–131
Emotional experience, corrective, 1–2, 4–5
Emotional processing
in GAD, 357, 373–375
healthy, 124–125

Emotional processing (*continued*)
  in imagery rescripting, 177
  in treatment of anxiety disorders, 122–123
Emotional schema therapy (EST), 288–309
  application of, 295–307
  assessment in, 297–299
  beliefs about duration and, 299–302
  empirical support for, 293–295
  future directions for, 307–308
  guilt and shame and, 305–306
  identifying problematic coping strategies and, 295–297
  incomprehensibility and, 302–304
  linking emotions to higher values and, 306–307
  model for, 292–293, 292f
  resources for, 308
  and social construction of emotion, 288–290
  theory of, 290–293
Emotional schemas
  assessing, 297–299
  maladaptive coping and, 297
Emotional-processing theory, of Foa and Kozak, 3, 85
Emotion-focused therapy (EFT), 4, 5, 239–262
  application of, 248–259
    with empty-chair exercise for unfinished business, 254–259
    with two-chair exercise for self-criticism, 248–254
  client needs in, 251–252, 257–258
  for couples, 245–246
  for depression, 245
  emotion schemes in, 240–244, 247–248, 250–251, 253–254, 257–258
  emotional arousal in, 246–247
  empirical evidence for, 244–248, 247f
  exposure-based cognitive therapy and, 134–135
  future directions for, 259–260
  in-session emotion conceptualization and, 241–244, 242f
  process orientation of, 239–240
  resources for, 260
Empathic bridging, 70
Empathic confrontation, 269, 274, 276–277
Empty-chair exercise
  Angry/Vulnerable Child mode and, 280–283
  child abuse/neglect and, 254–255

  with external *versus* internal "markers," 283
  for unfinished business, in emotion-focused therapy, 254–259
Encapsulated beliefs, in CT for social anxiety, 228–229
Envisioning opposite orientation practice, in emotion regulation therapy, 321
Equanimity, cultivating, in mindfulness practice, 13
Events, interpretations of, 105–106
Evolutionary context, in compassion-focused therapy, 60
Experience, defined, 312
Experiential avoidance, ACT and, 33f
Experiential techniques; *see also* Exposure therapy
  absence of research on, 400
  CBT and, 403
  in CT for social anxiety
    past-focused, 226–229
    present-focused, 222–226
  in emotion regulation therapy, 321–325
  empirical support and, 401–403
  next steps in, 399–403
Exposure
  in affect phobia therapy, 151–153
  mindfulness and, 17
Exposure and emotional processing, anxiety disorders and, 122–123
Exposure therapy, 83–104; *see also* Experiential techniques
  applications and illustration, 96–100
  versus behavioral experiments, 106–107
  challenges in, 87–89
  changing assessment of, 4
  and connection with emotion, 93–96, 95f
  death anxiety and, 90–91
  exposure-based cognitive therapy and, 125–126
  evidence supporting, 86–87
  exercises for, 85–86
  future directions for, 100–101
  historical bases and modern manifestations, 89–91
  new meanings *versus* emotion reduction and, 322
  for OCD, 97–98
  public relations problem of, 87–89
  resources for, 101
  for social anxiety, 220
  terror management theory and, 91–93
  theoretical basis of, 83–86
  in vivo, 5

Exposure-based cognitive therapy (EBCT)
  change process in, 126–127
  for depression, 123–126
    clinical application of, 127–142
  depressive network in, 127, 129–138
  emotional engagement in, 130–131
  emotional processing in, 131
  facets of the self session in, 136–138
  goals in, 140–141
  outcome evidence for, 126–127
  positive network and, 139–140
  self-acceptance and compassion in, 140
Extinction theory, 84
  versus imagery rescripting, 204
Eye movement desensitization and reprocessing (EMDR), 203

F

Focalism, 289–290
Freud, Sigmund, 90
Functional analytic psychotherapy (FAP), 6, 381–398
  application of, 384–395
    Rule 1 (watching for CRBs), 384–385
    Rule 2 (evoking CRBs), 385–390
    Rule 3 (reinforcing CRBs), 390–394
    Rule 4 (noticing impact), 394
    Rule 5 (interpreting behavior), 394–395
  avoiding exploitation in, 395
  clinical relevant behaviors in, 381–382
  as coping *versus* mastery model, 392
  evidence for, 382–383
  future directions for, 396
  precautions in, 395–396
  resources for, 396
  therapeutic loving in, 390–394
  therapist questions in, 384–385, 389–390
Functional Analytic Psychotherapy Rating Scale (FAPRS), 383
Fusion; *see* Cognitive fusion

G

Gay client, mindfulness-based therapy and, 19–23
Generalized anxiety disorder (GAD)
  approaches to, 6
  CBT for, 356–358
  characteristics of, 356–357
  emotional processing and, 372–375
  I/EP for, 356–380
  interpersonal factors in, 357–358
  new interpersonal strategies and, 368–372
Guilt, emotions and, 305

H

Happy Child mode, 266
Healthy Adult mode, 270, 281
  in confrontation with parental modes, 279–280
Heider, Fritz, 288, 289
Hopelessness, depression and, 122–124, 128–132, 135

I

Imagery
  in affect phobia therapy, 152–153
  mechanisms of, 280
  in schema therapy assessment, 277
  versus verbal cognition, 176–177
Imagery rescripting, 5
  in confrontation with parental modes, 279–280
  in CT for social anxiety, 228, 230–234
  imagined other in, 281–282, 281n3
  and therapist permission to enter, 280
Imagery rescripting for personality disorders, 175–202
  application of, 180–196
    with CBT, 196–198
    childhood memories in, 182–190
    in diagnosis, 180–182
    difficulties with, 195–196
    frequency of, 194
    general guidelines for, 190–192
    with imagery of safe place, 180
    patient rescripts in, 192–194
  childhood memory activation and, 177–178
  empirical evidence for, 178–180
  future directions for, 198–199
  mourning and, 191, 212
  patient dissociation and, 196
  and patient loyalty to parents, 196
  in present and future situations, 194–195
  rationale for, 176–179
  resources for, 199
  safe place imagery and, 180
  therapist's questions in, 182, 192
Imagery rescripting for PTSD, 203–215
  application of, 206–212
    with complex PTSD, 210
    difficulties with, 211–212
    with multiple traumas, 209–210
    with simple trauma, 206–209
  empirical evidence for, 204–206
  versus extinction, 204
  future directions for, 212–213
  indications for, 212

Imagery rescripting for PTSD (*continued*)
  mechanism of, 203–204
  rationale for, 203–204
  resources for, 213
  versus talk therapy, 207
  therapist's explanation of, 207–208
  therapist's questions in, 208–209
Imagery rescripting for social anxiety disorder, 216–236, 221; *see also* Cognitive therapy, for social anxiety disorder
Imaginal exposure, *versus* imagery rescripting, 205, 209
Imaginal exposure task, in emotion regulation therapy, 323
Imaginal exposure therapy exercises, 85–86
  clinical illustration of, 96–97
Immune neglect, 290
Impact bias, 290
Implosive therapy, 84
Impulsive/Undisciplined Child mode, 267
In vivo exposure therapy exercises, 85–86
Instrumental emotions, 241, 242f
Integrated self, in schema therapy, 283–284
Internal working models (IWMs), 335
Interoceptive exposure therapy, clinical illustration of, 96–97
Interpersonal and emotional processing therapy (I/EP), 356–380
  application of, 360–375
  background and theory of, 356–359
  case illustrations of, 362–365
  current interpersonal patterns and, 360–363
  and development of new interpersonal strategies, 368–372
  emotional processing in, 372–375
  evidence for, 359–360
  focus specificity in, 361
  future directions in, 375–377
  open process questioning in, 361–362
  overview of, 358–359
  past relationships and, 363–365
  present-moment focus in, 360–361
  therapeutic relationship and, 365–368
Interpersonal factors, in GAD, 357–358
Interpersonal psychotherapy, for social anxiety, 220–221
Interpersonal relationships
  developing new strategies in, 368–372
  in I/EP
    current, 360–363
    past, 363–365
Interpersonal theory, relational techniques and, 335

J

James, William, 147–148, 263

L

Language, and detachment from experience, 35–36
Leahy Emotional Schema Scale (LESS), 293–294, 297–298
Leahy Emotional Schema Scale--II (LESS-II), 298
Learning mechanisms, contextual
  in anxiety and depression, 313–314
  in emotion regulation therapy, 321–325
Letter writing, integrated self and, 284
Limited reparenting, 267–268, 270, 274, 280, 283
Love, therapeutic, 390–394
Loving-kindness meditation
  in functional analytic psychotherapy, 393
  impacts of, 67–68
  in mindfulness practice, 13

M

Major depressive disorder; *see* Depression
Maladaptive beliefs
  reinforcing, 117
  testing with behavioral experiments, 110–111
Maladaptive coping modes, 268–269
Maladaptive patterns, learning, 149–150
Maladaptive schemas, relational techniques and, 335–337
Meaning, child-level, changing, 177–178
Meditation; *see also* Mindfulness
  building and maintaining practice of, 23–25
  on courage and compassion, in ERT, 321
  with functional analytic psychotherapy, 388
  loving-kindness, 13, 393
    in functional analytic psychotherapy, 393
    impacts of, 67–68
  in mindfulness interventions, 22
  open presence, in emotion regulation therapy, 319
  psychotherapist practice of, 26
  research on, 26
  types of practice, 13
Memories
  childhood (*see* Childhood memories)
  in CT for social anxiety, 226–229
  trauma (*see* Imagery rescripting for PTSD; Trauma memories)

Metacognition, about therapist-client interactions, 366–368
Metacognitive awareness, mindfulness and, 17
Metacommunication
  in AFT, 341–344
  case example of, 345–351
  clinical discussion of, 351–352
  in relational techniques, 335–337
Metta meditation; *see* Loving-kindness meditation
Mindful belly breathing, in ERT, 319
Mindfulness, 11–31
  acceptance and compassion and, 14–15
  background and theory of, 12–15
  client attitude toward, 25–26
  in cognitive-behavioral therapy, 13–14
  definitions of, 12–13
  Pali term for, 13
  psychotherapist practice of, 26
  research on, 15–18, 16f, 26
  resources on, 27
  as transdiagnostic process, 18
Mindfulness exercises, in emotion regulation therapy, 318–321
Mindfulness meditation; *see also* Loving-kindness meditation; Meditation
  in depression, 128
  with functional analytic psychotherapy, 388
Mindfulness of emotions practice, in ERT, 319
Mindfulness practices, future directions for, 25–27
Mindfulness-based cognitive therapy (MBCT), 16
  clinician meditation practice and, 26–27
Mindfulness-based stress reduction (MBSR), 16
  clinician meditation practice and, 26–27
Mindfulness-based treatments
  applications of, 18–25
  clinical example of, 19–23
  mechanisms of action of, 17–18
  practices in, 19
  three-P model of, 20–23
Mode work
  application of, 273–283
  assessment in, 273–274
  common interventions in, 276–283
  conceptualization, 273–274
  future directions for, 284–285
  integrated self and, 283–284
  overview, 273
  resources for, 285
  as structural therapy, 274–276

Modes
  activation of, 270
  child, 266–267
  concept of, schema therapy and, 264–270
  coping, 268–269
  parental, 269–270
  as self-states, 265–266
  taxonomy of, 266–270, 271f
Motivational mechanisms, in anxiety and depression, 312–313
Mourning, imagery rescripting and, 191, 212

N

Naïve psychology, 288
Narcissistic client, mode work and, 276–277
Negative beliefs
  testing with behavioral experiments, 110–111
  updating, with CT, 222–226
New-brain psychology, *versus* old-brain psychology, 61–63, 62f
Nightmares, chronic, imagery rescripting and, 205–206
Nonverbal emotion, assessing, 298–299

O

Obsessive-compulsive disorder (OCD)
  behavioral experiments for identifying beliefs and assumptions in, 115–117
  exposure therapy for
    clinical illustration of, 97–98
    exercises in, 85–86
  and exposure *versus* behavioral experiments, 108–109
  extinction principle and, 84
Old-brain psychology, *versus* new-brain psychology, 61–63, 62f
Olivier, Laurence, 216
Open presence meditation, in ERT, 319

P

Pain
  chronic, ACT and, 37
  resistance and, 12
Panic disorder; *see also* Anxiety
  exposure therapy and, 96–97
Parental modes, 269–270
  confronting, 279–280
"Passengers on the Bus" metaphor, 40, 43–44
Person triangle, 149–150, 150f
  case example of, 157–159

Personality disorders
  affect phobia therapy and, 153–154
  changing perceptions of, 175
  imagery rescripting for (*see* Imagery rescripting for personality disorders)
  schema theory and, 175–176 (*see also* Imagery rescripting for personality disorders)
Personifications, 335
Phobias; *see also* Affect phobia
  cognitive mediation and, 109–110
  exposure-based cognitive therapy and, 125
Plato, 2
Positive blockade, 122
Posttraumatic stress disorder (PTSD)
  in ACT vignette 3, 48–53
  imagery rescripting for (*see* Imagery rescripting for PTSD)
Proactive valued action exercise, in emotion regulation therapy, 323–325
Psychoeducation, in emotion regulation therapy, 316–317
Psychological flexibility, ACT and, 34, 34f
Psychological rigidity, ACT and, 33–34, 33f
Psychology, naïve, 288
Psychopathology, maladaptive use of emotions and, 146
Psychotherapy
  functional analytic (*see* Functional analytic psychotherapy (FAP))
  interpersonal, for social anxiety, 220–221
  self-acceptance in, 15

R

Rationality, in Western culture, 2
Reality check, in compassion-focused therapy, 69–71
Reappraisal, mindfulness and, 17
Reattribution, in imagery rescripting, 177
Reframing, in emotion regulation therapy, 320–321
Regulatory mechanisms, in anxiety and depression, 313
Reinforcement, timing of, 391–392
Relational frame theory (RFT), ACT and, 32, 35–36, 40
Relational techniques, 333–355
  background and theoretical orientation, 335–339
  clinical applications of, 341–352
    case illustration of, 344–351
    discussion of, 351–352
  cognitive-interpersonal cycles in, 335–337
  complementarity and, 336
  empirical evidence for, 339–341
  future directions for, 352–353
  interpersonal theory and self-schemas in, 335
  maladaptive schemas in, 335–337
  metacommunication in, 335–337
  resources for, 353
  therapeutic alliance in, 338–339
  therapist self-examination in, 337, 342–343
  two-person approach in, 337
Relaxation therapy, for social anxiety, 220
Reparenting, limited, 267–268, 270, 274, 280, 283
Resistance, anxiety and, 11–12
Revenge, patient fantasies of, 188–189, 192, 211–213
Rogerian theory, 4
Rumination; *see also* Worry
  depression and, 123–126, 128, 130, 132, 136
  linking to emotion, 303–304

S

Sadness, self-compassion as antidote to, 22–23
Safe place, imagery of, 180
Safety and reward motivations, in anxiety and depression, 312–313
Safety behaviors, 107
  for challenging beliefs, 112
Safety-seeking behaviors, in social anxiety, 218
Schema theory, personality disorders and, 175–176; *see also* Imagery rescripting for personality disorders
Schema therapy, 5–6, 263–287; *see also* Emotional schema therapy (EST)
  chairwork in, 274–276
  imagery rescripting and, 179, 196, 198
  mode concept and, 264–270 (*see also* Mode work; Modes)
  research evidence for, 270–273
  theoretical basis of, 263–264
  versus transference-focused therapy, 271
Schemas, maladaptive, 335–337
Schumacher, Julie, 399
Seeking behaviors, 65
Self
  conceptualized, 33f
  integrated, in schema therapy, 283–284
Self-Aggrandizer mode, 276
Self Compassion Scale, 68
Self-acceptance, in psychotherapy, 15

Self-compassion
    as antidote to sadness/shame, 22–23
    loving-kindness meditation and, 68
    mindfulness and, 17
Self-criticism
    compassion-focused therapy and, 59–60 (see also Compassion-focused therapy (CFT))
    loving-kindness meditation and, 68–69
    negative effects of, 60
    two-chair exercise for, 248–254
Self-focused attention, 218
Self-images; see also Sense of self
    negative, 216–217
Self-interruption, two-chair exercise for, 259
Self-monitoring, in emotion regulation therapy, 317–318
Self-personification, 335
Self-schemas, relational techniques and, 335
Self-soothing, two-chair exercise for, 259
Self-states, modes as, 265–266
Sense of self
    in APT, 150–151
    flexible, mindfulness and, 17, 21–22
    in social anxiety, 216–217
Sentimentalism movement, 289
Sexual assault, imagery rescripting and, 205–206
Shame
    compassion-focused therapy and, 59–60 (see also Compassion-focused therapy [CFT])
    emotions and, 305
    loving-kindness meditation and, 68–69
    self-compassion as antidote to, 22–23
Skills building, in ERT, 311, 316–321
Social anxiety
    maintenance strategies in, 217–219, 219f
    prevalence of, 216–217
    treatment of, 216–217 (see also Cognitive therapy, for social anxiety disorder)
Somatic markers, 2
Soothing rhythm breathing, website for, 72
Spock, Benjamin, 289
Stimulus discrimination, in CT for social anxiety, 226–228
Stranded on a desert island exercise, in emotion regulation therapy, 323
Streisand, Barbra, 216
Stress management, in exposure-based cognitive therapy, 128–129
Stress-appraisal theory, 290–293

Suffering
    ACT and, 33 (see also Acceptance and commitment therapy (ACT))
    examples of, 70
Sullivan, Harry Stack, 335–337
Surveys, in cognitive therapy for social anxiety, 225
Symbolic events, reactions to, 63; see also Cognitive fusion
Symbolic relations, ACT and, 35–36

T

Teasdale, John D., 263
Terror management theory (TMT), 83, 86
    client and therapist reactions to, 100–101
    exposure therapy and, 91–96
Therapeutic alliance/relationship; see also Therapist-client relationship
    in ACT, 42–44
    in functional analytic psychotherapy, 382–395
        and awareness of CRBs, 384–385
        and evocation of CRBs, 385–390
    in relational techniques, 338–339
    ruptures in, 338–341
Therapeutic love, 393–394
Therapist
    exposure therapy and, 95f, 96–100
    as instrument of change, 389–390
    meditation practice of, 26–27
    overly directive, 43–44
    parallel processes for, 43
    as participant-observer, 336–337
    self-awareness practices for, 337, 342–343, 365–366, 385
Therapist-client relationship; see also Relational techniques; Therapeutic alliance/relationship
    in I/EP, 365–368
    metacognition about patterns in, 366–368
    methods for working with, 6
Therapist-directed attention training, 223–224
Thought
    interrelatedness with emotion and behavior, 1–2
    linking to emotion, 303–304
Threat, emotional response to, 64–65
Three P's (person, process, practice), clinical example of, 20–23
Time discounting, 290
Touch, patient's beliefs about, 299
Transference-focused therapy, versus schema therapy, 271

Trauma, unconditioned *versus* conditioned stimulus in, 204
Trauma memories, imagery rescripting and, 203–204, 207–208, 213, 221; *see also* Imagery rescripting for PTSD
Triangle of conflict, 148
Triggers
　activation of, 270
　defined, 267
　depressive, identifying, 129
　in emotion regulation therapy, 317–318
　interpretations of, 105–106
Two-chair dialogue in schema therapy, 274–276
Two-chair exercise for self-criticism, 248–254
Two-chair exercise for self-interruption, 259
Two-chair exercise for self-soothing, 259

U

Unconditioned stimulus, revaluation of, 204

V

Values
　acceptance and commitment therapy and, 34f, 47–48, 55
　client, in emotion regulation therapy, 322–325
　linking emotions to, 306–307
　meditation practice and, 24

Values clarification
　acceptance and commitment therapy and, 33f
　mindfulness and, 17
Video feedback, for updating negative beliefs, 222–223
Visualizations
　Compassion flowing in exercise, 73–75
　of compassionate self, 71–73
Vulnerable Child mode, 266–267
　empty-chair technique and, 280–283
　overcoming and bypassing, 276–278
　therapist response to, 283
　in two-chair dialogue, 275

W

Weber, Max, 288
Western philosophy, rationality in, 2
Worry; *see also* Rumination
　anxiety and, 107
　beliefs about, 292
　depression and, 123, 131
　emotion regulation therapy and, 315, 324
　GAD and, 356–358, 360, 363–364, 367, 370, 376–377
　guilt and shame and, 305
　metacognitive factors in, 294

Y

Young, Jeffery, 240–241, 264–265